Neuroscience Nursing

Assessment and Patient Management

edited by

Sue Woodward

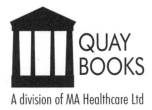

QUAY
BOOKS

A division of MA Healthcare Ltd

Quay Books Division, MA Healthcare Ltd, St Jude's Church, Dulwich Road, London SE24 0PB

British Library Cataloguing-in-Publication Data
A catalogue record is available for this book

© MA Healthcare Limited 2006
ISBN-10 1 85642 308 5
ISBN-13 978 1 85642 308 3

Printed in the UK by Cromwell Press Limited, Trowbridge, Wiltshire

Contents

Section 3 Management of patients with long-term neurological conditions

List of contributors

Thomas Aird is Principal Lecturer, Faculty of Health and Social Care, London South Bank University, London

Aimee Aubeeluck is Lecturer in Health Psychology, Faculty of Medicine and Health Sciences, School of Nursing University of Nottingham, Nottingham

Chris Beech is Nurse Consultant, Services for Older People, Highland Primary Care Trust, Inverness

Jonathan Birns is Clinical Lecturer in Stroke Medicine, Department of Stroke Medicine, King's College Hospital, London

Wendy Brooks is Stroke Nurse Consultant, Epsom and St Helier University Hospitals NHS Trust, Stroke Unit, St Helier Hospital, Carshalton, Surrey

Glynis Collis Pellatt is Senior Lecturer, Faculty of Health and Social Science, University of Luton

Diana De is Senior Lecturer, Adult Nursing, School of Care Science, University of Glamorgan, Wales

Maria Fitzpatrick is Clinical Nurse Specialist in Stroke, Department of Stroke Medicine, King's College Hospital, London

Helen Godfrey is Principal Lecturer, Faculty of Health and Social Care, University of the West of England, Bristol

Rosie Goulding is Nursing Research and Development Coordinator, Health and Social Services

Elizabeth Gray is Nurse Adviser, Innovex UK Ltd

Emily Harrison is Clinical Nurse Specialist, National Hospital for Neurology and Neurosurgery, University College London Hospitals NHS Foundation Trust, London

Christine Hayes is Epilepsy Specialist Nurse, Nottingham University Hospitals NHS Trust, Nottingham

Anne Jarvis is Nurse Specialist (SAH), Department of Neurosurgery, Hope Hospital, Salford

Lucy Johnson is Nurse Consultant in Pain Management, Pain Relief Unit, King's College Hospital, London

Ehsan Khan is Lecturer, Florence Nightingale School of Nursing and Midwifery, King's College London

Muili Lawal is Lecturer in Adult Health, Faculty of Health and Human Science, Thames Valley University, London

Rhona MacLean is Multiple Sclerosis Specialist Nurse, Leeds General Infirmary, Leeds

Roswell Martin is Consultant Neurologist, Gloucestershire Royal Hospital, Gloucestershire Hospitals NHS Foundation Trust, Gloucester

Michelle McIntosh is Senior Staff Nurse, Acute Brain Injury Unit, The National Hospital for Neurology and Neurosurgery, London

Anne McLeod is Lecturer in Critical Care, City University, St Bartholomew's School of Nursing and Midwifery, London

Kerry Mutch is Multiple Sclerosis Specialist Nurse, Walton Centre for Neurosurgery and Neuromedicine, NHS Trust, Liverpool

Mary O'Brien is Research Fellow, Centre of Health Research and Evaluation, Faculty of Health, Edge Hill, Ormskirk

Natalie Pattison is Nurse Researcher, Critical Care Nursing, Royal Marsden Hospital, London

Ian Peate is Associate Head of School, School of Nursing and Midwifery, Faculty of Health and Human Sciences, University of Hertfordshire

Bernadette Porter is Nurse Consultant Multiple Sclerosis, National Hospital for Neurology and Neurosurgery, University College London Hospitals NHS Foundation Trust, London

Andrew Russell is Multiple Sclerosis Specialist Nurse, Department of Neurosciences, York Hospital, York

Jane Skelton is Care Information Adviser, Motor Neurone Disease Association, Northampton

Louise Talbot is Macmillan Clinical Psychologist, Royal Manchester Children's Hospital, Manchester

Del Thomas is Multiple Sclerosis Specialist Nurse, Gloucestershire Royal Hospital, Gloucestershire Hospitals NHS Foundation Trust, Gloucester

Debbie Thompson is Associate Lecturer (Psychology), Open University

Richard Warner is Multiple Sclerosis Consultant Nurse, Gloucestershire Royal Hospital, Gloucestershire Hospitals NHS Foundation Trust, Gloucester

Sarah White is Multiple Sclerosis Specialist Nurse, St George's Healthcare NHS Trust, London

Gaynor Williams is Multiple Sclerosis Clinical Nurse Specialist, Neuro-inflammatory Unit, University Hospital of Wales, Cardiff

Sue Williams is Lecturer in Adult Nursing, School of Nursing and Midwifery, Cardiff University, Heath Park, Cardiff

Sue Woodward is Head of Section, Specialist and Palliative Care, Florence Nightingale School of Nursing and Midwifery, King's College, London

Preface

Sue Woodward

The last few years have been an exciting time for anyone working within the field of neuroscience nursing, with the profile of neuroscience services being raised nationally. There have been many initiatives impacting on practice, from the work undertaken through the NHS Modernisation Agency *Action on Neurology* project (Modernisation Agency, 2005) and the *Neurosciences Critical Care Report* (Modernisation Agency, 2004), to the publication of the *National Service Framework for Long-term Conditions* in March 2005 (Department of Health, 2005). Also, 2004 saw the inaugural conference from the newly formed Royal College of Nursing Neuroscience Forum, so there was much to be enthused about.

In April 2004 the *British Journal of Nursing* (*BJN*) re-launched in a new format, with a special focus on neuroscience nursing. As commissioning editor for this journal, I was in a position to be able to encourage authors to come forward from all fields of neuroscience nursing practice to publish within the journal. There was so much innovative work going on within this field, but at the time there was no neuroscience nursing journal in the UK. Very often potential authors from a neuroscience nursing background were unsure where to submit papers, with the net result that they did not submit at all. Once these authors became aware that the *BJN* was keen to publish neuroscience focused papers, the volume of manuscripts submitted increased, culminating in the launch of the *British Journal of Neuroscience Nursing* a year later.

This book brings together the best of the articles that have been published in the *BJN* since April 2004. Together they provide an essential reference for nurses working with people with neurological problems in a variety of settings from critical care and tertiary referral centres with specialist neuroscience units, through to stroke services and primary care teams to name a few. All the authors have had an opportunity to update their papers since their original publication in the *BJN* specifically for this book. In this way we are able to bring you a series of up-to-date, evidence-based papers from leading UK neuroscience nurses to underpin neuroscience nursing practice. This is the first time that such a collection of neuroscience articles has been brought together in one title for nurses practising in the UK.

The book is divided into three sections. The first section focuses on aspects of assessment relevant to neurological patients, the second covers a variety of issues in the management of patients with acute neurological conditions, including some key aspects of neuroscience critical care practice. The final section focuses on the management of patients with long-term neurological conditions.

The aim of this book is not to provide the definitive neuroscience nursing text, but rather to identify key areas of practice and evidence of current best care. The fact that such a wide range of papers has been published over such a short space of time in one generic nursing journal is testament to the importance of the subject for all practising nurses. With over 10 million people in the UK suffering from a neurological problem one can see the need for nurses everywhere to have access to resources to help them understand and implement appropriate care for these patients.

References

Department of Health (2005) *National Service Framework for Long-term Conditions*. Department of Health, London

Modernisation Agency (2004) *Neurosciences Critical Care Report: Progress in Developing Services*. Available from: http://www.modern.nhs.uk/criticalcare/5021/7117/20040%20DoH-Neurosciences.pdf. Accessed 2 March 2006

Modernisation Agency (2005) *Action on Neurology: Improving Neurology Services – a practical guide*. Available from: http://www.wise.nhs.uk/NR/rdonlyres/580E6AF8-38C7-4E38-BC6E-142BE325E3C4/1305/neurology032006.pdf. Accessed 2 March 2006

Section 1

Aspects of assessment in neuroscience nursing

Chapter 1

Intra- and extracranial causes of alteration in level of consciousness

Anne McLeod

Consciousness depends on effective interactions between the cerebral cortex and the brainstem. There are a variety of processes that can alter this exchange and, therefore, result in an altered level of consciousness. Level of consciousness is the most important aspect of neurological assessment as it is the earliest and most sensitive indicator of neurological deterioration (Hickey, 2002). Changes can occur rapidly over a few minutes or hours, or more slowly over weeks or even months. However, in the acute situation, nurses caring for patients outside designated neuroscience units must have knowledge of what can provoke an altered level of consciousness so that prompt action can be taken to resolve the problem, as it may be an indication of acute brain injury (Hickey, 2002).

Consciousness

Consciousness is a state of awareness of oneself and the surrounding environment and is particularly dependent on the functioning of the reticular activating system (RAS) (Hickey, 2002).

The RAS arises from the medulla oblongata within the brainstem, proceeds through the pons, midbrain and thalamus before it innervates the cerebral cortex as a diffuse network of neurones. This system controls the activity of the central nervous system (*Figure 1.1*).

Different sections of the RAS act in different ways: the

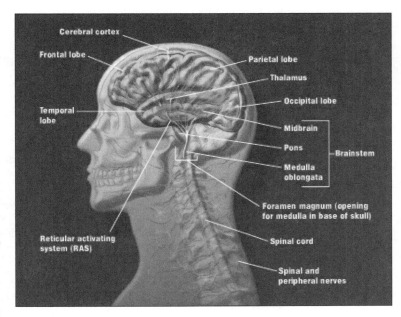

Figure 1.1: Diagrammatic representation of the brain

brainstem portion is believed to be involved with wakefulness, whereas the thalamic portion is believed to be involved with mental activity (Hickey, 2002). Therefore, consciousness, in terms of alertness and behaviour, relies on effective communication between the brainstem and the cerebral cortex.

A reduction or altered level of consciousness can be the result of lesions or metabolic disorders that directly affect either the cerebral hemispheres or the RAS. Therefore, altered level of consciousness can be defined as either a reduction in alertness or an alteration in behaviour (Vander et al, 2000); these changes may occur in isolation or in combination.

Intracranial pressure

Intracranial pressure (ICP) can be defined as the pressure exerted within the ventricles by the cerebrospinal fluid (CSF) (Hickey, 2002). Although a normal ICP is 0–10 mmHg (Lindsay et al, 1998), it is a fluctuating pressure influenced by respiratory movements and normal daily activities, such as coughing or the Valsalva manoeuvre (a technique for producing a transient increase in intrathoracic pressure) (Hickey, 2002; Porth, 2003) (*Table 1.1*).

The contents of the skull, which in adults is a rigid structure, fill the space available within the skull to capacity. The three essentially non-compressible contents of the skull are brain tissue (80%), blood (10%) and CSF (10%). In order to maintain a stable ICP, if one of the three volumes within the skull increases, another must decrease otherwise the ICP will rise. This concept is called the modified Monro–Kellie hypothesis (Hickey, 2002). An ICP above 15 mmHg is viewed as being raised (Hickey, 2002). Reciprocal compensation occurs among the three intracranial components to accommodate any increases in volume. Thus, if there is a rise in brain tissue volume, CSF can be displaced, CSF absorption can be increased and the low-pressure venous system can be compressed (Lindsay et al, 1998).

Table 1.1: Factors that elevate intracranial pressure

- Valsalva manoeuvre
- Coughing or sneezing
- Certain body positions (e.g. prone, neck flexion, extreme hip flexion)
- Emotional upset/pain
- Noxious stimuli
- Arousal from sleep
- Rapid eye movement sleep

From Hickey (2002)

Increases in volume over a longer period can be accommodated far more easily than a sudden increase in volume, such as is seen with a spontaneous intracranial bleed. This is clearly demonstrated by the pressure volume curve of ICP (*Figure 1.2*).

However, in either situation an altered level of consciousness will eventually occur if the source of the increase in volume does not dissipate.

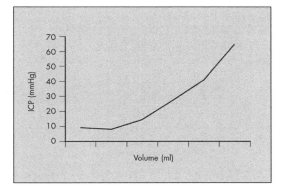

Figure 1.2:
Pressure–volume curve
of intracranial pressure

Assessment of level of consciousness

The Glasgow Coma Scale (GCS) (Teasdale and Jennett, 1974) (*Table 1.2*) is commonly used to assess level of consciousness in terms of providing a stimulus and observing the response. It was devised to assess depth of impaired consciousness with the aim of avoiding ambiguities and inconsistency between different assessors (Fairley and Cosgrove, 1999), thus providing an objective tool. With the GCS, level of consciousness is assessed in terms of eye opening and verbal and motor responses, with each aspect being assessed independently (Price, 2002), and the best response for each being documented.

These three responses provide information on the patient's awareness of the environment and stimuli within the environment. As consciousness is seen as a continuum from alertness to unconsciousness (Vander et al, 2000), the stimulation a patient requires to elicit a response is also on a continuum. The stimulation provided should begin with the minimal required to elicit a response, and allowing the stimulation to be increased as necessary. There is a range from not requiring any stimulation (or fully alert and aware) through auditory stimulation to painful stimulation, and finally to no response (or unconsciousness) (*Figure 1.3*).

Table 1.2: Glasgow Coma Scale

Eyes open

Spontaneous	4
To speech	3
To pain	2
None	1
C=eyes closed by swelling	

Verbal response

Oriented	5
Confused	4
Inappropriate words	3
Incomprehensible sounds	2
None	1
T=Endotracheal tube or tracheostomy	

Motor response

Obeys commands	6
Localizes to pain	5
Normal flexion	4
Abnormal flexion	3
Extension	2
None	1
Record best arm response	

From Teasdale and Jennett (1974)

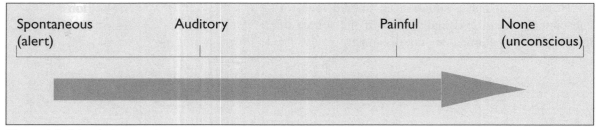

Figure 1.3: Stimulation continuum

Therefore, when assessing a patient's level of consciousness, the nurse must first observe any spontaneous response, and then use auditory stimulation if patient arousal is required. If no response is obtained, painful stimulation is used. A painful stimulus is usually required for patients who are unconscious or who have an obviously reduced level of consciousness (Hickey, 2002). If no response is obtained with this, 'none' is recorded on the neurological observation chart.

When using painful stimulation, it is generally advocated that 'central' pain should be used (Woodward, 1997; Addison and Crawford, 1999; Shah, 1999). A response to this implies that the neurones within the RAS and connecting neurones are still functioning to some extent (Price, 2002), rather than a spinal reflex being elicited and observed. Therefore, a response supposes interpretation within the cerebral cortex of the pain, with a resulting motor response. It is generally recommended that the source of central pain is either a trapezius muscle pinch or supraorbital pressure (Lowry, 1998; Addison and Crawford, 1999; Shah, 1999). Sternal rubs should be avoided as they cause bruising because of tissue damage (Price, 2002).

If not experienced in using the GCS, it can be a relatively complicated and time-consuming tool to use. The AVPU scale (A being Alert, V responds to Voice, P responds to Pain and U meaning Unresponsive) (*Table 1.3*) can give information quickly about the patient's level of consciousness, which can then be more formally assessed with the GCS as necessary (Smith, 2000; McNarry and Goldhill, 2004).

The AVPU scale assesses patients' responses on the continuum of consciousness:

- Are they alert?
- Do they respond to verbal stimulation?
- Do they respond to painful stimulation?
- Do they not respond at all?

Table 1.3: The AVPU scale

●	A	Alert
●	V	Voice
●	P	Pain
●	U	Unresponsive

From Smith (2000)

However, the AVPU scale only gives information about one aspect of the factors that contribute to awareness and, therefore, consciousness. It is used as an assessment strategy within primary survey or the initial assessment by the trauma/medical team when the patient arrives at the accident and emergency department following traumatic injury (Greaves et al, 2001). It can also be used in emergency situations or when a patient has had an acute deterioration by, for example, critical care outreach nurses (Smith, 2000; McNarry and Goldhill, 2004). However, it should not replace the GCS as an assessment tool.

Recent guidelines on head injury management continue to recommend the use of the GCS as the assessment tool to ensure that the three derivatives of consciousness are individually assessed (National Institute for Clinical Excellence, 2003). Therefore, a full, accurate assessment is achieved and behaviour can be described. In conjunction with level of consciousness, pupil reaction and limb power are also recorded with the use of the GCS. Pupil reactions provide information on the function of the third cranial nerve, or oculomotor nerve, which has its nucleus within the midbrain. If ICP is increasing, the only route for relief of the pressure is downwards through the foramen magnum at the base of the skull directly onto the brainstem (Lindsay et al, 1998). However, within the brainstem are essential physiological centres such as the respiratory and vasomotor centres (Tortora and Grabowski, 1996). Unrelieved pressure on these areas will lead to an inability to maintain respiratory and cardiovascular function. Additionally, the 12 cranial nerves arise from the brainstem and are involved with essential reflexes such as blinking and coughing. When pressure is increasing on the brainstem, the cranial nerves become compressed and cannot function normally.

As the third cranial nerve arises near the top of the brainstem and its function is easy to test through pupil reactions to light, dysfunction of this nerve is an early indicator of increasing pressure on the brainstem (Hickey, 2002). Oculomotor dysfunction is observed as pupils that react sluggishly to light or not at all and/or pupils that are dilated. Ipsilateral dilation occurs when pressure is increasing on one side of the brainstem; as cranial nerves do not cross over, the dilated pupil will be on the side of the increasing pressure.

Causes of a reduction in level of consciousness

Alteration in level of consciousness can be caused by a variety of processes that affect the interaction between the RAS and the cerebral cortex. These can easily be divided into intracranial and extracranial causes, or rather central nervous system structural abnormalities and metabolic imbalances (Hickey, 2002). For the nurse assessing a patient who does not have a known neurological insult, extracranial causes should be assessed and either excluded or treated.

Extracranial causes

The brain has extensive metabolic demands and depends on a continuous supply of oxygen and glucose for neuronal perfusion and, therefore, functioning. To deliver this, a 1500 g brain requires about 750 ml/min blood (Tortora and Grabowski, 1996). Therefore, if a patient who does not have a known neurological insult displays an altered level of consciousness such as confusion when previously he/she was alert and oriented, the following causes should be assessed and treated:

- Hypoxaemia
- Hypercapnia (above normal levels of carbon dioxide)/acidosis
- Hypotension
- Blood sugar level alterations (hypoglycaemia or hyperglycaemia).

These four factors can all contribute to a reduction of neuronal perfusion. The first three do so by influencing cerebral perfusion pressure (CPP). CPP is the blood pressure gradient across the brain and is derived by calculating the difference between the mean systemic arterial pressure and the ICP (Hickey, 2002). The average range of CPP in an adult is 80–100 mmHg, with a CPP of 60 mmHg being required for neuronal perfusion. If the CPP is below 60 mmHg, ischaemia will occur (Hickey, 2002). A reduction in CPP can be caused by either an increase in ICP or a reduction in mean systemic blood pressure. These alterations may occur individually or in combination, such as in a patient who has a head injury and who is also in hypovolaemic shock.

Hypoxaemia and hypercapnia both vasodilate the cerebral vasculature, therefore increasing the blood volume within the brain (Hickey, 2002); this then will increase ICP. Hypercapnia results from hypoventilation of a patient; situations when this may occur include during sleep, in a coma, following administration of sedation or during shallow breathing such as is seen in severe pain (Hickey, 2002).

Hypoventilation can also occur when a patient with chronic obstructive pulmonary disease is administered too high a concentration of oxygen. Hypercapnia will result in a respiratory acidosis, with a decrease in pH. Acidosis from other causes, such as the production of lactic acid from ischaemic tissue, will also lead to cerebral vessel vasodilation, resulting in an increase in ICP (Adam and Osbourne, 1997).

Hypoxaemia not only influences CPP but can also cause cerebral ischaemia and therefore neuronal hypoxia because of a lack of oxygen delivery. This may occur in combination with hypotension or as a consequence of poor gaseous exchange in the lungs. Causes of tissue hypoxia can generally be attributed to one of the following types of impaired oxygen supply (Adam and Osbourne, 1997):

- Hypoxic hypoxia, which can be viewed as the lack of oxygen within the blood (or hypoxaemia)
- Anaemic hypoxia, when the oxygen tension of arterial blood is normal, but the oxygen-carrying capacity of the blood is reduced either because of a lack of erythrocytes or a deficiency of the oxygen-carrying capacity of haemoglobin, such as in carbon monoxide poisoning or sickle cell crisis
- Circulatory hypoxia, which occurs when the oxygen tension and content of arterial blood is normal but the cardiovascular system is unable to meet the metabolic needs of the cells. This can be caused by a poor cardiac output or vascular insufficiency.

The factors that impair oxygen delivery should always be assessed if a patient displays an altered level of consciousness, such as confusion, and then treated with appropriate interventions such as administering oxygen or increasing intravascular volume through the use of a fluid challenge (Smith, 2000). If the hypoxia is sustained, neuronal cell death will occur. Thus, for example in situations of prolonged cardiac arrest, neurological dysfunction should always be assessed once the patient has been successfully resuscitated and has been stabilized in the intensive care setting (Adam and Osbourne, 1997).

Abnormal blood glucose levels can markedly alter the level of consciousness. Neurones require a steady supply of glucose to maintain their metabolic activity and cellular functions. However, they are sensitive to changes in glucose level and, therefore, level of consciousness can alter rapidly.

There are three main diabetic emergencies, all of which are associated with a decreased level of consciousness:

- Diabetic ketoacidosis
- Hyperosmolar, hyperglycaemic non-ketotic coma
- Hypoglycaemic coma.

Diabetic ketoacidosis (DKA)

A lack of insulin production results in hyperglycaemia and a metabolic acidosis following the use of free fatty acids released during lipolysis. A patient with DKA can rapidly become dehydrated because of the osmotic diuresis that results when the kidneys excrete glucose. Severe electrolyte imbalance also occurs. Many of the 'stress' hormones such as cortisol, adrenaline and noradrenaline that are also released can exacerbate the hyperglycaemia. Not all patients with DKA will be in a coma, but many will demonstrate an altered level of consciousness, with the severity of the DKA influencing the alteration (Adam and Osbourne, 1997).

Hyperosmolar, hyperglycaemic non-ketotic coma (HONK)

This occurs more commonly in patients with undiagnosed non-insulin dependent diabetes. It is associated with hyperglycaemia but ketosis is mild or absent. However, the incidence of coma is greater than in DKA and the period of time with a reduced level of consciousness is extended. Careful fluid resuscitation is required to avoid the development of cerebral oedema (Adam and Osbourne, 1997).

Hypogylcaemic coma

This can occur in diabetic patients who develop low blood glucose levels; this may be caused by an excessive insulin dose or inadequate food intake (or large alcohol ingestion). Although this is easy to diagnose at the bedside, rapid treatment with intravenous 50% dextrose may be required to avoid irreversible brain damage (Adam and Osbourne, 1997).

Liver dysfunction

Encephalopathy, or degeneration of the brain, may be associated with hepatic failure and can cause altered level of consciousness. Fulminant liver failure by definition includes encephalopathy, of which there are five grades (Adam and Osbourne, 1997) (*Table 1.4*). In grades III–IV, cerebral oedema is common, with 80% of patients with grade IV encephalopathy having cerebral oedema (Adam and Osbourne, 1997). Hepatic encephalopathy is a major cause of death in patients suffering from liver failure, with those having the higher grades and thus more cerebral impairment having a worse prognosis (Adam and Osbourne, 1997).

Table 1.4: Grades of hepatic encephalopathy

0	Normal awareness
I	Mood change, confusion
II	Drowsiness, inappropriate behaviour
III	Stuporous but rousable
IV	Unrousable to minimal stimuli or no response to noxious stimuli; decerebrate (arms stiffly extended, with possible extension of the legs) or decorticate (one or both arms in full flexion on the chest. Legs may be stiffly extended) posturing

From Adam and Osbourne (1997)

The pathogenesis of hepatic encephalopathy is unclear. It is thought that toxins normally cleared by the liver cause an increase in blood–brain barrier permeability, therefore allowing the movement of gamma-aminobutyric acid, electrolytes and plasma proteins into the CSF (Adam and Osbourne, 1997). The plasma proteins increase CSF oncotic pressure, which then further increases oedema formation. This will reduce cerebral perfusion pressure and increase ICP. Seizure activity may be obvious as a complication of the cerebral oedema (Adam and Osbourne, 1997); seizures should be controlled so that the metabolic demand (and therefore oxygen and glucose requirements) of the brain is not increased.

Fluid/electrolyte disorders

During both acute and chronic renal failure, cerebral function alterations may be apparent. In chronic renal failure, the uraemia that develops can cause confusion and thus an altered level of consciousness (Adam and Osbourne, 1997). In acute disorders, such as the neuroendocrine syndrome of inappropriate antidiuretic hormone secretion, antidiuretic hormone is secreted by the pituitary gland but inappropriately in relation to the serum osmolality (Woodrow, 2000). Therefore, there is reabsorption of water through the renal tubules creating a dilutional hyponatraemia.

Dilutional hyponatraemia occurs when the concentration of sodium in the blood reduces because of inappropriate fluid retention (Woodrow, 2000). This, if left untreated, can cause cerebral oedema through fluid overload and can initiate seizures and coma (Hickey, 2002).

Multi-organ dysfunction

Multi-organ dysfunction can have a marked effect on conscious level and may be attributed to the cardiovascular failure that is associated with multi-organ dysfunction. Therefore, cerebral perfusion is not maintained because of a reduction in mean systemic blood pressure and the reduced oxygenation of blood that may occur if there is respiratory involvement such as acute lung injury (Adam and Osbourne, 1997). Additionally, liver and renal failure that can be seen in multi-organ dysfunction will have similar consequences as previously outlined, such as the effects of uraemia and electrolyte imbalance. Situations that can result in multi-organ dysfunction include sepsis, shock, pancreatitis and trauma (Adam and Osbourne, 1997).

Disequilibrium syndrome

This occurs when, during haemofiltration, urea and uraemic toxins are removed too rapidly. This then creates an osmotic gradient between CSF and blood, which results in water moving from the blood into brain tissue (Woodrow, 2000), thus forming cerebral oedema. Although careful observation of exchange rates during haemofiltration and judicious monitoring of serum urea can avoid this, the neurological effects can be distressing to both the patient and his/her family. Neurological complications include confusion, aggression and a reduction in level of consciousness (Woodrow, 2000).

Drug effects

A number of drugs can alter the level of consciousness. Benzodiazepines have hypnotic (sleep-inducing) and anxiolytic (anxiety-reducing) properties, which can reduce the patient's level of consciousness (Neal, 2002). Opioid analgesics have a sedatory effect, thereby also altering the level of consciousness. Anticonvulsants, neuroleptics and antidepressants all have sedatory effects and some may cause hyponatraemia (Neal, 2002). Recreational drugs, such as heroin, can mimic the effects of opioid analgesics; others, such as cocaine and LSD, also cause a 'high' during which altered behaviours may be exhibited (Neal, 2002). Additionally, alcohol can lead to an altered level of consciousness, and alcohol ingestion can lead to falls and thus possible head injuries.

Excessive administration of dextrose-containing intravenous solutions can also lead to an alteration in level of consciousness. Generally, the rationale for their administration is for cellular rehydration. However, if given excessively, cerebral oedema can result.

Excessive use of diuretics can cause hyponatraemia through the loss of sodium in the urine (Hudak et al, 1998). This can also lead to neurological complications of confusion, a decreased level of consciousness and potentially coma.

Intracranial causes

Once extracranial causes have been excluded as causative factors of a reduced level of consciousness, then potential intracranial causes should be sought. Depending on the patient's primary diagnosis, intracranial effects may be initially assessed. However, it is likely that in these instances the patient will have a history of neurological pathology such as a cerebral trauma, which may now be causing a rise in ICP. However, cerebral trauma can be associated with alcohol ingestion (Greaves et al, 2001). It may be difficult to differentiate between an altered level of consciousness being the result of a cerebral injury, the effects of the alcohol or a combination of both.

The intracranial causes can be divided into three main groups (*Table 1.5*):

- Space-occupying lesions
- Cerebral oedema
- Increases in cerebrospinal fluid.

Table 1.5: Intracranial causes of altered level of consciousness

Space-occupying lesions	Cerebral oedema	Increases in cerebrospinal fluid
Tumours	Vasogenic	Non-communicating hydrocephalus
Haemorrhages/ haematomas	Cytotoxic	Communicating hydrocephalus
Contusions	Interstitial	
Abscesses		

Space-occupying lesions

Space-occupying lesions are conditions when there is a proportion of brain tissue that has been compressed by a tumour, a haematoma/bruise or collection of infection that is literally taking up space within the intracranial contents (Lindsay et al, 1998). The additional volume within the skull not only increases ICP but also can cause localized dysfunction, which is then manifested as, for example, seizures or a hemiparesis (weakness affecting one side of the body) (Lindsay et al, 1998). If a patient has a seizure, there is usually a period following the seizure during which the patient will have a decreased level of consciousness — this is usually referred to as the post-ictal phase (Hickey, 2002).

Benign cerebral tumours tend to be meningomas. These are tumours arising from the meninges that surround the brain and the spinal cord. These tumours tend to be slow growing so clinical signs of the tumour are not usually obvious until the tumour is fairly large; until that time the intracranial contents compensate for the additional mass (Hickey, 2002).

Malignant cerebral tumours can be either primary brain tumours or metastases. Primary brain tumours arise from the connective tissue between neurones and are, therefore, classified under the umbrella term of glioma (Hickey, 2002). Following biopsy, the actual connective tissue type can be identified and hence classified, for example as an astrocytoma. These brain tumours are highly malignant with a poor prognosis (Lindsay et al, 1998).

Cerebral haemorrhages are differentiated by their location in relation to the meninges (*Figure 1.4*). An extradural haematoma occurs between the skull and the outermost meningeal layer, or dura mater, and is seen to be a neurosurgical emergency as it is caused by arterial bleeding (Hickey, 2002). A bleed between the dura mater and the arachnoid layer is a subdural bleed, which is a venous bleed.

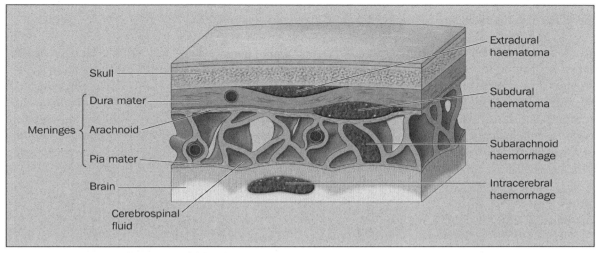

Figure 1.4: Location of intracranial bleeds

Below the arachnoid layer is a space containing cerebrospinal fluid; it is into this space that a subarachnoid haemorrhage is located. Any bleed below the fine, tissue-like pia mater is within the brain tissue itself and is hence an intracerebral bleed (Hickey, 2002). Depending on the size, location and neurological consequences (such as significantly raised ICP), these bleeds could have fairly mild effects on the patient, but they can also be devastating.

If a patient has a significant intracranial bleed or has a condition that is of concern, such as a GCS <8 or persistent, unexplained confusion, he/she should be referred to a specialist neurosurgical centre so that the neurosurgeons can advise about medical management and possible transfer to that centre (National Institute for Clinical Excellence, 2003). A GCS <8 suggests that the patient is in a coma and may, therefore, have a significant neurological deficit (Hickey, 2002).

A contusion is bruising within the brain and can result from a traumatic injury. Contusions tend to worsen after 48 hours as swelling develops around the contusion, causing an increase in ICP (Lindsay et al, 1998).

Abscesses are collections of infection and pus within the brain tissue. They can be caused by a variety of processes, which can be systemic or involving head/neck infections. Systemic infections include, for example, subacute bacterial endocarditis, whereas head/neck infections include chronic ear infections, frontal sinusitis and skull fractures (Lindsay et al, 1998). Abscesses are usually multiple and tend to be treated conservatively with intravenous antibiotics (Lindsay et al, 1998).

Other cerebral infective processes can cause an altered level of consciousness. Bacteria, viruses and fungi can cause meningitis or inflammation of the meninges. Bacterial meningitis, especially when caused by the meningococcal bacterium, can cause a rapid deterioration in neurological status and needs to be treated promptly with broad-spectrum antibiotics until the exact bacterium is identified (Lindsay et al, 1998).

The cardinal signs and symptoms of bacterial meningitis are neck stiffness, photophobia, altered level of consciousness, vomiting, fever and possibly a purpuric rash (Hickey, 2002). Encephalitis is a generalized inflammation of the brain and is usually caused by a viral infection, such as herpes simplex (Lindsay et al, 1998). Again, an altered level of consciousness is observed accompanied by, for example, headache and fever. Additionally, seizures may develop.

Cerebral oedema/swelling

Cerebral oedema can occur around traumatic or ischaemic injury such as following prolonged cardiac arrest or around lesions. There are three types of oedema. First, vasogenic oedema occurs around traumatic/ischaemic injury and is formed by protein-rich fluid moving from the cerebral vascular system across capillary walls into the extracellular space. Second, cytotoxic oedema occurs around tumours and is formed by fluid accumulating within cells. Last, there can be interstitial cerebral oedema that usually occurs during hydrocephalus (the accumulation of CSF within the cerebral ventricular system and subarachnoid space) when CSF is forced out of the ventricles by pressure (Hickey, 2002).

Increases in CSF

Hydrocephalus can be a consequence of a number of situations, but falls into two categories depending on whether there is flow of CSF between the ventricles and the subarachnoid space. Obstructive (or non-communicating) hydrocephalus occurs when there is obstruction of the flow of CSF. This can result from, for example, brainstem tumours, cerebellar haemorrhages or blood clots within the fourth ventricle (Lindsay et al, 1998).

Communicating hydrocephalus occurs when there is a build-up of CSF but the cause of this is outside of the ventricles. There is flow of CSF between the ventricles and the subarachnoid space but the flow becomes sluggish or obstructed within the subarachnoid space. This can occur, for example, following meningitis and subarachnoid haemorrhage (Lindsay et al, 1998). Patients with long-term hydrocephalus will probably have had a ventriculoperitoneal shunt inserted to allow for drainage of the CSF. However, the shunt may become blocked, for example by exudate, or may become infected (Hickey, 2002). Should this occur, the patient will demonstrate the signs of raised ICP, one of which is an altered level of consciousness as the hydrocephalus reoccurs.

Conclusion

There are many different reasons why a patient may display an altered level of consciousness. It is essential that nurses are able to assess accurately a patient with an altered level of consciousness and to identify likely causes of the alteration. If the patient does not have a known neurological pathophysiology, such as a haematoma or cerebral infection, it is recommended that extracranial causes be excluded. Therefore, questions to ask are:

- Is the patient hypoxaemic and/or anaemic, which may limit cerebral oxygenation?
- Is the patient hypoventilating, thereby causing a hypercapnia, which will alter the cerebral vasculature?
- Is the patient's blood pressure high enough to perfuse his/her brain?
- Does the patient have a normal blood glucose level?

By using a systematic approach and with the use of an assessment tool, neurological deterioration can be identified. Specific organ dysfunctions that can result in cerebral dysfunction can be excluded in relation to the patient's known medical history, such as liver disease, chronic renal dysfunction or drug therapy. By using a systematic approach and problem solving, care can be rationalized. Even so, whatever the cause of the altered level of consciousness, interventions must be implemented quickly so that permanent brain damage is avoided.

References

Adam S, Osbourne S (1997) *Critical Care Nursing Science and Practice*. Oxford Medical Publications, Oxford

Addison C, Crawford B (1999) Not bad, just misunderstood. *Nurs Times* **95**(43): 52–3

Fairley D, Cosgrove J (1999) Glasgow Coma Scale: improving nursing practice through clinical effectiveness. *Nurs Crit Care* **4**(6): 276–9

Greaves I, Porter K, Ryan J (2001) *Trauma Care Manual*. Arnold, London

Hickey JV (2002) *The Clinical Practice of Neuromedical and Neurosurgical Nursing*. 5th edn. Lippincott, Williams & Wilkins, Philadelphia

Hudak CM, Gallo BM, Gonce Morton P (1998) *Critical Care Nursing: A Holistic Approach*. 7th edn. Lippincott, Williams & Wilkins, Philadelphia

Lindsay KW, Bone I, Callender R (1998) *Neurology and Neurosurgery Illustrated*. 3rd edn. Churchill Livingstone, London

Lowry M (1998) Emergency nursing and the Glasgow Coma Scale. *Accid Emerg Nurs* **6**(3): 143–8

McNarry AF, Goldhill DR (2004) Simple bedside assessment of level of consciousness: comparison of two simple assessment scales with the Glasgow Coma Scale. *Anaesthesia* **59**(1): 34–7

National Institute for Clinical Excellence (2003) *Head Injury: Triage, Assessment, Investigation and Early Management of Head Injury in Infants, Children and Adults*. NICE, London

Neal MJ (2002) *Medical Pharmacology at a Glance*. 3rd edn. Blackwell Science, Oxford

Porth CM (2003) *Essentials of Pathophysiology: Concepts of Altered Health States*. Lippincott, Williams & Wilkins, Philadelphia

Price T (2002) Painful stimuli and the Glasgow Coma Scale. *Nurs Crit Care* **7**(1): 19–23

Shah S (1999) Neurological assessment. *Nurs Stand* **13**(22): 49–56

Smith G (2000) *ALERT: Acute Life-threatening Events Recognition and Treatment*. 1st edn. University of Portsmouth, Portsmouth

Teasdale G, Jennett B (1974) Assessment of coma and impaired consciousness. *Lancet* **2**: 81–4

Tortora GJ, Grabowski NP (1996) *Principles of Anatomy and Physiology*. 8th edn. Harper Collins, London

Vander AJ, Sherman JH, Luciano DS (2000) *Human Physiology: The Mechanisms of Body Function*. 7th edn. McGraw-Hill, London

Woodrow P (2000) *Intensive Care Nursing: A Framework for Practice*. Routledge, London

Woodward S (1997) Neurological observations: 1. Glasgow Coma Scale. *Nurs Times* **93**(45): 46–8

Chapter 2

Nursing tools and strategies to assess cognition and confusion

Thomas Aird, Michelle McIntosh

How often have nurses used the following expression to describe a patient's mental status:

'Thomas appears to be acting a bit confused today'?

Objectively, what does that statement mean and how often does it actually serve to cause confusion among staff involved with caring for the patient? Patients with neurological dysfunction present with a complex range of problems. Physical impairments, because of their observable, measurable and frequently predictable clinical course, often overshadow more subtle cognitive deficits. Yet cognitive impairment may in fact contribute to the severity of physical impairment, and cognitive and behavioural changes are likely to place more stress on the family than is experienced by those families of patients with physical disability.

The social impact of cognitive impairment is discussed by Benner and Wrubel (1989) who state that:

'... people with neurological illness sustain damage to their "selves" in a way that people with no other illness do.'

Reference is made to the changes in personality and the impact that this can have when patients become strangers to their friends and families. Similarly, Rose and Johnson (1996) stress the role of the brain in defining our individuality and uniqueness. The integration of sensory data with mood, feelings, skills and memories is essential when interaction with the environment and communication with others is our key goal.

Florence Nightingale wrote in 1860 that:

'... if you do not get into the habit of observation one way or another (including taking notes) you had better give up being a nurse, for it is not your calling' (Baly, 1991).

This statement is particularly relevant to nurses working with patients experiencing neurological dysfunction where astute observational skills are necessary in order to detect discrete and ever-changing problems experienced by patients. The purpose of this chapter is to discuss cognitive assessment appropriate to bedside nursing, identifying tools and strategies used to assess patients.

Problems of definition

Terms such as 'confusion', 'dementia', 'delirium' and 'disorientation' are often used to describe a patient's mental status. Geary (1994) argues that acute confused states are not clearly and consistently defined and this leads to ambiguity. There are over 30 separate terms to define delirium. Some common terms used include intensive care unit (ICU) psychosis or ICU syndrome.

Simpson (1984) used a questionnaire to elucidate what doctors and nurses meant when they described a patient as confused. The sample included 58 physicians, 74 patients, 69 registered nurses and 73 psychiatric nurses. Simpson states that the word confused, although widely used in the English language, has many different definitions. These include disorientation to time and place, and a condition in which there is a disturbance of consciousness, among other things. Simpson concluded that there is a wide discrepancy in the understanding of the word confusion, to such an extent that its meaning is ambiguous.

Yeaw and Abdate (1993) warn that the term confused 'encompasses an amorphous group of symptoms', stressing the need to include behavioural and cognitive data. They also stress that the focus of assessment:

'... should be on how confusion interferes with patients' ability to function rather than on interference with nurses' function.'

This highlights two major nursing goals — the need to maintain the safety and the dignity of a compromised and vulnerable patient.

Cognition includes perception, thinking, remembering and organizing information (Hannegan, 1989). Hickey (1997) states that cognitive functioning includes several domains of intellectual ability such as language, visuospatial ability, abstract reasoning, attention and mental tracking, set shifting and memory. *Table 2.1* lists the key elements of cognitive assessment (Hickey, 1997).

Such functions require awareness of self and environment, and it is at this point that consciousness and cognition are considered one and the same. Awareness is traditionally considered as a component of consciousness, and alterations in awareness reflect an altered conscious state. This is often described in terms of confusion or disorientation.

Cognition, therefore, requires the blending of many types of sensory input, previous experience, learning and recall. Grzankowski (1997) states that:

'The symptoms for which nurses should assess a patient include changes in the patient's ability to filter out irrelevant stimuli, learn new information, comprehend the evidence of what is happening in a specific situation, apply old solutions to new situations, generate different solutions for specific problems, direct his or her own behaviour and follow through on a plan.'

Table 2.1: Cognitive functioning

- Orientation
- Memory
- Attention
- Ability to evaluate
- Affect and mood
- Abstract reasoning
- Insight
- Behaviour

From Hickey (1997)

Cook and Thigpen (1993) define cognition as a process that allows a patient to understand and retain instructions, solve problems and begin tasks.

Tess (1991) makes reference to a number of studies that describe acute confusional states as characterized by widespread cerebral dysfunction involving cognitive functions of perception, thought and memory, disturbed sleep–wake cycles and impaired attention.

Birkland and Dyck (1993) differentiate between the terms dementia and delirium. Dementia is described as a long-term, non-reversible loss of both short-term and long-term memory. Delirium is defined as an acute confusional state, usually as a result of a physical cause. The transient nature of delirium is further emphasized by Hodges (1994). Transient not only refers to the total duration of the period of delirium, but also the fluctuations that may take place over a 24-hour period. Although the syndrome has certain core characteristics, features may vary between patients.

Dementia, on the other hand, reflects structural changes in the cerebral cortex. Holden (1995) believes that dementia is not a disease in its own right, rather, it is deterioration in social behaviour and intellectual functioning. Crucial to this perspective is the progressive nature of dementia and the impact that the process has on the individual and his/her family. Holden (1995) makes some interesting distinctions between the two syndromes stating that:

> '... the defining characteristics of delirium are ... disturbed attention abilities and disordered thinking, which are not seen in dementia.'

Historically, cognitive impairment and ageing have been considered synonymous. Foreman and Grabowski (1992) believe that cognitive impairment should not be perceived as a benign and inevitable part of ageing, but as a condition that warrants prompt and aggressive action. Cognitive impairment is a significant health problem for the critically ill older patient and is associated with severe negative consequences, higher morbidity and mortality and a diminished capacity to care for oneself (Foreman and Grabowski, 1992; Matthiesen et al, 1994; Scherubel and Tess, 1994; Heath and Vink, 1999). The quality of incoming data is vital in determining perceptual quality. Cognitive functioning, therefore, requires intact cortical and subcortical structures necessary for the interpretation and integration of information. It must be remembered that significant changes take place to sensory systems as we age that will subsequently affect the quality of sensory data available for processing (Holden, 1995) (*Table 2.2*).

Table 2.2: Age-related changes in the senses

Vision	Reduction in the number of rods and cones; loss of elasticity of the lens; changes to the autonomic nervous system resulting in reduced ability of the pupil to dilate
Olfaction	Degeneration of neurones of the olfactory bulb
Taste	Reduction in the number of taste buds and reduction of saliva production
Hearing	Loss of neurones in auditory area; stiffening of ear drum; ear wax build-up
Touch	Reduced ability to perceive tactile stimuli through loss of peripheral receptors

From Holden (1995)

Delirium is a clinical diagnosis based primarily on the patient's behaviour. It is generally agreed that nursing management must focus on the safety of patients, as delirious patients have an increased risk of unintentional self-harm, such as dislodging life-support and monitoring equipment. Tess (1991) undertook a literature review into confusional states in intensive care settings. She concluded that confused patients are 2–5 times more likely to die than non-confused patients, and they are more likely to become permanently cognitively impaired and to require institutionalization.

Rockwood et al (1999) believe there is a strong correlation between delirium, dementia and death. They report a higher incidence of dementia in patients experiencing delirium, compared with those without delirium. They conclude that delirium is an important marker of risk of dementia. Although they acknowledge that the pathology is unclear, they suggest two possible reasons for the strong association:

- Delirium may give rise to brain damage, which results in predisposition or initiation of dementia
- Delirium may serve as a marker for a subclinical dementing process.

Assessment of a patient's cognitive functioning as well as physical health is an important consideration for long-term planning. Palmateer and McCartney (1985) suggest that the elderly patient with a reduced cognitive capacity, which has been compensated for with established habits of daily living supported in a variety of ways outside the hospital, may be perceived on admission to hospital as retaining overall adaptive functioning. Preservation of a patient's social amenities can lead clinicians to believe the individual to be cognitively intact and, as a consequence of adaptation, the assessment of cognitive capacity may not be pursued.

Langdon and Thompson (1996) refer to the adaptation that is necessary after a physical injury, such as a fractured leg. Movement such as getting into a car requires a great deal of concentration such as guarding against pain. The cognitively impaired individual may have the added difficulty of performing such activities with impaired problem-solving abilities. Guin and Freudenberger (1992) highlight the impact uncorrected visual deficits, glaring lights and frequent changes in nursing staff can have on maintaining the orientation of elderly patients.

Assessment

Merluzzi (1993) stresses that, from a clinical perspective, cognitive assessment does not necessarily refer to intelligence testing or neuropsychological assessment. Although an important aspect of cognitive functioning, intelligence testing may be included in more formal neuropsychological testing. The association of cognitive assessment with mental status, however, can have a profound negative impact on the patient. Leary (1990) believes there is a strong correlation between test performance and anxiety. He concludes that:

> *'Cognitive appraisal precipitates subjective anxiety, which disposes people to ruminate further and may interfere with ongoing behaviour. As behavioural performance is degraded, intrusive thinking escalates, which results in increased anxiety and additional interference.'*

A simple but effective method of assessing a patient's mental state is proposed by Holden (1995). By giving the patient a magazine or newspaper, information can be gathered about a number of different functions. These include memory for what has been read and associated events, recognition of pictures, comprehension, attention, speech, apraxias (pointing to items, picking up the magazine), ability to read and presence of unilateral neglect. Although this appears to be a simplistic approach, it could highlight the need for a more formal and comprehensive assessment. The assessor should consider carefully the need to be aware of the content of the material used if an objective assessment is to take place.

In her novel *Regeneration*, Pat Barker (1991) highlights this point. Detailing the first meeting between Siegfried Sassoon, the First World War poet who was suffering from shell shock, and neuropsychologist WHR Rivers, she describes the scene in the office during the serving of afternoon tea:

> *'His hands, doing complicated things with cup, saucer, plate, sandwiches, cake, sugar tongs and spoon, were perfectly steady...One of the nice things about serving afternoon tea to newly arrived patients was that it made so many neurological tests redundant.'*

The key message is the value of careful observation of the patient during the performance of normal activities of living.

The Glasgow Coma Scale (GCS) is probably the best known and most widely used neurological assessment tool. Jennett and Teasdale introduced it in 1974 as a simple means of providing a uniform method of assessing a patient's level of consciousness. Jennett (1986) described the main purpose of the GCS as a tool to provide a common language in order to improve communication for the wide range of personnel involved in patient care.

Teasdale (1975) placed the GCS into context by stating that, in spite of advances in monitoring patients by machines, this is one of the circumstances in which a record of nurses' observations is greatly superior to anything that can be produced by connecting the patient to a machine.

The GCS measures three modes of behaviour independently:

- Eye opening
- Verbal response
- Motor response.

Each mode is arranged in a scale of increasing dysfunction, and all three are combined to produce a level of consciousness (Frawley, 1990). The scale consists of ratings for eye opening based on a 4-point scale, verbal response on a 5-point scale and motor response on a 6-point scale. Altered consciousness consists of abnormal behaviour in one or more of the three functional areas: eye opening (arousal), verbal response (awareness) and motor response (activity). Arousal is considered to be a prerequisite to awareness. Awareness itself reflects the cognitive component of consciousness. What the patient says gives insight into the content of his/her consciousness. Orientation is the recognition of one's position in relation to time and space. Using the GCS, a person who is oriented knows who they are (name), where they are (for example, in hospital), and when it is (month and year). If these three questions are answered correctly, the patient is said to be oriented.

Segatore and Way (1992) consider the psychometric properties of the GCS to be weak. They argue that the GCS lacks the subtleties necessary to describe in appropriate detail patients with discrete disturbances of intellectual function. Indeed, as early as 1975, Jennett and Bond acknowledged that individuals with significant brain damage may show evidence of behavioural, cognitive and long-term memory deficits beyond what can be elicited by the GCS.

One of the most often referred to assessment tools is the Mini-Mental Status Examination (MMSE) (*Table 2.3*) (Folstein et al, 1975).

Table 2.3: Mini-Mental Status Examination (MMSE)

Record response to each question

Orientation	
Year, month, day, date, season	-/5
Country, county (district), town, hospital, ward (room)	-/5
Registration	
Examiner names three objects (tree, flag, ball)	
Patient asked to repeat three names	
Score one for each correct answer	-/3
Then ask patient to repeat all three names three times	
Attention	
Subtract 7 from 100, then repeat from result (i.e. 100, 93, 86, etc.)	
Stop after 5 (do not correct if errors made)	
(Alternatively, if unable to perform serial subtraction:	
spell 'world' backwards: D L R O W)	
Score the best performance on either task	-/5
Recall	
Ask for the names of the three objects learned earlier	-/3
Language	
Show the patient and ask him/her to name a pencil and a watch	-/2
Repeat 'No ifs, ands, or buts'	-/1
Give a three-stage command. Score one for each stage	-/3
(e.g. 'Take this piece of paper in your right hand, fold it in half and	
place it on the chair next to you')	
Ask the patient to read and obey a written command on a piece of paper, stating:	-/1
'Close your eyes'	
Ask the patient to write a sentence. Score if it is sensible, and has a subject and a verb	-/1
Copying	
Ask the patient to copy two intersecting pentagrams	-/1
Total score	-/30

From Folstein et al (1975); Hodges (1994)

The MMSE was originally developed to evaluate the cognitive abilities of psychiatric patients. It has found favour within elderly care settings where it is used extensively. The MMSE measures orientation, attention, registration, calculation, recall, ability to follow a three-part command and the use of language. The tool consists of 11 open-ended questions, which are designed to evaluate an individual's orientation, recall and ability to carry out simple visuospatial commands.

Folstein et al (1975) stressed that the MMSE is not intended to diagnose cognitive problems, rather it is used to rule out or confirm cognitive impairment. The MMSE is considered to be a simple and easy tool to use, taking approximately 10 minutes to complete. Each item is given a weighted score. All the scores are added together to give a total score, the maximum score possible being 30. Iliffe et al (1990) group the scores into three bands: 0–18, cognitive impairment; 19–24, possible cognitive impairment; 25–30, no cognitive impairment.

Geary (1994) believes that the MMSE is useful as a baseline assessment, but it is not always practical for use in high-dependency areas where patients may not be able to speak or pay attention for an extended period. Likewise, Cimprich (1995) found the MMSE to be a valid and reliable bedside screening tool in detecting global cognitive impairment (e.g. delirium), but it may not be able to detect the more subtle impairments in attention and concentration. Grzankowski (1997) recommends that nurses include family members when reviewing the patient's previous level of cognitive ability, as some behaviour may be normal for the patient. A cautionary note is necessary, however, in terms of adaptation. Changes occurring over a period of time require adaptation of the patient and of those close to them. How much this may mask the actual deficits is questionable.

Foreman and Zane (1996) caution that scores on mental status questionnaires can be misleading. The type of cognitive impairment, level of formal education and test environment may all influence performance. This is supported by Hodges (1994), who cautions about the vulnerability of the test to age, education level and socioeconomic status. Hodges suggests the following age-related cut-offs when applying the test: 40s–29; 50s–28; 60s–28; 70s–28; 80s–26. It is suggested, therefore, that the MMSE should be used as an adjunct to other nursing observations. Hilton (1991) believes that the MMSE does not test spatial-perceptual skills and argues that the MMSE favours left-sided brain functions at the exclusion of right-sided functions. Localized cognitive functions are listed in *Table 2.4*.

Table 2.4: Localized cognitive functions

Dominant hemisphere (usually left cerebral cortex)

Language: most aspects of spoken language, plus reading and writing
Calculation
Praxis (higher motor control)

Non-dominant hemisphere (usually right cerebral cortex)

Spatially directed attention
Complex visual-perceptual skills
Constructional abilities
Prosodic components of language (tone, melody, intonation)
Attention/concentration and vigilance

Adapted from Hodges (1994)

Implications for nursing

Nurses are in a unique position to observe and evaluate continually the patient's level of cognitive functioning. Evidence, however, suggests that cognitive impairment remains undetected in a significant number of patients. Matthiesen et al (1994) found assessments to be informal, incomplete, based on overt deficits and influenced by how the patient responded socially. They also add that patients may be oriented to person, place and time on admission, but still have problems with attention, memory and thinking.

Rockwood (2003) suggests that when a healthcare professional encounters a patient with delirium, he/she should conclude that the patient is sick, and that a delirious patient is likely to be sick as a result of factors that usually cause acute illness in old age. These include medications, infections, heart failure, metabolic abnormalities, some combination or something else. Worryingly, Young and George (2003) report that delirium was only recorded in 26% of the nursing notes and 50% of the medical notes of 211 patients entered into their study.

When implementing care and treatment plans for neurologically impaired patients, Harrison (2000) believes that a care plan should be created that aims to maximize personal autonomy and quality of life. Woodrow (1998) argues, however, that for most people the ability to make their own choices enables them to make the most of their lives. Woodrow believes that those patients suffering from confusional states are at risk of being robbed of a state of autonomy. Even if the cognitive limitations can be overcome, the label 'confused' invites others to ignore and dismiss the patient's request.

Cook and Thigpen (1993) discuss the management of patients with cognitive deficits within a rehabilitation setting. They stress the importance of ascertaining why a patient may not carry out routine tasks or may be labelled as non-compliant. They state that once the nurse ascertains why a patient is not benefiting from instruction;

'The nurse needs to find an appropriate teaching technique to accommodate the cognitive or perceptual impairment demonstrated by the patient.'

Common sense would dictate that there is no logic in providing patients with information they cannot process.

Brewin and Lewis (2001) undertook a phenomenological study of patients' perspectives of cognitive deficits and identified six themes that had an impact on daily activities:

- Communication
- Social
- Domestic
- Driving and using transport
- Hobbies.

The authors raise some concern in that no patients reported being given any warning with regard to driving ability. Hemingway and McAndrew (1997) also caution that the impact of cognitive deficits may only become apparent when the patient returns home. Cognitive impairment will often restrict the person's prospects of returning to his/her previous lifestyle. The person's role within the family can change with catastrophic effects, leading to a shift in responsibilities between partners, and old friends may drift away leaving the individual more isolated and dependent on others.

The question remains, however, as to how often cognitive assessment should be performed. Foreman and Zane (1996) advocate that it should be carried out routinely, for example on each shift. Testing can be simple if the patient is alert and oriented, but a more comprehensive test can be performed if the patient demonstrates any change. Dellasega and Morris (1993) question using the MMSE as a single measure of cognitive impairment. The often reversible nature of delirium necessitates regular testing of the mental state. Dellasega and Morris (1993) propose that testing should take place in different environments at different times of the day.

Arguably then, cognitive assessment should be carried out routinely and should be given the same status as the GCS. Given the relationship of impaired attention associated with anxiety, the resultant data collected may be inaccurate. This reflects the sensitive approach necessary when performing cognitive assessment and its association with mental status.

Many authors have mixed beliefs regarding nursing assessment of cognitively impaired patients. Hemingway and McAndrew (1997) suggest that, following acute brain injury, people are expected to follow a pattern of grief whereby they go through stages of shock, denial and anger. Feelings of grief and hopelessness are normal and usually transient in the adjustment phase. Adjustment problems are common in people who are physically ill and this can present the clinical team with difficulties when attempting to distinguish between normal and abnormal responses to illness.

Harrison (2000) suggests that, as a direct result, both medical and surgical nursing staff generally tend to ignore the psychological needs of those experiencing physical illness. Flannery (1998) defends this lack of nursing assessment, arguing that it is not generally the nurse's responsibility to assess the cognitive level of these patients in the acute setting. She believes that the data routinely collected as a basis for nursing care provide the necessary baseline to make such an assessment, but nurses who are not rehabilitation practitioners do not know how to interpret this information to develop cognitive rehabilitation plans for such patients.

Ludwick and O'Toole (1996) carried out a study into nurses' knowledge and interventions of the confused patient. They reported that most nurses in the study used verbal behaviours, such as orientation of the patient, to define confusion. Physical behaviours such as poor eye contact, restlessness and getting out of bed were also reported, but by fewer nurses in the sample group.

Conclusion

This chapter has considered the difference between confusion and cognition. The dilemma surrounding the use of terminology has been explored and some of the key differences highlighted. Nurses working within acute general clinical areas do not routinely perform assessment of a patient's mental state. The patient's priorities in terms of physical needs are often paramount and overshadow the subtleties manifest in cognitive impairment. Ways of assessing cognitive status at the bedside have been identified through informal and formal testing. Although testing may indicate some degree of cognitive impairment, formal neuropsychological testing may be necessary in order to evaluate the true extent of the problem. Nurses need to be aware of the potential complications of cognitive impairment and initiate strategies that ensure the safety and dignity of the patient.

References

Baly M, ed (1991) *As Miss Nightingale Said: Florence Nightingale Through Her Sayings — a Victorian Perspective.* Scutari Books, London

Barker P (1991) *Regeneration.* Penguin Books, London

Benner P, Wrubel J (1989) *The Primacy of Caring. Stress and Coping in Health and Illness.* Addison-Wesley, New York

Birkland P, Dyck E (1993) 'Psychiatric' or 'medical'? Assessing confusion in the elderly patient. *J Emerg Nurs* **19**(5): 408–11

Brewin J, Lewis P (2001) Patients' perspectives of cognitive deficits after head injury. *Br J Ther Rehabil* **8**(6): 218–27

Cimprich B (1995) Symptom management: loss of concentration. *Semin Oncol Nurs* **11**(4): 279–88

Cook EA, Thigpen R (1993) Identification and management of cognitive and perceptual deficits in the rehabilitation patient. *Rehabil Nurs* **18**(5): 310–13

Dellasega C, Morris D (1993) The MMSE to assess the cognitive state of elders. *J Neurosci Nurs* **25**(3): 147–52

Flannery J (1998) Using the levels of cognitive functioning assessment scale with patients with traumatic brain injury in an acute care setting. *Rehabil Nurs* **23**(2): 88–94

Folstein MF, Folstein SE, McHugh PR (1975) Mini-mental state: a practical method for grading the cognitive state of patients for the clinician. *J Psychiatr Res* **12**: 189–98

Foreman MD, Grabowski R (1992) Diagnostic dilemma: cognitive impairment in the elderly. *J Gerontol Nurs* **18**(9): 5–12

Foreman MD, Zane D (1996) Nursing strategies for acute confusion in elders. *Am J Nurs* **96**(4): 44–52

Frawley P (1990) Neurological observations. *Nurs Times* **86**(35): 29–34

Geary SM (1994) Intensive care unit psychosis revisited: understanding and managing delirium in the critical care setting. *Crit Care Nurs Q* **17**(1): 51–63

Grzankowski J (1997) Altered thought processes related to traumatic brain injury and their nursing implications. *Rehabil Nurs* **22**(1): 24–9

Guin PR, Freudenberger K (1992) The elderly neuroscience patient: implications for the critical care nurse. *AACN Clin Issues* **3**(1): 98–105

Hannegan L (1989) Transient cognitive changes after craniotomy. *J Neurosci Nurs* **21**(3): 165–70

Harrison A (2000) Psychological problems in the neurology setting. *Prof Nurse* **15**: 706–9

Heath DL, Vink R (1999) Secondary mechanisms in traumatic brain injury: a nurse's perspective. *J Neurosci Nurs* **34**(2): 97–103

Hemingway S, McAndrew S (1997) Acquired brain injury: identifying emotional and cognitive needs. *Nurs Stand* **12**(10): 40–5

Hickey JV (1997) *The Clinical Practice of Neurological and Neurosurgical Nursing.* 4th edn. Lippincott, New York

Hilton G (1991) Review of neurobehavioural assessment tools. *Heart Lung* **20**(5): 436–42

Hodges JR (1994) *Cognitive Assessment for Clinicians.* Oxford University Press, Oxford

Holden U (1995) *Ageing, Neuropsychology and the New Dementias.* Chapman and Hall, London

Iliffe S, Booroff A, Gallivan S, Goldenberg E, Morgan P, Haines A (1990) Screening for cognitive impairment in the elderly using the mini-mental state examination. *Br J Gen Pract* **40**: 277–9

Jennett B (1986) Altered consciousness and coma. In: Crockard A, Hatward R, Hoff JT, eds. *Neurosurgery: The Scientific Basis of Clinical Practice.* Blackwell Science, Oxford: 117–26

Jennett B, Bond M (1975) Assessment of outcome after severe brain damage. *Lancet* **1**: 480–4

Jennett B, Teasdale G (1974) Assessment of coma and impaired consciousness. A practical scale. *Lancet* **2**: 81–4

Langdon D, Thompson A (1996) Cognitive problems in multiple sclerosis. *MS Management* **3**(2): 5–9

Leary MR (1990) Anxiety, cognition, and behaviour: in search of a broader perspective. *Soc Behav Pers* **5**(2): 39–44

Ludwick R, O'Toole AW (1996) The confused patient: nurses' knowledge and interventions. *J Gerontol Nurs* **22**(1): 44–9

Matthiesen V, Sivertsen L, Foreman MD, Cronin-Stubbs D (1994) Acute confusion: nursing interventions in older patients. *Orthop Nurs* **13**(2): 21–7, 29

Merluzzi TV (1993) Cognitive assessment: clinical applications of self-statement assessment. *J Couns Dev* **71**: 539–45

Palmateer LM, McCartney JR (1985) Do nurses know when patients have cognitive deficit? *J Gerontol Nurs* **11**(2): 6–7, 10–12

Rockwood K (2003) Need we do so badly in managing delirium in elderly patients? *Age Ageing* **32**: 473–4

Rockwood K, Cosway S, Carver D, Jarrett P, Stadnky K, Fisk J (1999) The risk of dementia and death after delirium. *Age Ageing* **28:** 551–6

Rose D, Johnson D (1996) *Brain Injury and After. Towards Improved Outcome*. John Wiley and Sons, Chichester

Scherubel JC, Tess MM (1994) Measuring clinical confusion in critically ill patients. *J Neurosci Nurs* **26**(3): 146–50

Segatore M, Way C (1992) The Glasgow Coma Scale: time for change. *Heart Lung* **21**(6): 548–57

Simpson CJ (1984) Doctors' and nurses' use of the word confused. *Br J Psychiatry* **145**(10): 441–3

Teasdale G (1975) Acute impairment of brain function. 1: Assessing 'conscious level'. *Nurs Times* **71**(24): 914–17

Tess MM (1991) Acute confusional states in critically ill patients: a review. *J Neurosci Nurs* **23**(6): 398–402

Woodrow P (1998) Interventions for confusion and dementia. 1: Quality of life. *Br J Nurs* **7:** 891–4

Yeaw EMJ, Abdate JH (1993) Identification of confusion among the elderly in an acute care setting. *Clin Nurse Spec* **7**(4): 192–7

Young LJ, George J (2003) Do guidelines improve the process and outcomes of care in delirium? *Age Ageing* **32:** 525–8

Chapter 3

Assessment of chronic neuropathic pain and the use of pain tools

Sarah White

In the UK it is estimated that there are about 550 000 people suffering from neuropathic pain (Jameson, 1996). Chronic neuropathic pain is often identified as a significant problem by patients with neurological conditions. There is a prolific amount written in the literature about pain assessment, but most is not specific to neuropathic pain. This chapter examines the evidence base for the assessment of chronic neuropathic pain. The literature was reviewed from 1992–2002 and, for the purpose of this publication, updated to March 2006. The key words used in the search were: 'neuropathic pain', 'chronic pain', 'assessment' and 'measurement of pain'. Databases used were British Nursing Index, Journals@Ovid, CINAHL and Medline.

Neuropathic pain

Neuropathic pain occurs as a result of damage in the peripheral or central nervous system as a result of a primary lesion or disease. The injured nerve abnormally processes stimuli, and pain is felt by the individual (Munafo and Trim, 2000). Allodynia is one example where a non-painful stimulus, such as touch, feels painful. The characteristics of neuropathic pain are usually described as burning, shooting, tingling or electric in nature. It is often chronic and difficult to treat as the pain does not respond to conventional analgesia (Jameson, 1996; McCaffery and Pasero, 1999; Munafo and Trim, 2000).

Unlike acute pain, chronic pain does not have a predictable ending and serves no useful purpose (O'Hara, 1996). In the literature there is a discrepancy in the duration the pain needs to be experienced before it is termed chronic. Maloni (2000) defines it as a pain that lasts longer than 1 month. Davis (2000) states that it is pain from disease that persists for more than 3 months. However, McCaffery and Pasero (1999) describe chronic non-malignant pain as pain that has continued for at least 6 months and has not been resolved with treatment.

Chronic neuropathic pain can affect the patient physically, psychologically and socially. A study by Walker and Sofaer (1998) demonstrated that 60% of patients suffering with chronic pain had emotional problems owing to psychosocial factors either because of, or secondary to, their pain. These problems included fears about the future, loss of social life and relationship problems.

Nurse assessment of pain

Davis (2000) believes that the nurse has an important role to play in identifying the consequences of chronic pain and implementing appropriate interventions to improve the patient's quality of life. It is well documented how vital it is for the nurse to assess the patient's pain so that a treatment plan for both the pain, and related problems, can be devised (Simon, 1996; Davies and McVicar, 2000a). The initial assessment can also be used as a baseline to measure improvement or deterioration (Simon, 1996; Munafo and Trim, 2000) and can be the basis for setting rehabilitation goals.

However, even though the importance of detailed assessment is emphasized in much of the literature, McCaffery and Ferrell (1997) state that many studies indicate that nurses are not assessing pain adequately. In the studies that Simon (1996) examined, she found that a large proportion of the nurses lacked knowledge about chronic pain and that detailed assessments were not being performed. Hamilton and Edgar (1992) conducted a survey of nurses' knowledge of pain control, which demonstrated that a large majority did not know the clinical differences between acute and chronic pain.

Assessment in practice

It was the challenging nature of assessing and treating chronic neuropathic pain successfully within the author's area of practice that led to this review being undertaken. At the time of writing the author practised as a specialist nurse in a neurological rehabilitation community team within intermediate care. The team comprised physiotherapists, occupational therapists, speech and language therapists, therapy assistants, specialist nurses and administrative staff.

Before the review, when a patient was referred to the team an initial holistic assessment was performed to gather information using past medical history, current function and how it was affecting activities of living. Goals were set with the patient and scored on a numerical rating scale to describe how much each problem was interfering with his/her everyday activities.

If chronic neuropathic pain was identified as a problem it was rated at the initial assessment and at evaluation on discharge. Pain was also recorded on the Dartmouth Cooperative (COOP) Function and Health Status Measure (Dartmouth Cooperative Project, 1995). This is one of nine charts used as an outcome measure by the team. It was identified that the scores obtained at initial assessment were often unchanged at discharge. Both of these measures used were unidimensional, not sensitive to small changes in pain levels following treatment and did not conform to the evidence base to assess the multifaceted nature of neuropathic pain.

When selecting a management option, each professional discipline asked more specific questions about the pain relevant to their area of practice. This conformed with the evidence base in relation to interdisciplinary care (Davies and McVicar, 2000b) and aimed to address the impact that chronic pain has on many areas of an individual's life (Fordham and Dunn, 1994; McCaffery and Pasero, 1999). However, a standardized tool was not used, and care was reliant on the professional's knowledge of neuropathic pain and appropriate treatment options.

Pain assessment tools

There are many different pain assessment tools. Some only measure one aspect of pain, such as a numerical rating scale measuring pain intensity (*Figure 3.1*), while others are multidimensional (Munafo and Trim, 2000).

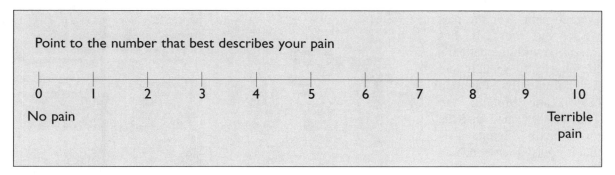

Point to the number that best describes your pain

0 1 2 3 4 5 6 7 8 9 10

No pain   Terrible pain

Figure 3.1: A numerical rating scale

Numerical Rating Scale

The Numerical Rating Scale is easy and quick to use (McCaffery and Pasero, 1999). It can also be used verbally with a patient when it is not available in its written form or if the patient is visually impaired. The tool is available in different languages and is appropriate for use with patients from different cultures (McCaffery and Pasero, 1999). However, it only measures pain intensity, and McCaffery and Pasero (1999) recommend that the initial pain assessment is multidimensional because by nature chronic pain is complex and can affect many different areas of a person's life. An accurate and detailed history and assessment is vital in being able to develop an individual treatment care plan (Simon and McTier, 1996).

Some of the main multidimensional tools are discussed below, and their suitability for assessing neuropathic pain will be explored.

Initial Pain Assessment Tool

The Initial Pain Assessment Tool (McCaffery and Beebe, 1989) collects details on the location, intensity and quality of the pain. It also records what increases or relieves the pain and the effects of the pain on the patient's quality of life. It is in a simple format and could be completed in a relatively short period. There is no intensity scale included in the form, which gives the nurse the choice of using the most appropriate one for the individual; however, this may cause problems with the same scale not being used at subsequent recordings.

Brief Pain Inventory

The Brief Pain Inventory (Cleeland, 1991) (*Figure 3.2*) assesses the pain by scoring on a scale of 0–10 the patient's worst and average pain over the past week and how it has interfered with the patient's life physically, socially and psychologically. Pateman (1996) and Munafo and Trim (2000) agree that the tool's main advantage is that it is easy to use and can be completed by the patient unaided. If a particular problem is identified on initial assessment, just this part of the questionnaire can be used for regular reassessment to measure i m p r o v e m e n t s / deteriorations in relation to management and treatment.

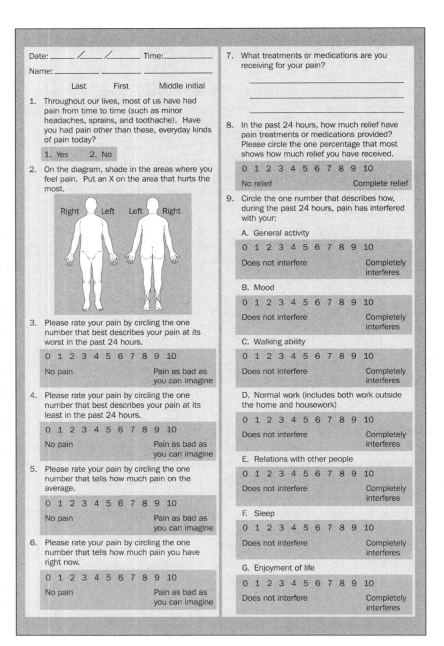

Figure 3.2: The Brief Pain Inventory (short form) (Cleeland, 1991). Diagram adapted from McCaffery and Pasero (1999).

McGill Pain Questionnaire

Munafo and Trim (2000) advocate the McGill Pain Questionnaire (Melzack, 1983) as an excellent tool for chronic pain assessment. It has been widely used in research and in its shorter form in clinical practice. The shorter form has 15 descriptive words to describe pain, which the patient rates and then achieves an overall score. It also includes a visual analogue scale and a present pain intensity scale.

Munafo and Trim acknowledge that the patient needs explanation on how to score and that it takes considerable time to complete. However, O'Hara (1996) views the shorter form as quick and easy to use, which has the advantage for reassessment purposes. Pateman (1996) observes that this tool may be limited for use with patients who have a good understanding of the vocabulary used in the tool. This has significance in patients with a neurological diagnosis where there may be cognitive impairment. Richardson (2001) also argues that this tool, along with other measurement tools, can be unreliable as it depends on the patient's memory when scoring.

Chronic Pain Assessment Tool

Simon and McTier (1996) state that tools such as those described so far are appropriate for initial assessment, but that a more comprehensive tool is needed for patients with unresolved or inadequately managed chronic pain. They developed a Chronic Pain Assessment Tool for this purpose. It is divided into six sections, which include pain and medication history, how the pain is affecting various areas of the patient's life and the impact the pain has had on personal relationships and goals. Examining the effect the pain is having on the individual's life helps the patient to identify rehabilitation goals. The fifth section measures the nurses' observations of the client's pain. This part of the tool may only be suitable for patients in an inpatient setting as it requires the nurse to note indicators, such as verbal and non-verbal complaints and body language, which would be difficult to record in the limited amount of time the patient would be observed in a community setting. The last section of the tool gives space for the nurse to add any further comments.

This tool is comprehensive and is suitable for the rehabilitation setting. However, it has only been tried in an inpatient environment, and the nurse's observation section would need to be adapted for community use. It is also time consuming to complete. Simon and McTier (1996) record that it takes between 45–90 minutes, which may be a disadvantage if fatigue is a problem, such as in multiple sclerosis. To overcome this, the patient could complete it in several shorter blocks of time. An advantage of the tool is that it is easy to understand and can mostly be completed by the patient unaided.

Neuropathy Pain Scale

Galer and Jensen (1997) noted that there was not an assessment tool that specifically measured neuropathic pain. They recognized that the McGill Pain Questionnaire contained descriptive words that described the nature of neuropathic pain but did not measure the level to which it was felt. They also observed that the existing tools were not sensitive enough to identify individual groups of people who, by the way they describe their pain, may benefit from a particular treatment.

Galer and Jensen (1997) acknowledge that this theory has not been well studied and further research is needed. Based on their clinical experience they identified the words commonly used to describe neuropathic pain as 'sharp', 'hot', 'dull', 'cold', 'sensitive', 'itchy', 'deep' and 'surface pain'. These were then used in the development of the Neuropathy Pain Scale (Galer and Jensen, 1997) (*Figure 3.3*).

The Neuropathy Pain Scale has eight descriptive qualities of neuropathic pain, which the patient scores from 0–10 using a numerical rating scale. It also includes a measure for how unpleasant or

Date: _____ / _____ / _____   Name: _____

There are several different aspects of pain which we are interested in measuring: pain sharpness, heat/cold, dullness, intensity, overall unpleasantness and surface versus deep pain.

The destinction between these aspects of pain might be clearer if you think of taste. For example, people might agree on how *sweet* a piece of pie might be (the *intensity* of sweetness), but some might enjoy it more if it were sweeter, while others might prefer it to be less sweet. Similarly, people can judge the loudness of music and agree on what is more quiet and what is louder, but disagree on how it makes them feel. Some prefer quiet music and some prefer it louder. In short, the *intensity* of a sensation is not the same as how it makes you feel. A sound might be unpleasant and still be quiet (think of someone grating their fingernails along a chalkboard). A sound can be quiet and "dull" or loud and "dull".

Pain is the same. Many people are able to tell the difference between many aspects of their pain: for example, *how much* it hurts and *how unpleasant* or annoying it is. Although often the intensity of pain has a strong influence on how unpleasant the experience of pain is, some people are able to experience more pain than others before they feel very bad about it.

There are scales for measuring different aspects of pain. For one patient, a pain might feel extremely hot, but not at all dull, while another patient may not experience any heat, but feel like their pain is very dull. We expect you to rate very high on some of the scales below and very low on others. We want you to use the measures that follow to tell us exactly what your experience of pain has been, on average, *during the past week*.

- -

Instructions: Please think about each sensation listed below and rate that sensation as the *average* you have experienced *during the past week*. Place an "X" through the number that best describes this.

1. Please use the scale below to tell us how intense your pain has been on average during the past week.

No pain | 0 | 1 | 2 | 3 | 4 | 5 | 6 | 7 | 8 | 9 | 10 | The most intense pain sensation imaginable

2. Please use the scale below to tell us how sharp your pain has felt on average during the past week. Words used to describe "sharp" feelings include: "like a knife", "like a spike", "jabbing", or "like jolts".

No pain | 0 | 1 | 2 | 3 | 4 | 5 | 6 | 7 | 8 | 9 | 10 | The most sharp sensation imaginable ("like a knife")

3. Please use the scale below to tell us how hot your pain has felt on average during the past week. Words used to describe very hot pain include: "burning" and "on fire".

Not hot | 0 | 1 | 2 | 3 | 4 | 5 | 6 | 7 | 8 | 9 | 10 | The most hot sensation imaginable ("on fire")

4. Please use the scale below to tell us how dull your pain has felt on average during the past week. Words used to describe very dull pain include: "like a dull toothache", "dull pain", "aching", and "like a bruise".

Not dull | 0 | 1 | 2 | 3 | 4 | 5 | 6 | 7 | 8 | 9 | 10 | The most dull sensation imaginable

5. Please use the scale below to tell us how cold your pain has felt on average during the past week. Words used to describe very cold pain include: "like ice" and "freezing".

Not cold | 0 | 1 | 2 | 3 | 4 | 5 | 6 | 7 | 8 | 9 | 10 | The most cold sensation imaginable ("freezing")

6. Please use the scale below to tell us how sensitive your skin has been to light touch or clothing on average during the past week. Words used to describe sensitive skin include: "like sunburned skin" and "raw skin".

Not sensitive | 0 | 1 | 2 | 3 | 4 | 5 | 6 | 7 | 8 | 9 | 10 | The most sensitive sensation imaginable ("raw skin")

7. Please use the scale below to tell us how itchy your pain has felt on average during the past week. Words used to describe itchy pain include: "like poison oak" and "like a mosquito bite".

Not itchy | 0 | 1 | 2 | 3 | 4 | 5 | 6 | 7 | 8 | 9 | 10 | The most itchy sensation imaginable ("like poison oak")

8. Which of the following best describes the time quality of your pain on average during the past week?

Please check only one: a, b, or c

a ☐ I felt background pain **all of the time** and occasional flare-ups (break-through pain) **some of the time**

Describe the background pain: _____

Describe the flare-up (break-through pain): _____

b ☐ I felt a single type of pain **all of the time.** Describe this pain: _____

c ☐ I felt a single type of pain **only sometimes**. Describe this pain: _____

9. Now that you have told us the different physical aspects of your pain, the different types of sensations, we want you to tell us overall how unpleasant your pain has been. Words used to describe very unpleasant pain include: "miserable" and "intolerable". Remember, pain can have a low intensity, but still feel extremely unpleasant, and some kinds of pain can have a high intensity but be very tolerable. Please use the scale below to tell us how unpleasant your pain has felt on average during the past week.

Not unpleasant | 0 | 1 | 2 | 3 | 4 | 5 | 6 | 7 | 8 | 9 | 10 | The most unpleasant sensation imaginable ("intolerable")

10. Lastly, we want you to give us an estimate of the severity of your deep versus surface pain. We want you to rate each location of pain separately. We realise that it can be difficult to make these estimates, and most likely it will be a "best guess", but please give us your best estimate.

HOW INTENSE HAS YOUR DEEP PAIN BEEN ON AVERAGE DURING THE PAST WEEK?

No deep pain | 0 | 1 | 2 | 3 | 4 | 5 | 6 | 7 | 8 | 9 | 10 | The most intense deep pain sensation imaginable

HOW INTENSE HAS YOUR SURFACE PAIN BEEN ON AVERAGE DURING THE PAST WEEK?

No surface pain | 0 | 1 | 2 | 3 | 4 | 5 | 6 | 7 | 8 | 9 | 10 | The most intense surface pain sensation imaginable

Figure 3.3: The Neuropathy Pain Scale (Galer and Jensen, 1997). Diagram adapted from McCaffery and Pasero (1999).

intolerable the pain is and whether it is surface or deep pain. The researchers report that the studies they performed to check the validity of the tool to assess the specific pain qualities of neuropathic pain were favourable. They note that the tool does not measure pain induced by standing or walking, which they plan to include in a revised version. McCaffery and Pasero (1999) state that there are several advantages to this tool. It is easy to use and may only take approximately 5 minutes to complete. It can be used at reassessment as it is sensitive to the effects of treating and managing the pain. The tool also has useful instructions at the beginning to help both the nurse and patient.

Neuropathic Pain Questionnaire

Since this article was originally published one further tool has been developed which is worth examining. Krause and Backonja (2003) noted that although Galer and Jenson's (1997) Neuropathy Pain Scale was a good general measure of neuropathic pain it did not discriminate neuropathic pain from non-neuropathic pain. The Neuropathic Pain Questionnaire was developed as a tool that would provide both a general assessment of neuropathic pain as well as help in discriminating between neuropathic and non-neuropathic pain (Krause and Backonja, 2003).

The questionnaire has 12 items which the patient has to score their most severe or disturbing site of pain on numerical rating scales. The items include assessing shooting pain, numbness, and electric and squeezing pain which are not included in the Neuropathic Pain Scale (Krause and Backonja, 2003). The tool has clear simple instructions and would only take the patient a few minutes to complete. One disadvantage of the tool is that calculating the score, which determines neuropathic or non-neuropathic pain, is a lengthy procedure and it would be relatively easy to make a mistake. However, the score could be calculated at the initial assessment to identify the type of pain and, when the tool is subsequently used as an outcome measure, a reduction in specific numerical rating scales would indicate a response to treatment. This would eliminate the need to recalculate the overall score. The questionnaire records the location, intensity and quality of the pain but does not measure the effect pain has on quality of life, making it less useful in a rehabilitation setting. It has the advantage over some of the other frequently used tools in the sensitivity and specificity of the questions (Krause and Backonja, 2003).

Advantages and disadvantages of tools

It is recognized that people of varying cultures express and experience pain in different ways (Carr and Mann, 2000). The cultural bias of the tools discussed in this chapter has not been addressed. Assessment tools play their part, but Davies and McVicar (2000a) maintain that they may limit patients' descriptions of their pain experience. The authors suggest that it is more important that the nurse facilitates the patient to tell his/her story by using good interview techniques such as open questions and active listening.

All the tools reviewed measure chronic pain and have advantages and disadvantages. Careful consideration needs to be made when selecting a pain assessment tool to ensure it is appropriate for the client group with whom it is intended to be used (Carr and Mann, 2000). There also needs to be examination as to how easy it is to complete the tool, what aspects of the pain are being assessed, such as site, intensity, qualities and effects, and the length of time it takes to record the information.

The Chronic Pain Assessment Tool (Simon and McTier, 1996) is a comprehensive tool, but is disadvantaged by the length of time it takes to complete. Some tools only measure the quality and intensity of the pain such as the short-form McGill Questionnaire and the Neuropathy Pain Scale (see *Figure 3.3*). Other tools also record the effect the pain has on quality of life, such as the Initial Pain Assessment Tool and the Brief Pain Inventory (see *Figure 3.2*).

The Brief Pain Inventory does not record the quality of the pain, but has an advantage over the Initial Pain Assessment Tool in that the effect of pain on physical, psychological and social aspects of life are measured using a numerical rating scale. This is beneficial in a rehabilitation setting as goals can be set using these scales to measure the success of management and treatment. The Neuropathy Pain Scale's distinct advantage is that, at the time this article was originally published, it was the only tool that specifically measured the different qualities of neuropathic pain. However, it does not assess the impact the pain has on quality of life.

Pain diary

Much of the literature advocates the use of a pain diary by the patient as part of ongoing assessment (de Rond et al, 1999; de Wit et al, 1999; Carr and Mann, 2000). This involves recording pain intensity on a numerical rating scale several times each day. Other information can also be recorded, such as activities of living, medication and other treatments or coping strategies the patient is using. This information can then be used to see if there is an emerging pattern in the correlation between pain intensity and activity, and to assess the outcome of treatment and management strategies. de Rond et al (2001) state that inadequate treatment of pain is as a result of nurses failing to assess pain daily.

Several studies have shown that both the patient and nurse valued daily pain assessment and that it improved the management of the pain (Johnstone, 1998; de Wit et al, 1999; de Rond et al, 2001). These studies were all carried out in the hospital setting. It is much easier to monitor and record the pain of patients in hospital or care facilities than it is to record the pain of patients at home. Nurses in a clinical setting are with the patient throughout the day and can incorporate recording pain experienced by the patient when they are taking the patients' vital signs (de Rond et al, 1999). In the community setting it is therefore even more important that the patient participates in recording this information in a diary (de Wit et al, 1999).

The use of a pain diary was evaluated by de Wit et al (1999) in a randomized control trial of 313 patients with chronic cancer pain in the home setting. Sixty per cent of the group thought it had helped them gain insight into their pain. The researchers report that patient compliance was high; it was more sensitive to changes in pain intensity than pain reported retrospectively and was a valuable tool in assessing treatment effects. These benefits would also be of value when managing neuropathic pain. The majority of the experimental group was female, which could have caused a bias in the results as the level of compliance may have been higher. The participants were also only required to complete the pain diary for 8 weeks. Pateman (1996) maintains that recording in a pain diary can become less reliable with time and can draw the patient's attention to his/her pain and the limitations it causes to daily activities.

Nurses' knowledge and attitudes to pain assessment

Pain is a subjective experience and it is therefore vital that the nurse believes the patient's report of pain (Davies and McVicar, 2000a). McCaffery's (1968) definition of pain is often quoted:

'Pain is whatever the experiencing person says it is, existing whenever he says it does.'

This is particularly important for the nurse to remember when assessing neuropathic pain, as the intensity of pain reported may not correlate to physical findings (McCaffery and Pasero, 1999). McHugh and Thoms (2001) conducted a study of patient's satisfaction with management of their chronic pain using focus groups. The research showed that patients often thought that the healthcare professionals did not believe their reports of pain.

For successful assessment to take place, the nurse must have adequate knowledge of pain management. McCaffery and Ferrell (1997) conducted a study comparing similar surveys of nurses' knowledge of pain assessment from 1988 and 1995. They identified that there had been some improvements in knowledge of pain assessment, but there were still areas where nurses lacked knowledge, such as the importance of the patient's self-report of pain and the inadequate use of analgesics. It must be noted that the nurses' sample was probably not a true representation of a national sample as the surveys were completed by nurses attending study days on pain. The authors remark that these nurses were more likely to have an interest in pain and therefore a better knowledge of the subject.

A more recent review by de Rond et al (1999) found that pain assessment is still not being performed adequately by nurses. This is vital if a nurse's practice is to be evidence based. Davies and McVicar (2000a) raise the question:

- If nurses have a poor understanding of pain, how can they use the information collected at assessment appropriately?

Role of the nurse within multidisciplinary pain assessment

During pain assessment the nurse needs to gather information relating to the pain from interventions tried in the past. Patients with chronic pain have often been seen by several different health professionals and may have already tried some treatments unsuccessfully (McCaffery and Pasero, 1999). It may be necessary for the nurse to restore the patient's confidence in the health service, particularly if treatments have been used inappropriately (Munafo and Trim, 2000). Although nurses are responsible for the assessment and evaluation of pain they are not autonomous in implementing treatment. Davies and McVicar (2000b) suggest that nurses need to be confident in discussing a management or treatment plan, particularly if there is disagreement between healthcare professionals.

During the assessment it is important that the patient is given an explanation of what causes neuropathic pain and is involved in selecting management options (McCaffery and Pasero, 1999).

This may not be possible if there is significant cognitive impairment, in young children or if the patient is unconscious (Carr and Mann, 2000). It is crucial that the patient and family are aware that neuropathic pain cannot always be resolved and that the overall aim will be to reduce the pain and improve functional, psychological and social consequences (McCaffery and Pasero, 1999; Tripp, 1999). One purpose of the pain assessment is to set goals with the patient, which must be meaningful, realistic and time-framed (Fordham and Dunn, 1994; McCaffery and Pasero, 1999).

Nursing practice needs to be evidence-based to be clinically effective (Benton, 1999). Extending knowledge of the pathophysiology of chronic neuropathic pain and suitable management options is vital when assessing the patient to ensure the best outcome. This could be achieved by inservice training, attending suitable study days, providing a resource file that is regularly updated and reading relevant literature. Roberts (1999) maintains that where patient care is delivered by a multidisciplinary team, evidence-based practice is not the responsibility of an individual practitioner, but a team responsibility.

Change in practice

An examination of the evidence overwhelmingly recommended that chronic pain needs to be assessed using a multidimensional assessment tool (Simon, 1996; McCaffery and Pasero, 1999; Carr and Mann, 2000).

The Brief Pain Inventory (see *Figure 3.2*) and the Neuropathy Pain Scale (see *Figure 3.3*) appeared to be the most appropriate tools currently available:

- The Brief Pain Inventory addresses the physical, psychological and social factors of pain
- The Neuropathy Pain Scale has an advantage in that it is the only tool that specifically measures the different aspects of neuropathic pain and therefore may be more sensitive to changes in the pain when treatments are evaluated. However, this tool does not address how the pain is affecting activities of living, which is important when measuring outcomes in a rehabilitation setting (Smith, 1999). This is vital as the impact pain is having on daily living can be used to set meaningful goals.

The effectiveness of these tools within the author's rehabilitation setting was evaluated through team discussion. The Brief Pain Inventory was chosen as the preferred tool. Although it does not record the descriptive qualities of the pain, such as burning, sharp or shooting, team members decided to document this next to the body diagrams on the tool. In addition, a pain diary is now used as part of ongoing assessment. The evidence suggested that there is a value to assessing chronic pain daily. Using a pain diary in the community setting appears to be the only way of achieving this where patients are not always seen daily by healthcare professionals.

A care pathway is a map that outlines how care is to be delivered and highlights what action to take when expected outcomes are not achieved (Lowe, 1998). Ideally, it should be patient-focused, multidisciplinary and not restricted to organizational boundaries (Benton, 1999). Within the author's neurological rehabilitation team a pain care pathway was developed by three team members — a physiotherapist, occupational therapist and specialist nurse — to be used by all members of the neurological rehabilitation team when a patient identifies pain as a problem.

A care pathway helps to ensure that the care is systematically organized, each patient is appropriately assessed and that management options are tried within a set timeframe. It also guides referral to other agencies as necessary. Ignatavicius and Hausman (1995) maintain that an interdisciplinary clinical pathway improves communication and teamwork and benefits the patient by informing him/her about what to expect. In order to use the pain pathway effectively the nurse or therapist needs to listen, believe and document the patient's own report of his/her pain and have a good knowledge of pain management (Davies and McVicar, 2000a).

A formal evaluation of the changes made as a result of this review is planned later this year. However, the pain pathway does seem to ensure that patients identifying pain are properly assessed using a multidimensional tool, management options tried and patients referred onto other agencies when appropriate. Staff seem more confident in addressing the challenging nature of chronic neuropathic pain and are more aware of alternative treatment options.

Conclusion

The overall aim in rehabilitation is to restore maximum possible independence in all activities of living (Smith, 1999). It is vital that the patient participates in setting goals and choosing treatment options. In order to achieve this, patients need to be well informed of the causes of neuropathic pain and different treatments available. Smith (1999) states that the rehabilitation nurse plays an important role in educating the patient. McHugh and Thoms's (2001) research into patient satisfaction with chronic pain management found that patients wanted more information on specific treatments and an explanation of what was causing their pain.

Chronic neuropathic pain can have a detrimental effect on the life of the individual and his/her family. For the management of the pain to be successful, detailed ongoing assessment is necessary. The Code of Professional Conduct (Nursing and Midwifery Council, 2002) states that nurses have a responsibility to ensure that their knowledge and skills are up to date. With this evidence-based knowledge, nurses are ideally placed to assess and evaluate pain (Davies and McVicar, 2000a). The evidence base strongly recommends that chronic neuropathic pain should be assessed using a multidimensional tool. This is to ensure that the holistic consequences of the pain are identified, so that treatment plans devised are effective.

The Brief Pain Inventory (see *Figure 3.2*) was chosen as the preferred tool in the author's clinical setting. This was selected as it records site, intensity and how the pain is affecting the patient's quality of life, which was considered important in a rehabilitation setting. The changes made following the recommendations of this review appear to have improved patient care and clinical effectiveness in the author's area of practice.

The author would like to acknowledge Sue Woodward, Head of Specialist and Palliative Care, Florence Nightingale School of Nursing and Midwifery, King's College, London, for her help in editing this chapter.

References

Benton D (1999) Clinical effectiveness. In: Hamer S, Collinson G, eds. *Achieving Evidence-based Practice. A Handbook for Practitioners*. Baillière Tindall, Edinburgh: 87–108

Carr E, Mann E (2000) *Pain: Creative Approaches to Effective Management*. Palgrave Macmillan, New York

Cleeland C (1991) *The Brief Pain Inventory*. Pain Research Group, Department of Neurology, University of Wisconsin-Madison

Dartmouth Cooperative Project (1995) COOP function and health status measure. Dartmouth Medical School, Butler Building, HB 7265 Hanover, NH 03755. (www.dartmouth.edu/~coopproj/index.html) (accessed 19 March 2004)

Davies J, McVicar A (2000a) Issues in effective pain control. 1: Assessment and education. *Int J Palliat Nurs* **6**(2): 58–65

Davies J, McVicar A (2000b) Issues in effective pain control. 2: From assessment to management. *Int J Palliat Nurs* **6**(4): 162–9

Davis B (2000) *Caring for People in Pain*. Routledge, London

de Rond M, De Wit R, Van Dam F et al (1999) Daily pain assessment: value for nurses and patients. *J Adv Nurs* **20**(2): 436–44

de Rond M, De Wit R, Van Dam F (2001) The implementation of a pain monitoring programme for nurses in daily clinical practice: results of a follow-up study in five hospitals. *J Adv Nurs* **35**(4): 590–8

de Wit R, Van Dam F, Hanneman M et al (1999) Evaluation of the use of a pain diary in chronic cancer pain patients at home. *Pain* **79**: 89–99

Fordham M, Dunn V (1994) *Alongside the Person in Pain. Holistic Care and Nursing Practice*. Baillière Tindall, London

Galer B, Jensen M (1997) Development and preliminary validation of a pain measure specific to neuropathic pain: the neuropathic pain scale. *Neurology* **48**(2): 332–8

Hamilton J, Edgar L (1992) A survey examining nurses' knowledge of pain control. *J Pain Symptom Manage* **7**(1): 18–26

Ignatavicius D, Hausman K (1995) *Clinical Pathways for Collaborative Practice*. WB Saunders, Philadelphia

Jameson P (1996) Neuropathic pain. In: Dolin S, Padfield N, Pateman J, eds. *Pain Clinic Manual*. Butterworth-Heinemann, Oxford: 38–47

Johnstone E (1998) Pain by numbers. *Nurs Times* **94**(35): 34–5

Krause S, Backonja M (2003) Development of a neuropathic pain questionnaire. *Clin J Pain* **19**(5): 306–14

Lowe C (1998) Care pathways: have they a place in 'the new NHS'? *J Nurs Manage* **6**: 303–6

McCaffery M (1968) *Nursing Practice Theories Related to Cognition, Bodily Pain and Man-environment Interactions*. University of California at Los Angeles Students' Store, Los Angeles

McCaffery M, Beebe A (1989) *Pain: Clinical Manual for Nursing Practice*. CV Mosby, St Louis

McCaffery M, Ferrell BR (1997) Nurses' knowledge of pain assessment and management: how much progress have we made? *J Pain Symptom Manage* **14**(3): 175–86

McCaffery M, Pasero C (1999) *Pain Clinical Manual*. 2nd edn. Mosby, Missouri

McHugh G, Thoms G (2001) Patient satisfaction with chronic pain management. *Nurs Stand* **15**(51): 33–8

Maloni H (2000) Pain in multiple sclerosis: an overview of its nature and management. *J Neurosci Nurs* **32**(3): 139–44

Melzack R (1983) The McGill Pain Questionnaire: major properties and scoring methods. *Pain* **1**: 277–99

Munafo M, Trim J (2000) *Chronic Pain: A Handbook for Nurses*. Butterworth-Heinemann, Oxford

Nursing and Midwifery Council (2002) *Code of Professional Conduct*. NMC, London

O'Hara P (1996) *Pain Management for Health Professionals*. Chapman and Hall, London

Pateman J (1996) Measurement of pain. In: Dolin S, Padfield N, Pateman J, eds. *Pain Clinic Manual*. Butterworth-Heinemann, Oxford: 11–16

Richardson C (2001) Chronic pain and coping: a proposed role for nurses and nursing models. *J Adv Nurs* **34**(5): 659–67

Roberts R (1999) *Information for Evidence-based Care*. Radcliffe Medical Press, Abingdon

Simon J (1996) Chronic pain syndrome: nursing assessment and intervention. *Rehabil Nurs* **21**(1): 13–9

Simon J, McTier C (1996) Development of a chronic pain assessment tool. *Rehabil Nurs* **21**(1): 20–4

Smith M (1999) The nature of rehabilitation. In: Smith M, ed. *Rehabilitation in Adult Nursing Practice*. Churchill Livingstone, Edingburgh: 1–30

Tripp S (1999) Providing psychological support. In: Smith M, ed. *Rehabilitation in Adult Nursing Practice*. Churchill Livingstone, Edinburgh: 105–37

Walker J, Sofaer B (1998) Predictors of psychological distress in chronic pain patients. *J Adv Nurs* **27**(2): 320–6

Chapter 4

Neuropathic pain: Recognition and assessment

Lucy Johnson

Neuropathic pain has been defined as pain initiated or caused by a primary lesion or dysfunction in the nervous system (Merskey and Bogduk, 1994), or pain owing to a primary lesion of the peripheral or central nervous system (Hansson et al, 2001). Neuropathic pain is suffered by approximately 1% of the UK population — around 500 000 people (Karlsten and Gordh, 1997). It has an enormous socioeconomic impact, because of unemployment and expenditure on medical and social services (Hall, 2003). It is likely to become more common as people are living longer with diseases that precipitate neuropathic pain, such as human immunodeficiency virus (HIV) and cancer (Hall, 2003).

However, neuropathic pain continues to present a major therapeutic challenge to healthcare professionals as it can be difficult to recognize and difficult to treat. Difficulty in recognizing neuropathic pain may be attributed to the manifestation of coexisting symptoms, such as numbness, weakness, pins and needles or changes to nails, skin and hair, which may appear peculiar to those unfamiliar with neuropathic pain. Also, the pain and associated symptoms may be more severe and longer lasting than expected in relation to the perceived level of injury.

Difficulty in treating neuropathic pain is partly caused by the complex mechanisms of neuropathic pain, which make it often refractory to conventional analgesic drugs and interventions (Sindrup and Jensen, 1999). Although some individuals may respond well to anti-neuralgic treatments initiated in general healthcare settings, other patients will require referral to a specialized pain service. Improving the prognosis for reducing neuropathic pain depends on early recognition and aggressive therapy (Lipman, 1998).

This chapter sets out to: equip nurses with the skills to identify neuropathic pain through pain assessment; support patients and their families by understanding the basic causes and effective treatments of neuropathic pain; expedite pain relief through appropriate intervention and referral within the multidisciplinary team.

Background

Pain is a universal experience. It is also the most likely reason for people to seek health care (Hall, 2003). The type of pain that results from normal activation of pain-sensitive nerves, often called nociceptive or inflammatory pain, serves to warn us of imminent or actual tissue damage (Woolf and Mannion, 1999). Mechanical, thermal or chemical receptors are activated and pain messages are carried via an intact nervous system to the spinal cord and the conscious level in the brain (Besson, 1999). Protective responses are elicited, which on an everyday basis may involve withdrawing a hand from a sharp knife or hot water or, after an accident or surgery, may involve resting and taking painkillers. Once the injury or disease process has healed, the nervous system usually resumes its normal function. Problems can occur if inflammatory processes cause permanent nerve damage, for example as a result of proinflammatory cytokines such as tumour necrosis factor (Pappagallo, 2002). Pain persists but is deemed to have progressed from acute to chronic when it outlasts the normal tissue healing time (assumed to be 3 months) (International Association for the Study of Pain, 1986).

Chronic pain serves no useful purpose as it does not provide a warning to change a behaviour that is causing bodily damage; therefore, the suffering is needless. As Woolf and Mannion (1999) state:

'Persistent pain syndromes offer no biological advantage and cause suffering and distress.'

The persistence of chronic pain can have a devastating impact on a person's quality of life because of associated depression and disability. Indeed, patients with chronic pain use the health service up to five times more frequently than the rest of the population (Elliott et al, 1999).

A wide range of processes that lead to damage in the peripheral or central nervous system can cause neuropathic pain. Some conditions in which neuropathic pain may manifest are shown in *Table 4.1*, while others have no associated diagnosis or apparent cause.

Table 4.1: Causes of neuropathic pain and associated conditions

Mechanical	Spinal cord injury/nerve compression; spinal canal stenosis; syringomyelia; nerve entrapment, e.g. carpal tunnel syndrome; amputation (phantom pain/stump pain); complex regional pain syndrome (after fracture)
Metabolic	Diabetes mellitus (painful diabetic neuropathy); alcoholism; malnutrition; niacin/thiamine deficiency
Toxicity	Drugs, e.g. chemotherapy, isoniazid, phenytoin; poisons, e.g. lead, arsenic, mercury
Ischaemic	Stroke; polyarteritis nodosa; lupus erythematosus; ischaemic neuropathy
Post-inflammatory changes	Herpes zoster infection (trigeminal neuralgia); Guillain-Barré syndrome; human immunodeficiency disease (neuropathy)
Degenerative	Multiple sclerosis; motor neurone disease
Inherited	Charcot–Marie tooth disease; porphyria
Cancer-related	Infiltration/compression by tumour/metastases; nerve damage by radiotherapy or chemotherapy, e.g. vincristine

From Attal et al (2000)

Despite the diversity of these conditions, most research into mechanisms and treatment of neuropathic pain has examined either postherpetic neuralgia or painful diabetic neuropathy (Dworkin, 2002). Common symptoms are described in *Table 4.2*.

Table 4.2: Symptoms of neuropathic pain

Paraesthesias	Spontaneous, intermittent painless abnormal sensations, e.g. pins and needles, tingling
Dysaesthesias	Spontaneous or evoked unpleasant sensations, e.g. numbness, burning, cramping
Allodynia	Pain evoked by a non-painful stimulus, e.g. light touch
Hyperalgesia	An exaggerated pain response evoked by a painful stimulus

Adapted from Dworkin (2002)

Classification

It is useful to classify neuropathic pain to guide management. Traditionally, it has been classified according to presumed diagnosis or anatomical distribution (central or peripheral) (Hansson et al, 2001). However, evidence demonstrates that multiple pathophysiological mechanisms underlie neuropathic pain (Dickenson et al, 2001). An integrated approach to recognition and treatment of neuropathic pain, accounting for aetiology, anatomy and possible mechanisms, is considered to lead to more effective outcomes (Nicholson, 2000). For example, in a patient with pain after a stroke, it is important to consider carefully his/her description of symptoms, the distribution of pain and the site of the lesion in determining whether the pain is caused by the central lesion or by conditions affecting the paralysed extremity (Widar et al, 2002).

Pain assessment

Pain is a complex and highly subjective experience. The only way to gain an objective understanding of individuals' pain and plan appropriate intervention is to ask them about their pain as part of a systematic assessment. Despite a plethora of valid and reliable pain assessment tools, healthcare professionals tend to underestimate pain (Solomon, 2001). In general, the pain assessment process is accepted to lie within nurses' remit (Wilson, 2002). However, while pain is frequently identified as a problem on patients' care plans, nurses often fail to assess it routinely and, therefore, to treat it (Schafheutle et al, 2004). This is particularly apparent for non-surgical patients, who are also more likely to suffer neuropathic pain (Johnson et al, 2003).

Since neuropathic pain is often unexpected, unpredictable and unfamiliar, recognizing it requires finely tuned communication and observation skills. Assessment tools can be honed to suit specific healthcare settings, and information collected can be used to measure the quality of patient outcomes such as reduction in pain, improvement in mood or increase in physical function. Nurses are particularly well placed to listen to individuals' accounts of how their pain began, how they sought and experienced healthcare intervention, how they are coping and how the pain impacts on their quality of life. A core pain assessment chart is an invaluable framework to document every pain assessment process. The basic parameters, as they relate to neuropathic pain, are outlined below.

Diagnosis

Pain assessment starts with building up a picture of the likely cause of pain. This includes considering previous test results and suggested diagnoses in relation to the patient's story and current symptoms. History of a precipitating neural injury is suggestive of neuropathic pain (Woolf and Mannion, 1999). Peripheral nerve injuries tend to be the most common because the nerves are more accessible, such as carpal tunnel syndrome in which the median nerve passing through the wrist becomes entrapped or peripheral neuropathies associated with diabetes and renal failure (Ellis, 2003). Any injury involving the nervous system causes inflammatory responses, adding to the complexity of the process (Backonja, 2003). Central pain syndromes may be caused by direct spinal cord injury or lesions within the spinothalamic pain and temperature pathways, which may be caused by stroke and demyelinating conditions, such as Guillain–Barré syndrome (Gill and Oaklander, 2001). It is often difficult to determine a definitive diagnosis in neuropathic pain conditions; however, patients tend to benefit from a broad explanation of their type of pain.

Distribution

Patients can draw the site of their main pain and any radiation to other body parts on a picture of the human body. This picture can be included on a self-assessment form and may be enhanced by dermatome markings, which depict the segments innervated by the spinal nerves. It may help the patient to see why his/her pain is projected to certain areas. Pain shown to be in a neuroanatomical distribution correlating with the site of a suspected or confirmed nerve lesion is indictive of neuropathic pain (Ellis, 2003).

There may be a mixed pain pattern; for example nerve root compression from a prolapsed intervertebral disc usually gives rise to a combination of localized, nociceptive pain in the area of the ruptured disc and radicular, neuropathic pain in the dermatomal distribution corresponding to the affected root (Hansson et al, 2001). Sciatica from lumbar disease is easily recognized as pain running down the back of the leg and numbness in the big toe (i.e. symptoms in the distribution of the sciatic nerve; Ellis, 2003), but compression of nerve roots at other spinal levels can produce radicular pain in the genitals, thorax, head, arms or abdomen (Gill and Oaklander, 2001).

Duration

The pattern and frequency of pain can reveal the presence of neuropathic pain. Patients may find it useful to record the timing of their pain and any changes in a diary — subtle changes in frequency of flashes of trigeminal neuralgia pain are more likely to be noticed when they are catalogued. Episodes of pain and periods of pain relief may be shown to correlate with specific activities or therapeutic interventions.

Descriptors

Whereas descriptions of somatic and visceral pain are sometimes vague, neuropathic pain is classically described as burning, pricking, tingling, being like an electric shock, cold and itching (Boureau et al, 1990). Patients may liken their pain to something else, such as 'a toothache in the buttock' in sciatica, or 'insects crawling over the skin' in Guillain–Barré syndrome. Adjectives consistent with abnormal sensations are indicative of neuropathic pain, such as 'cold water running down' an affected limb (Attal et al, 2000). The importance of a detailed description of the pain is borne out in situations where different types of pain coexist, for example in stump pain, which is mainly nociceptive and inflammatory, and in phantom limb pain, which is neuropathic.

Pain severity

Pain intensity is one of the most basic factors in any pain assessment and almost all patients are able to score their pain. Unfortunately, nurses rarely use the standardized tools available (de Rond et al, 1999). The following psychometric instruments are widely used and have been validated by de C Williams (1995):

- Numerical rating scale (NRS) — patients are asked to rate their pain from 0–10, 'if 0 is no pain and 10 is the worst pain imaginable'
- Visual analogue scale (VAS) — patients are asked to visualize their pain severity on a 100 mm line with 'no pain' at one end and 'worst pain imaginable' at the other
- Verbal rating scale (VRS) — patients are asked to describe their pain as 'none, mild, moderate or severe'.

The VAS and NRS are approximately equal in sensitivity to changes in pain intensity (Breivik et al, 2000). The VRS is useful for patients unable to ascribe a number to their pain, such as with dementia. Pain scales in different languages can be found on the Pain Society's website (www.painsociety.org/pain_scales.html).

Associated symptoms

Symptoms suggestive of sensory or motor deficits, such as a leg giving way, or sensory dysfunction, such as a cold sensation around a scar, are often synonymous with neuropathic pain (Attal et al, 2000). Symptoms are often unfamiliar and some may be alarming, such as skin temperature and colour changes owing to injured autonomic nerves in complex regional pain syndrome (Janig and Baron, 2001). Reassurance that these symptoms are normal for the neuropathic pain condition can greatly relieve anxiety.

Aggravating and relieving factors

Determining what, if anything, makes the pain better or worse is paramount in understanding the pain generator; for example pain on light touch with a history of shingles suggests postherpetic neuralgia (Johnson, 2003). Furthermore, aggravating and palliative factors hint at the usefulness of particular treatments; for example if rubbing the painful area relieves pain, transcutaneous electrical nerve stimulation (TENS) may be effective. Patients' behavioural responses can also demonstrate their coping skills; for example whether an individual whose headache is made worse by noise becomes intolerant and withdrawn, or adopts yoga and self-hypnosis.

Interventions

The success, failure and side-effects associated with previous analgesic interventions are useful in establishing the most important component of a person's pain and appropriate types of treatment; for example pain that persists despite increasing doses of opioid may point to another class of drug being tried. Assessing an individual's understanding of his/her analgesic dosing will indicate his/her need for verbal and written information and may highlight safety issues such as inadvertent overdose of paracetamol when taken regularly with a co-analgesic containing paracetamol. Patients' expectations of treatments may also need to be tempered; for example they need to know that TENS may have little carry-over effect when the machine is off or that intermittent top-up acupuncture may be required after a course (Moore et al, 2003). The outcome of any previous invasive procedures may highlight a cause for pain; constant back pain in the same distribution 4–6 months after a lumbar discectomy may indicate epidural fibrosis or scar tissue formation (La Tourette, 2002).

Medications

Tolerability, interactions, contraindications or allergies relating to any of the patient's medications should be assessed so remedial action can be taken. The patient's current medications will also highlight existing medical problems that the patient may have omitted to mention, indicating which analgesics may be contraindicated because of interactions or health risk. For example, if a patient is prescribed anticonvulsants, further questioning would be needed to ascertain whether this was for epilepsy or neuropathic pain; tramadol would be contraindicated if the patient suffered from epilepsy (British Medical Association and Royal Pharmaceutical Society of Great Britain, 2004).

Systems review

As some painful neuropathies are related to systemic diseases, consideration should be given to the following:

- Existing conditions, such as diabetes mellitus, hypothyroidism and chronic renal failure
- Observable characteristics, such as joint swelling, tremors and unsteady gait
- General health, such as eating patterns and use of alcohol and illicit drugs.

System problems will also identify which analgesics should be avoided because of potential risks; cardiovascular problems, such as tachyarrhythmias or uncontrolled hypertension, would preclude the use of tricyclic antidepressants for neuropathic pain (British Medical Association and Royal Pharmaceutical Society of Great Britain, 2004).

Family/social history

An individual's pain experience is modified by mood, coping mechanisms and social and cultural background (Thomas and Rose, 1991). People are more likely to suffer if the extent of their pain puts their physical, psychological, occupational and social integrity in jeopardy (Turk and Okifuji, 1999). Support mechanisms are a key determinant in successful rehabilitation (La Tourette, 2002); therefore, it is useful to establish the patient's level of independence, enjoyment of social life, finances, ability to work, and responses of family and health staff.

Quality-of-life measures

There are many recognized, appropriate quality-of-life questionnaires to quantify the effect of pain on activities of living. The Brief Pain Inventory (Cleeland and Ryan, 1994) (*Figure 4.1*) is a multidimensional tool that demonstrates pain severity at various intervals and interference with physical and psychosocial

Name_____ Date_____

Brief Pain Inventory Assessment

Please circle your response or ask for help if you are having problems

1. Please rate your pain by circling the one number that best describes your pain at its WORST in the past week

| 0 | 1 | 2 | 3 | 4 | 5 | 6 | 7 | 8 | 9 | 10 |
No pain   Pain as bad as you can imagine

2. Please rate your pain by circling the one number that best describes your pain at its LEAST in the past week

| 0 | 1 | 2 | 3 | 4 | 5 | 6 | 7 | 8 | 9 | 10 |
No pain   Pain as bad as you can imagine

3. Please rate your pain by circling the one number that best describes your pain on AVERAGE

| 0 | 1 | 2 | 3 | 4 | 5 | 6 | 7 | 8 | 9 | 10 |
No pain   Pain as bad as you can imagine

4. Please rate your pain by circling the one number that best describes your pain RIGHT NOW

| 0 | 1 | 2 | 3 | 4 | 5 | 6 | 7 | 8 | 9 | 10 |
No pain   Pain as bad as you can imagine

5. Circle the number that describes how, during the past week, PAIN HAS INTERFERED with your:

A. General activity

| 0 | 1 | 2 | 3 | 4 | 5 | 6 | 7 | 8 | 9 | 10 |
Does not interfere   Completely interferes

B. Mood

| 0 | 1 | 2 | 3 | 4 | 5 | 6 | 7 | 8 | 9 | 10 |
Does not interfere   Completely interferes

C. Walking ability

| 0 | 1 | 2 | 3 | 4 | 5 | 6 | 7 | 8 | 9 | 10 |
Does not interfere   Completely interferes

D. Normal work

| 0 | 1 | 2 | 3 | 4 | 5 | 6 | 7 | 8 | 9 | 10 |
Does not interfere   Completely interferes

E. Relationships with other people

| 0 | 1 | 2 | 3 | 4 | 5 | 6 | 7 | 8 | 9 | 10 |
Does not interfere   Completely interferes

F. Sleep

| 0 | 1 | 2 | 3 | 4 | 5 | 6 | 7 | 8 | 9 | 10 |
Does not interfere   Completely interferes

G. Enjoyment of life

| 0 | 1 | 2 | 3 | 4 | 5 | 6 | 7 | 8 | 9 | 10 |
Does not interfere   Completely interferes

Figure 4.1: Brief Pain Inventory (short form). Adapted from Cleeland (1991)

functioning. It is easy for patients to understand and complete independently, easy to score, sensitive to change and is endorsed by the Pain Society (Griffiths et al, 2003). It can be included on a patient's self-assessment form. The Short Form Health Survey (SF-36) (Ware et al, 1993) is more in-depth, containing items such as physical and social functioning and general and mental health, and has been deemed reliable and relevant to patients with chronic peripheral neuropathic pain (Meyer-Rosberg et al, 2001).

Neuropathic pain scale

Neuropathic pain can be identified by using a specific neuropathic pain scale to clarify the relative contribution of neuropathic symptoms to the assessment process. The Leeds Assessment of Neuropathic Symptoms and Signs (LANSS) Pain Scale (Bennett, 2001) is a validated tool for isolating patients in whom neuropathic mechanisms dominate their symptoms. It is based on analysis of sensory description and examination of nerve dysfunction, through basic sensory testing. It is easily incorporated into the clinical context and has been used to distinguish effectively between neuropathic and nociceptive pain (Martinez-Lavin et al, 2003).

The LANSS is divided into two sections:

- The first is completed by patients
- The second is a straightforward clinical assessment that nurses and community health professionals could complete after some basic training in its use.

The Neuropathic Pain Scale (Galer and Jensen, 1997) includes items for specifically evaluating descriptors of neuropathic pain (sharp, dull, hot, cold, sensitive, itchy, deep and surface pain), as well as intensity and unpleasantness.

The short-form McGill Pain Questionnaire (Melzack, 1987) is not specifically for neuropathic pain and is more complicated for patients, but has demonstrable ability to discriminate between different pain syndromes (Turk and Okifuji, 1999). The short-form McGill Pain Questionnaire can also be used by nurses with minimal experience in assessing neuropathic pain to enable it to be identified more readily.

Investigations

Once the core assessment and pain questionnaires have identified the potential for neuropathic pain, a more detailed inspection by an appropriately qualified professional is likely to be needed. Pain in a dermatomal distribution of spinal nerves will require neurological examination of tone, power, flexion, extension, sensation and reflexes (Attal et al, 2000). Other conditions will require inspection of symptomatic body parts, such as for classic symptoms of complex regional pain syndrome, hypertrophy and specific 'signs' of temperature changes and sweating. Various sensations can be produced such as dynamic allodynia by moving some gauze over the skin, static allodynia by blunt pressure with a finger, light punctate allodynia with von Frey filament and thermal allodynia by brief application of ice (Dworkin, 2002). Qualitative sensory testing, aimed at quantifying the amount of stimulation required to evoke specific sensations, is becoming more commonplace among pain specialists.

Useful information regarding the likely cause and appropriate treatments for the pain can be gleaned from the reports of previous investigations, such as magnetic resonance imaging, nerve conduction studies and blood tests. Further tests should be arranged swiftly, as patients may often be required to wait.

Treatment

Once neuropathic pain is suspected, appropriate interventions should be initiated as soon as possible. The aim of pain management is usually to reduce pain and help patients cope, rather than eradicate their pain completely. Additional aims may be to alleviate psychological and behavioural dysfunction and distress, reduce disability and dependence and restore function, rationalize medications and attend to social, family and occupational issues (Royal College of Anaesthetists and Pain Society, 2003). Nurses can assist patients in setting realistic goals by explaining some hard facts about pain management; for example that options may be limited and may only achieve partial or short-term relief.

Evidence of effective treatments to prevent neuropathic pain developing is lacking, although a reduction in future pain may be achieved; for example, pre-emptive administration of low-dose amitriptyline has been shown to reduce pain prevalence by half (Bowsher, 1997). Nurses are well placed to identify patients who are likely to develop neuropathic pain so that early treatment can be initiated. Examples of common practice include commencing anti-viral treatment and anti-neuralgics early in patients with shingles with the aim of shortening the duration of postherpetic neuralgia, and running an epidural infusion and starting anti-neuralgics in patients before leg amputation to minimize the intensity of phantom limb pain (Wood et al, 1996). Neuropathic pain tends to respond poorly to conventional analgesics, such as non-steroidal anti-inflammatory drugs and paracetamol (Karlsten and Gordh, 1997). An effective analgesic regimen usually involves a combination of treatments with various modes of action. Common neuropathic pain treatments are detailed below.

Antidepressants

Tricyclic antidepressants, such as amitriptyline and prothiaden, remain the superior drugs for neuropathic pain (Rowbotham, 2002). Nurses should tell patients that these drugs are also used for depression and it will take a few weeks for them to notice a beneficial reduction in pain. Doses usually start at 10–25 mg (Sindrup and Jensen, 2001) and are increased gradually. Anticholinergic side-effects are common, including dry mouth and constipation (Ashburn and Staats, 1999). Drowsiness is also common, hence tricyclics for pain are normally prescribed at night, which can be useful for patients who sleep poorly because of chronic pain (Ashburn and Staats, 1999).

Anticonvulsants

The newer anti-epileptics are frequently used alone or in conjunction with tricyclics in the management of neuropathic pain (Moore et al, 2003). Gabapentin has been shown to reduce pain in patients with a wide range of neuropathic pain syndromes and induce better sleep, mood and quality of life (Rice et al, 2001; Serpell and Neuropathic Pain Study Group, 2002). Doses are usually commenced at 300 mg per day and titrated up to 1800–2400 mg per day (Rice et al, 2001). Side-effects tend to be uncommon, transient, mild and related to central nervous system depression, including dizziness, headache, confusion and ataxia (Rice et al, 2001). Pregabalin is a more recent follow up to gabapentin, which, due to its greater potency, could potentially achieve efficacy at lower doses, and with fewer dose-related side-effects (Rosenstock et al, 2004). Topiramate has been studied to a lesser degree, but there is growing evidence to support its role in neuropathic pain (Chong and Libretto, 2003). Carbamazepine, an older anti-epileptic, has been reported to be beneficial in various neuropathic pain conditions (Sindrup and Jensen, 1999), but is associated with greater adverse effects (Ashburn and Staats, 1999).

Opioids

Tramadol has both weak opioid agonistic and monoaminergic effects, is effective for neuropathic pain and is considered to have a low addiction potential (Sindrup and Jensen, 1999). Pure opioids, such as morphine, levorphanol and oxycodone, are being used more for neuropathic pain because of mounting evidence of their efficacy (Gimbel et al, 2003; Rowbotham et al, 2003). They are particularly useful in conjunction with tricyclics and/or anticonvulsants (Zochodne and Mitchell, 2003). However, use of opioids in non-malignant pain remains controversial in general healthcare settings, and patients must be regularly reassessed in line with the Pain Society's (2003) recommendations.

Topical drugs

Capsaicin cream is derived from chilli peppers and causes a depletion of the neurotransmitter, substance P, from sensory nerves (Mason et al, 2004). It has demonstrated some efficacy, particularly in diabetic neuropathy and osteoarthritis (Sindrup and Jensen, 1999) and has few systemic side-effects (Mason et al, 2004). It should be applied sparingly four times a day, but concordance can be limited by a burning sensation when applied (Mason et al, 2004). Nurses can play an important role in educating and reassuring patients about its correct application. Lidocaine patches are also showing promising results (Newton et al, 2004), but are largely unavailable in the UK.

Non-pharmacological treatments

TENS and acupuncture, in the hands of experienced practitioners, represent safe therapies with broad anecdotal evidence of efficacy in neuropathic pain. For most complementary therapies, there is no scientific evidence of efficacy in relieving pain, arguably reflecting the nature of the therapists as predominantly non-scientific. However, patients with neuropathic pain that responds poorly to other treatments may want to explore all available options. Nurses can encourage patients to be realistic about the likely outcomes and assist them in accessing treatments they feel will help aspects of their quality of life, such as mood. Since stress and anxiety exacerbate pain (Hadjistavropoulos et al, 2004), it makes sense for nurses to offer patients reassurance and support with relaxation, distraction and breathing techiques.

Invasive treatments

There is a sound basis for some procedures, such as epidural steroid injections in sciatica and coeliac plexus block in pancreatic cancer (McQuay and Moore, 1998), with the benefits deemed to outweigh the side-effects (Moore et al, 2003). Since much of the evidence is contradictory, neural blockade and spinal cord stimulation should form part of a comprehensive multidisciplinary approach, where the benefits and risks have been carefully assessed (Justins and Siemaszko, 2002).

Appropriate referral

The multidisciplinary team may need to be engaged in determining the likely cause and appropriate investigations and treatments. When and whether to enlist the help of pain specialists and therapists will depend on their availability in the healthcare setting and the local team's own expertise. Regular pain assessment will demonstrate the need to refer the patient. Pain specialists may be required for more detailed physical assessment and sensory testing, more effective neuropathic pain interventions and reassurance of both patients and staff. Patients with poor coping, weak social support and a tendency to catastrophize are likely to need support from a psychologist or other psychological health professional (Hinnant, 2002). Physiotherapists and occupational therapists can show patients strengthening exercises, help them to pace their activities and administer physical treatments. Some patients may need to be assessed by a surgeon or neurologist.

Conclusion

Neuropathic pain is not an uncommon condition, with at least 500 000 people suffering from it in the UK alone (Karlsten and Gordh, 1997). In the past it has been difficult to treat, but with the advent of new and effective medications, the prognosis for patients can be significantly improved by early recognition, aggressive therapy and substantial psychological support. To this end, when neuropathic pain is suspected, a straightforward but comprehensive assessment of patients, using tried-and-tested tools, coupled with appropriate referral, can lead to much better patient outcomes and associated quality of life.

References

Ashburn MA, Staats PS (1999) Management of chronic pain. *Lancet* **353**: 1865–9

Attal N, Nicholson B, Serra J (2000) *New Directions in Neuropathic Pain: Focusing Treatment on Symptoms and Mechanisms*. Royal Society of Medicine, London

Backonja M (2003) Defining neuropathic pain. *Anesth Analg* **97**(3): 785–90

Bennett M (2001) The LANSS pain scale: the Leeds assessment of neuropathic symptoms and signs. *Pain* **92**: 147–57

Besson J (1999) The neurobiology of pain. *Lancet* **353**: 1610–15

Boureau F, Doubrere J, Luu M (1990) Study of verbal description in neuropathic pain. *Pain* **42**: 145–52

Bowsher D (1997) The management of chronic pain: a review. In: Arnoff G, ed. *Evaluation and Treatment of Chronic Pain*. Williams and Wilkins, Baltimore

Breivik E, Björnsson G, Skovlund E (2000) A comparison of pain rating scales by sampling from clinical trial data. *Clin J Pain* **16**: 22–8

British Medical Association and Royal Pharmaceutical Society of Great Britain (2004) *British National Formulary*. Number 47. British Medical Association and Royal Pharmaceutical Society of Great Britain, London

Chong M, Libretto S (2003) The rationale and use of topiramate for treating neuropathic pain. *Clin J Pain* **19**: 59–68

Cleeland C (1991) *The Brief Pain Inventory*. Pain Research Group, Department of Neurology, University of Wisconsin-Madison

Cleeland C, Ryan K (1994) Pain assessment: global use of the Brief Pain Inventory. *Ann Acad Med Singapore* **23**(2): 129–38

de C Williams AC (1995) Pain measurement in chronic pain management. *Pain Reviews* **2**: 39–63

de Rond M, de Wit R, van Dam F et al (1999) Daily pain assessment: values for nurses and patients. *J Adv Nurs* **29**: 436–44

Dickenson AH, Matthews EA, Suzuki R (2001) Central nervous system mechanisms of pain in peripheral neuropathy. In: Hansson P, Fields H, Hill R, Marchettini P, eds. *Neuropathic Pain, Pathophysiology and Treatment*. IASP Press, Seattle: 85–106

Dworkin R (2002) An overview of neuropathic pain: syndromes, signs and several mechanisms. *Clin J Pain* **18**: 343–9

Elliott A, Smith B, Penny K, Smith W, Chambers W (1999) The epidemiology of chronic pain in the community. *Lancet* **354**: 1248–52

Ellis S (2003) How the nervous system works. *Relay* **16**: 10–13

Galer B, Jensen M (1997) Development and preliminary validation of a pain measure specific to neuropathic pain: the Neuropathic Pain Scale. *Neurology* **48**: 332–8

Gill J, Oaklander A (2001) Ten most commonly asked questions about neuropathic pain. *Neurologist* **7**(4): 263–9

Gimbel J, Richards M, Portenoy M (2003) Controlled-release oxycodone for pain in diabetic neuropathy: a randomized controlled trial. *Neurology* **60**: 927–34

Griffiths D, Noon J, Campbell F, Price C (2003) Clinical governance and chronic pain: towards a practical solution. *Anaesthesia* **58**(3): 243–8

Hadjistavropoulos H, Asmundson G, Kowalyk K (2004) Measures of anxiety: is there a difference in their ability to predict functioning at three-month follow-up among pain patients? *Eur J Pain* **89**(1): 1–11

Hall M (2003) *Target Pain*. Association of the British Pharmaceutical Industry, London

Hansson P, Lacerenza M, Marchettini P (2001) Aspects of clinical and experimental neuropathic pain: the clinical perspective. In: Hansson P, Fields H, Hill R, Marchettini P, eds. *Neuropathic Pain, Pathophysiology and Treatment*. IASP Press, Seattle: 1–18

Hinnant D (2002) Psychological evaluation and assessment of pain. In: Tolliston C, Satterthwaite J, Tolliston J, eds. *Practical Pain Management*. Lippincott Williams and Wilkins, Philadelphia

International Association for the Study of Pain (1986) Classification of chronic pain: descriptions of chronic pain syndromes and definitions of pain terms. *Pain* **3**(Suppl): S1–S226

Janig W, Baron R (2001) The role of the sympathetic nervous system in neuropathic pain: clinical observations and animal models. In: Hansson P, Fields H, Hill R, Marchettini P, eds. *Neuropathic Pain, Pathophysiology and Treatment*. IASP Press, Seattle: 125–149

Johnson L (2003) Effective pain management of post-herpetic neuralgia. *Nurs Times* **99**(10): 32–34

Johnson L, Regaard A, Herrington N (2003) Pain in general medical patients: an audit. In: Dostrovsky J, Carr D, Koltzenburg M, eds. *Progress in Pain Research and Management*. IASP Press, Seattle: 577–86

Justins D, Siemaszko O (2002) Rational use of neural blockade for the management of chronic pain. In: Giamberardino M, ed. *Pain 2002: An Updated Review*. Refresher Course Syllabus. IASP Press, Seattle

Karlsten R, Gordh T (1997) How do drugs relieve neurogenic pain? *Drugs Aging* **11**: 398–412

La Tourette P (2002) Focused evaluation of the pain patient. In: Tolliston C, Satterthwaite J, Tolliston J, eds. *Practical Pain Management*. Lippincott Williams and Wilkins, Philadelphia

Lipman A (1998) Pharmacological approaches to pain management: non-traditional analgesics and analgesic adjuvants. In: Ashburn M, Rice L, eds. *The Management of Pain*. Churchill Livingstone, New York

McQuay H, Moore A (1998) *An Evidence-based Resource for Pain Relief*. Oxford University Press, Oxford

Martinez-Lavin M, Lopez S, Medina M, Nava A (2003) Use of the Leeds assessment of neuropathic pain symptoms and signs questionnaire in patients with fibromyalgia. *Semin Arthritis Rheum* **32**(6): 407–11

Mason L, Moore R, Derry S, Edwards J, McQuay H (2004) Systematic review of topical capsaicin for the treatment of chronic pain. *Br Med J* **328**: 991

Melzack R (1987) The short-form McGill pain questionnaire. *Pain* **30**: 191–7

Merskey H, Bogduk N, eds (1994) *Classification of Chronic Pain*. 2nd edn. IASP Press, Seattle: 222

Meyer-Rosberg K, Burchhardt C, Huizar K, Kvarnström A, Nordfors L, Kristofferson A (2001) A comparison of the SF-36 and Nottingham Health Profile in patients with chronic neuropathic pain. *Eur J Pain* **5**: 391–403

Moore A, Edwards J, Barden J, McQuay H (2003) *Bandolier's Little Book of Pain: An Evidence-based Guide to Treatments*. Oxford University Press, Oxford

Newton W, Collins L, Fotinos C (2004) What is the best treatment for diabetic neuropathy? *J Fam Pract* **53**(5): 403–8

Nicholson B (2000) Taxonomy of pain. *Clin J Pain* **16**(Suppl 3): S114–S17

Pappagallo M (2002) Neuropathic pain in peripheral neuropathies. In: Tollison C, Satterthwaite J, Tollison J, eds. *Practical Pain Management*. Lippincott Williams and Wilkins, Philadelphia

Pain Society (2003) *Provisional Recommendations for the Appropriate Use of Opioids in Patients with Chronic Non-cancer Related Pain*. Pain Society, London

Rice A, Maton S, Postherpetic Neuralgia Study Group (2001) Gabapentin in postherpetic neuralgia: a randomized, double-blind, placebo controlled study. *Pain* **94**: 215–24

Rosenstock J, Tuchman M, La Moreaux L, Sharma U (2004) Pregabalin for the treatment of painful diabetic peripheral neuropathy: A double-blind, placebo-controlled trial. *Pain* **110**(3): 628–38.

Rowbotham M (2002) Neuropathic pain: from basic science to evidence-based treatment. In: Giamberardino M, ed. *Pain 2002: An Updated Review*. Refresher Course Syllabus. IASP, Seattle

Rowbotham M, Twilling L, Davies P, Reisner L, Taylor K, Mohr D (2003) Oral opioid therapy for chronic peripheral and central neuropathic pain. *N Engl J Med* **348**: 1223–32

Royal College of Anaesthetists and Pain Society (2003) *Pain Management Services. Good Practice*. Royal College of Anaesthetists/Pain Society, London

Schafheutle E, Cantrill J, Noyce P (2004) The nature of informal pain questioning by nurses — a barrier to postoperative pain management? *Pharm World Sci* **26**(1): 12–17

Serpell M, Neuropathic Pain Study Group (2002) Gabapentin in neuropathic pain syndromes: a randomized, double-blind, placebo-controlled trial. *Pain* **99**: 557–66

Sindrup S, Jensen T (1999) Efficacy of pharmacological treatments of neuropathic pain: an update and effect related to mechanism of drug action. *Pain* **83**: 389–400

Sindrup S, Jensen T (2001) Antidepressants in the treatment of neuropathic pain. In: Hansson P, Fields H, Hill R, Marchettini P, eds. *Neuropathic Pain, Pathophysiology and Treatment*. IASP Press, Seattle

Solomon P (2001) Congruence between health professionals' and patients' pain ratings: a review of the literature. *Scand J Caring Sci* **15**(2): 174–80

Thomas V, Rose F (1991) Ethnic differences in the experience of pain. *Soc Sci Med* **32**: 1063–6

Turk D, Okifuji A (1999) Assessment of patients' reporting of pain: an integrated perspective. *Lancet* **353**: 1784–8

Ware J, Kosinski M, Kellar S (1993) *Health Survey, Manual and Interpretation Guide*. Health Institute, Boston, MA

Widar M, Samuelsson L, Karlsson-Tivenius S, Ahlerstrom G (2002) Long-term pain conditions after a stroke. *J Rehabil Med* **34**: 165–70

Wilson M (2002) Overcoming the challenges of neuropathic pain. *Nurs Stand* **16**(33): 47–53

Wood M, Kay R, Dworkin R, Soong S, Whitley R (1996) Oral acyclovir therapy accelerates pain resolution in patients with herpes zoster: a meta analysis of placebo-controlled trials. *Clin Infect Dis* **22**: 341–47

Woolf CJ, Mannion RJ (1999) Neuropathic pain: aetiology, symptoms, mechanisms and management. *Lancet* **353**: 1959–1964

Zochodne D, Mitchell M (2003) An old acquaintance: opioids in neuropathic pain. *Neurology* **60**(6): 894–95

Section 2

Management of patients with acute neurological conditions

Chapter 5

An examination of the blood–brain barrier in health and disease

Ehsan Khan

The brain is the most well-protected organ in the body. This protection is a result of a number of features: externally, the brain is protected by its hard bony encasing, the cranium; internally, the brain is protected from bloodborne, potentially toxic, substances by the blood–brain barrier (BBB) (Bradbury, 1984). The presence of a barrier between the blood and the brain became apparent in the 19th century. The notion of a BBB is popularly attributed to Paul Ehrlich, a German scientist (Ehrlich, 1902); however, his understanding of this structure was not complete. It was not until 1933 that Spatz proposed a cerebral vascular system and nutrient delivery system similar to the contemporary model of the blood–brain barrier (Spatz, 1933). Finally, in 1967, Reese and Karnovsky verified this model of the BBB using electron microscopy.

What is the BBB?

The BBB is the result of interactions between capillary endothelium and glial cells that, together with a basement membrane, form the neurovascular unit (Begley, 2004) and constitute the microvascular

capillaries that ramify (branch) within the brain substance. The microstructure of these cells is primarily responsible for the unique features of the BBB (Begley, 2004). Although our understanding of cells involved in forming the BBB is far from complete, it appears that at least four different cell types are needed to form this structure:

- Endothelial cells
- Astrocytes
- Pericytes
- Neurons (Khan, 2002).

These cells are represented in a schematic diagram in *Figure 5.1*.

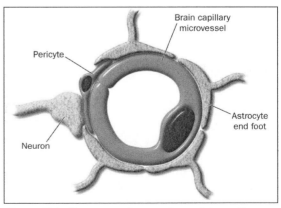

Figure 5.1: Current understanding of the cell types involved in production of the blood–brain barrier

Endothelial cells

Endothelial cells cover all blood-facing surfaces of the cardiovascular system. Endothelium is a layer of endothelial cells. Although endothelium is present throughout the body, a number of specific features differ between brain and peripheral endothelium. These characteristics include:

- Lack of fenestrations (openings in the endothelial membrane) and folds in the endothelium. This largely reduces the surface area of the brain capillary, and a lack of fenestrations also makes it impermeable to plasma proteins (Tamai and Tsuji, 2000)
- Presence of tight cell-to-cell junctions. Although all cells have junctions of varying tightness, the tight junctions found in the BBB endothelium are particularly strong and occlusive (Mitic and Anderson, 1998), preventing transfer of solutes between the cells
- Specific membrane transport channels and proteins. These allow selective entry to nutrients and actively remove potentially hazardous substances (Khan, 2002)
- Presence of a large number of mitochondria (Bradbury and Lightman, 1990). The quantity of these cell organelles suggests that the brain endothelium requires a large amount of energy (adenosine triphosphate; ATP) for its function.

These features in brain and peripheral endothelium are compared schematically in *Figure 5.2*.

The presence of the above characteristics allows the brain microvessel (synonym for capillary) endothelium to form a more restrictive endothelial barrier than most other endothelial barriers in the body. The exact causes for the differences between brain and peripheral endothelium are yet to be determined; however, the presence of the aforementioned cells appears to have a strong influence on the development of BBB-like characteristics in the endothelium (Begley, 2004). Of these, astrocytes at present appear to be one of the main contributors (Begley, 2004).

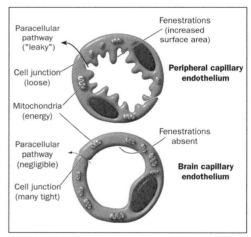

Figure 5.2: Differences between peripheral and blood–brain barrier capillary endothelium

Astrocytes

Astrocytes are neuroglial cells found in the central nervous system. Astrocytic processes cover almost the entire outer surface of the brain capillary, as a fine lattice (Kacem et al, 1998). Although it has long been known that astrocytes promote the formation and complexity of brain endothelium tight junctions *in vitro* (Tao-Cheng et al, 1987), the contribution of astrocytes to the expression of tight junctions remains unclear. Interestingly, the presence of astrocytes confers BBB endothelial-like properties to other non-brain endothelial cells when the two are grown together (co-cultured) in close proximity to each other (Isobe et al, 1996).

Pericytes and neurons

Pericytes are connective tissue cells found above blood vessels. The effect of pericytes and neurons on the BBB remains to be clarified. Pericytes may have a role to play in capillary integrity and organization (Ballabh et al, 2004). Evidence supporting this includes:

- Mature BBB capillaries are surrounded by pericytes (Dore-Duffy et al, 2000)
- Newly formed or growing capillaries have a reduced number of pericytes compared with mature capillaries (Katychev et al, 2003)
- Capillaries that are inflamed or diseased also have fewer pericytes (Dore-Duffy et al, 2000; Minagar and Alexander, 2003)
- Growing endothelial cells, astrocytes and pericytes together (tricultures) result in the formation of capillary-like structures (Ramsauer et al, 2002).

As a result of these characteristics, the brain capillary endothelial cells form a continuous and restrictive barrier between the blood and the brain. Thus, for any substance to enter the brain it needs to pass through the brain capillary cell. As cell membranes are made up largely of lipid (phospholipids), the only way a substance can diffuse through the membrane is if the substance is lipid-soluble. Many nutrients, including salts, glucose and many amino acids, are water-soluble. Therefore, they cannot pass through the capillary wall by passive diffusion. To facilitate transport of essential nutrients across the capillary wall into the brain, the capillary endothelium possesses many specialized transport proteins and channels, examples of which are given in *Table 5.1*.

Table 5.1: Examples of transport proteins and channels present in the brain capillary endothelium

Name	Form	Carries	In/out of the brain	Driving force
Glut-1	Transport protein	Glucose	In	Concentration gradient
y^+ system	Transport protein	Positively charged amino acids	In	Concentration gradient
L system	Transport protein	Large, neutral amino acids	In	Concentration gradient
Na^+ channel	Ion channel	Sodium	In	Concentration gradient
P-glycoprotein	Transport protein	Lipid-soluble substances	Out	ATP

From Khan (2002); ATP=adenosine triphosphate

It can be seen from *Table 5.1* that water-soluble nutrients are carried through the BBB by a number of transport proteins. These proteins may be BBB-specific or found in capillaries in the periphery. The Glut-1 glucose transport protein is found in great abundance in the BBB endothelium (Virgintino et al, 2000). The presence of a large number of these transport proteins is crucial to maintain adequate levels of glucose, as the brain cannot synthesize glucose from other sources (Dienel, 2002).

The Glut-1 transporter is equilibrative in nature, i.e. it transports glucose into the brain according to the plasma glucose concentration gradient. As the Glut-1 transporter provides the sole source of central nervous system (CNS) glucose, even mild changes in plasma glucose levels have an observable effect on CNS function (Messier, 2004). Similarly, transport of amino acids is dependent on BBB membrane transport proteins (see *Table 5.1*). Large, neutral amino acids compete for transport across the BBB via the L-type amino acid carrier (see *Table 5.1*).

In inherent metabolic diseases the levels of a number of amino acids are raised, such as in phenylketonuria (Weglage et al, 2002). As a result of an increased plasma phenylalanine concentration in phenylketonuria, the L system transporter is effectively taken over by phenylalanine transport. This occurs at the expense of not loading other large, neutral amino acids into the brain, resulting in a depletion of these amino acids and the characteristic abnormalities in brain development seen in infants who suffer from this disease (Pietz et al, 1999).

Thus, for something to enter the brain it either needs to be lipid-soluble, so that it can diffuse through the BBB capillary membranes into the brain, or if the substance is water-soluble then it needs to be carried through the BBB by a transport protein. There are some substances that need to enter the brain that are neither lipid-soluble nor small enough to be transported by a transport protein, such as other proteins or hormones. Protein entry into the brain takes a different pathway — transcytosis (*Figure 5.3*).

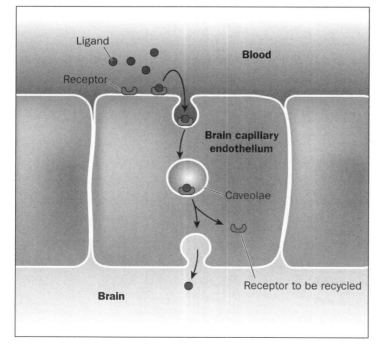

Figure 5.3: A simplified schematic of movement of a substance (ligand) by receptor-mediated transcytosis. A ligand binds to its receptor, which causes the cell membrane to envelop the ligand-receptor complex to form a vesicle (caveolae) within the cell. The contents of this caveolae are then transported through the cell and liberated on the other side into the brain. The receptor is then recycled

In transcytosis the protein attaches to the inner luminal (blood-side) endothelial wall (Khan, 2002). This attachment may or may not be mediated by a receptor. The protein then becomes enveloped by the membrane such that the membrane forms a small sphere (caveolae) inside the endothelial cell. This caveolae then enters the cell and is either carried to the other side of the cell where the process is reversed, so that the protein is transported out of the cell on the abluminal (brain-side) of the capillary, or the contents of the caveolae are liberated within the cell to be used up within the cell (Khan, 2002). Important examples of transcytosis include entry of insulin initially into the endothelial cell and then the brain by an insulin receptor, and iron initially into the endothelial cell and then the brain by a transferrin receptor-mediated transcytosis (Bradbury, 1997).

The BBB can also keep lipid-soluble substances out of the brain; it does this largely by two different mechanisms — efflux and drug metabolism. As these mechanisms use enzymatic-like processes to keep drugs out of the brain, they collectively constitute the enzymatic BBB (*Figure 5.4*).

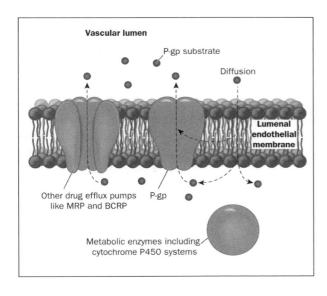

Figure 5.4: The enzymatic blood–brain barrier. This consists of the drug efflux proteins P-glycoprotein (P-gp) and multidrug resistance-related protein (MRP) that remove lipid-soluble drugs from the cell. It also includes the drug-metabolizing enzyme cytochrome P450 system. BCRP=breast cancer resistance protein

Efflux

Lipid-soluble compounds can diffuse through the lipid membranes of the BBB endothelium; however, they can be removed from the endothelial cell or membrane back into the bloodstream by a number of proteins present in the luminal endothelial cell surface. These proteins include P-glycoprotein (P-gp) and multidrug resistance-related protein (MRP). These proteins 'eject' lipid-soluble substances from the cell membrane (Gottesman and Pastan, 1993) (see *Figure 5.4*). As these proteins have to push the substance against its concentration gradient, they need energy in the form of ATP to do this (Ambudkar et al, 2003). These proteins are highly effective in reducing lipid-soluble drug entry into the brain (Khan et al, 1998; Khan, 2002).

Metabolism

Just as substances are metabolized in the liver, in the same way they are also metabolized in the brain and brain epithelium. A number of metabolic enzymes can be found in the BBB (Chat et al, 1998; Rieder et al, 2000). Here, these enzymes can either destroy the substance or convert it in such a way that it cannot enter the brain (Wacher et al, 1998).

Together BBB-based drug efflux and metabolism reduce the entry of drug into the neuronal parenchyma (brain matter), thus protecting the brain from the toxic effects of many drugs (Khan, 2002). Intracerebral distribution of P-gp has also been implicated in the pathogenicity and treatment outcomes of a number of diseases including Alzheimer's disease and Parkinson's disease (Lee and Bendayan, 2004). Increased numbers (overexpression) of P-gp units in epilepsy foci (areas where epileptic nerve discharges originate) are suggested to be, at least in part, the cause of long-term resistance to pharmacotherapy in this illness (Rogawski, 2002; Sisodiya et al, 2002).

The protective nature of the BBB can be used beneficially in treating some CNS illnesses. A common example of this is the use of a combination of levodopa and carbidopa in patients with Parkinson's disease. Parkinson's disease is characterized by a deficit in functional doperminergic neurons leading to a reduction in dopamine secretion in the brain. Replacement of dopamine can be an effective way of treating this deficiency (Rang et al, 2003). Dopamine cannot cross the BBB; therefore, although neuronal dopamine remains in the CNS and does not cause peripheral side-effects, dopamine cannot be administered orally or intravenously to treat Parkinson's disease (Rang et al, 2003). Levodopa, the natural precursor of dopamine, is given to overcome this problem.

Levodopa is transported via the L-type amino acid transport system across the BBB into the brain (Begley, 2004), where it is converted to dopamine by the enzyme dopa decarboxylase. As dopa decarboxylase is also present in the peripheral organs, the administered levodopa also gets converted into dopamine in the systemic circulation, leading to generation of the adverse effects of increased plasma dopamine levels such as cardiovascular excitation, and nausea and vomiting (Rang et al, 2003). To overcome this situation, a dopa decarboxylase inhibitor, carbidopa, is administered. Carbidopa cannot cross the BBB; therefore, it only inhibits peripheral dopa decarboxylase, resulting in a reduction in peripheral dopamine production, but leaving CNS levodopa conversion unchanged (Rang et al, 2003). Clinically, these two compounds are available as a combined preparation, Madopar.

The BBB can also act as a delivery system for substances produced in the brain. P-gp can efflux physiologically important substances from the brain — an example of this is the transport of opioids (morphine, beta-endorphin) from the brain to the bloodstream (King et al, 2001).

The BBB and disease

The BBB influences and is influenced by disease. The BBB inhibits entry of drugs into the brain. P-gp is one of the major mechanisms responsible for the reduction in drug entry of lipid-soluble drugs into the brain (Khan, 2002; Potschka et al, 2002; Rittierodt and Harada, 2003; Begley, 2004). The amount of P-gp produced in brain capillaries increases with an increase in drug concentration or exposure; this has been found using anti-epileptics and anti-cancer drugs (Potschka et al, 2002; Rittierodt and Harada, 2003). Similar increases in P-gp are seen in cancer, where the overexpression of P-gp in cancerous cells is a major obstacle to establishing effective cancer chemotherapy (Ueda et al, 1986; Rittierodt and Harada, 2003). The major consequence of an increased P-gp content in the BBB is that it will make patients refractory to treatments that may initially have been effective (Khan, 2002).

The BBB allows entry of the human immunodeficiency virus (HIV) and the simian immunodeficiency virus (SIV) into the brain via receptor-mediated endocytosis (Banks et al, 1998; Strelow et al, 2002). Initially, it was reported that virus entry had little effect on BBB integrity (Strelow et al, 2002). However, it has now been shown that in primates SIV infections do initially reduce BBB integrity (Stephens et al, 2003). Using bloodborne fibrinogen, a substance not able to penetrate the BBB, Stephens et al (2003) found that during the acute phase of SIV infection (2 weeks) there was a deposition of fibrinogen in the area of the brain infected by the virus. This finding was associated with a lack of one of the main cell-to-cell junctional proteins — zonula occludens 1 (ZO-1) — in the area of fibrinogen deposition, suggesting a breakdown in endothelial cell tight junction architecture.

These findings were not found in primate brains with endstage disease or in primates infected with gene-deleted non-pathogenic virus over a year later (Stephens et al, 2003). Thus, although during the acute phase of the infection the BBB is disrupted, this disruption is later 'repaired'. As many HIV therapies are excluded from the brain by the BBB, the virus is consequently protected from influence of drugs in later stages of the disease, possibly when it first clinically manifests. Thus, the brain can become a sanctuary for the HIV virus (Kim, 2003).

Conversely, inflammation influences BBB integrity and permeability via a number of cytokines and inflammatory mediators including bradykinin, histamine and free radicals (Abbott and Romero, 1996; Abbott, 2000; Dore-Duffy et al, 2000). Breakdown of the BBB results in the entry of a large number of toxins into the brain (Lossinsky and Shivers, 2004), causing toxicity and detrimental effects to the CNS. At present it is difficult to assess the degree of BBB breakdown *in vivo*; development of biochemical markers would prove to be beneficial. One such marker is the astrocytic protein S100 beta (Marchi et al, 2004), which may be found in the peripheral bloodstream following breakdown of the BBB.

BBB breakdown is found in a number of CNS diseases. These include cerebral hypoxia and ischaemia, septic encephalopathy, brain tumours and HIV-induced dementia, multiple sclerosis and Alzheimer's disease (Ballabh et al, 2004). All these diseases have an element of inflammation to them (Ballabh et al, 2004). BBB breakdown also allows leukocyte entry into the brain, leading to an activation of the inflammatory cascade, which further reduces BBB endothelial cell junctions (Bolton et al, 1998) and thus increasing BBB permeability.

Summary

The BBB forms a barrier between the cerebral blood flow and the brain tissue. This barrier, although primarily made up of brain microcapillary endothelium, is produced by the collective effects of a number of cell types including the brain microcapillaries, astrocytes, pericytes and nerves. This results in a tight occlusive lipid barrier and provides an enzymatic barrier that inhibits the passage of substances into the brain. The BBB protects the brain from bloodborne toxins, and also presents difficulties when developing pharmacological treatments for many CNS diseases.

References

Abbott NJ (2000) Inflammatory mediators and modulation of blood–brain barrier permeability. *Cell Mol Neurobiol* **20:** 131–47

Abbott NJ, Romero IA (1996) Transporting therapeutics across the blood–brain barrier. *Mol Med Today* **2:** 106–13

Ambudkar SV, Kimchi-Sarfaty C, Sauna ZE, Gottesman MM (2003) P-glycoprotein: from genomics to mechanism. *Oncogene* **22:** 7468–85

Ballabh P, Braun A, Nedergaard M (2004) The blood–brain barrier: an overview: structure, regulation and clinical implications. *Neurobiol Dis* **16**(1): 1–13

Banks WA, Akerstrom V, Kastin AJ (1998) Adsorptive endocytosis mediates the passage of HIV-1 across the blood–brain barrier: evidence for a post-internalization coreceptor. *J Cell Sci* **111:** 533–40

Begley DJ (2004) Delivery of therapeutic agents to the central nervous system: the problems and the possibilities. *Pharmacol Ther* **104**(1): 29–45

Bolton SJ, Anthony DC, Perry VH (1998) Loss of the tight junction proteins occludin and zonula occludens-1 from cerebral vascular endothelium during neutrophil-induced blood–brain barrier breakdown *in vivo*. *Neuroscience* **86:** 1245–57

Bradbury MW (1984) The structure and function of the blood–brain barrier. *Fed Proc* **43:** 186–191

Bradbury MW (1997) Transport of iron in the blood–brain–cerebrospinal fluid system. *J Neurochem* **69:** 443–54

Bradbury MW, Lightman SL (1990) The blood–brain interface. *Eye* **4:** 249–54

Chat M, Bayol-Denizot C, Suleman G, Roux F, Minn A (1998) Drug metabolizing enzyme activities and superoxide formation in primary and immortalized rat brain endothelial cells. *Life Sci* **62:** 151–63

Dienel GA (2002) Energy generation in the central nervous system. In: Edvinsson L, Krause DN, eds. *Cerebral Blood Flow and Metabolism*. Lippincott, Williams and Wilkins, Philadelphia: 140–61

Dore-Duffy P, Owen C, Balabanov R, Murphy S, Beaumont T, Rafols JA (2000) Pericyte migration from the vascular wall in response to traumatic brain injury. *Microvasc Res* **60:** 55–69

Ehrlich P (1902) Uber die Beziehungen von chemischer constitution, Vertheilung, und pharmakologischer Wirkung. Reprinted and translated in: *Collected Studies in Immunity*. (1906) John Wiley, New York: 567–97

Gottesman MM, Pastan I (1993) Biochemistry of multidrug resistance mediated by the multidrug transporter. *Annu Rev Biochem* **62:** 385–427

Isobe I, Watanabe T, Yotsuyanagi T et al (1996) Astrocytic contributions to blood–brain barrier (BBB) formation by endothelial cells: a possible use of aortic endothelial cell for *in-vitro* BBB model. *Neurochem Int* **28:** 523–33

Kacem K, Lacombe P, Seylaz J, Bonvento G (1998) Structural organization of the perivascular astrocyte endfeet and their relationship with the endothelial glucose transporter: a confocal microscopy study. *Glia* **23:** 1–10

Katychev A, Wang X, Duffy A, Dore-Duffy P (2003) Glucocorticoid-induced apoptosis in CNS microvascular pericytes. *Dev Neurosci* **25:** 436–46

Khan EU (2002) The role of P-glycoprotein at the blood–brain barrier. PhD thesis, King's College, London

Khan EU, Reichel A, Begley DJ, Roffey SJ, Jezequel SG, Abbott NJ (1998) The effect of drug lipophilicity on P-glycoprotein-mediated colchicine efflux at the blood–brain barrier. *Int J Clin Pharmacol Ther* **36**(2): 84–6

Kim RB (2003) Drug transporters in HIV therapy. *Top HIV Med* **11:** 136–9

King M, Su W, Chang A, Zuckerman A, Pasternak GW (2001) Transport of opioids from the brain to the periphery by P-glycoprotein: peripheral actions of central drugs. *Nat Neurosci* **4:** 268–74

Lee G, Bendayan R (2004) Functional expression and localization of P-glycoprotein in the central nervous system: relevance to the pathogenesis and treatment of neurological disorders. *Pharm Res* **21:** 1313–30

Lossinsky AS, Shivers RR (2004) Structural pathways for macromolecular and cellular transport across the blood–brain barrier during inflammatory conditions. *Histol Histopathol* **19:** 535–64

Marchi N, Cavaglia M, Fazio V, Bhudia S, Hallene K, Janigro D (2004) Peripheral markers of blood–brain barrier damage. *Clin Chim Acta* **342:** 1–12

Messier C (2004) Glucose improvement of memory: a review. *Eur J Pharmacol* **490**(1–3): 33–57

Minagar A, Alexander JS (2003) Blood–brain barrier disruption in multiple sclerosis. *Mult Scler* **9**(6): 540–9

Mitic LL, Anderson JM (1998) Molecular architecture of tight junctions. *Annu Rev Physiol* **60:** 121–42

Pietz J, Kreis R, Rupp A et al (1999) Large neutral amino acids block phenylalanine transport into brain tissue in patients with phenylketonuria. *J Clin Invest* **103:** 1169–78

Potschka H, Fedrowitz M, Loscher W (2002) P-glycoprotein-mediated efflux of phenobarbital, lamotrigine and felbamate at the blood–brain barrier: evidence from microdialysis experiments in rats. *Neurosci Lett* **327**: 173–6

Ramsauer M, Krause D, Dermietzel R (2002) Angiogenesis of the blood–brain barrier in vitro and the function of cerebral pericytes. *FASEB J* **16**: 1274–6

Rang HP, Dale MM, Ritter JM, Moore PK (2003) *Pharmacology*. 5th edn. Churchill Livingstone, Edinburgh, London

Reese TS, Karnovsky MJ (1967) Fine structural localization of a blood–brain barrier to exogenous peroxidase. *J Cell Biol* **34**: 207–17

Rieder CR, Parsons RB, Fitch NJ, Williams AC, Ramsden DB (2000) Human brain cytochrome P450 1B1: immunohistochemical localization in human temporal lobe and induction by dimethylbenz(a) anthracene in astrocytoma cell line (MOG-G-CCM). *Neurosci Lett* **278**: 177–80

Rittierodt M, Harada K (2003) Repetitive doxorubicin treatment of glioblastoma enhances the PGP expression: a special role for endothelial cells. *Exp Toxicol Pathol* **55**: 39–44

Rogawski MA (2002) Does P-glycoprotein play a role in pharmacoresistance to antiepileptic drugs? *Epilepsy Behav* **3**: 493–5

Sisodiya SM, Lin WR, Harding BN, Squier MV, Thom M (2002) Drug resistance in epilepsy: expression of drug resistance proteins in common causes of refractory epilepsy. *Brain* **125**(1): 22–31

Spatz H (1933) Die Bedeutung der vitalen Farbung fur die Lehre vom stoffaustausch zwischen dem Zentralnervensystem und dem ubrigen korper. *Arch Psychiat Nervenkr* **101**: 267–358

Stephens EB, Singh DK, Kohler ME, Jackson M, Pacyniak E, Berman NE (2003) The primary phase of infection by pathogenic simian-human immunodeficiency virus results in disruption of the blood–brain barrier. *AIDS Res Hum Retroviruses* **19**(10): 837–46

Strelow L, Janigro D, Nelson JA (2002) Persistent SIV infection of a blood–brain barrier model. *J Neurovirol* **8**: 270–80

Tamai I, Tsuji A (2000) Transporter-mediated permeation of drugs across the blood–brain barrier. *J Pharm Sci* **89**: 1371–88

Tao-Cheng JH, Nagy Z, Brightman MW (1987) Tight junctions of brain endothelium *in vitro* are enhanced by astroglia. *J Neurosci* **7**: 3293–9

Ueda K, Cornwell MM, Gottesman MM et al (1986) The mdr1 gene, responsible for multidrug-resistance, codes for P-glycoprotein. *Biochem Biophys Res Commun* **141**: 956–62

Virgintino D, Robertson D, Benagiano V et al (2000) Immunogold cytochemistry of the blood–brain barrier glucose transporter Glut-1 and endogenous albumin in the developing human brain. *Brain Res Dev Brain Res* **123**: 95–101

Wacher VJ, Silverman JA, Zhang Y, Benet LZ (1998) Role of P-glycoprotein and cytochrome P450 3A in limiting oral absorption of peptides and peptidomimetics. *J Pharmceutical Sci* **87**: 1322–30

Weglage J, Wiedermann D, Denecke J et al (2002) Individual blood–brain barrier phenylalanine transport in siblings with classical phenylketonuria. *J Inherit Metab Dis* **25**: 431–6

Chapter 6

Understanding pain: Physiology of pain

Helen Godfrey

Pain is a common problem and affects people of all ages, socioeconomic groups and ethnicities. A survey in the UK of 1037 adults indicated that 11% of respondents had suffered recurring pain for over 3 months before the study (Rigge, 1990). Another survey, conducted in Europe, in which 46 000 people were interviewed from 16 countries, revealed that the overall prevalence of chronic pain was 19% and the prevalence of chronic pain in the UK was 13% (Fricker, 2003). Estimates of the prevalence of chronic pain vary considerably, reflecting differences in definitions, populations studied and research methods (Smith et al, 2001; Stannard and Johnson, 2003). In a Swedish study, 28% of patients visiting a GP over 1 year had some kind of medically defined pain problem (Hasselstrom et al, 2002). In a questionnaire survey in the UK, 14.1% of patients in the sample (*n*=3065) reported significant chronic pain, defined as pain that has persisted for at least 3 months and for which painkillers have been taken and treatment sought recently and frequently (Smith et al, 2001).

Pain is a common experience in many groups of hospitalized patients. In a 3-year study, 59% of patients admitted to a single hospital in Chicago experienced pain, with 28% experiencing severe pain (Whelan et al, 2004). Pain has a significant impact on health, employment and daily life (Latham and Davis, 1994; Smith et al, 2001).

Patients and health professionals continue to report that pain is often inadequately managed in hospital and community settings (Yates et al, 1998; Drayer et al, 1999; McHugh and Thoms, 2001; Whelan et al, 2004). In a survey of GPs (*n*=504), most of them (81%) felt that the management of chronic pain was unsuccessful in over half of the patients seeking help (Stannard and Johnson, 2003). The authors suggest that further education of all health professionals who manage pain is required to elicit improvements in the management of pain (Stannard and Johnson, 2003).

Nurses are in a unique position to contribute to successful pain management as they have many opportunities to identify patients in pain, assess pain and its effects, instigate action to control the pain and evaluate the efficacy of these actions and any adverse effects. While pain management is an integral aspect of nursing care it could be argued that it is often not tangible in terms of accounting for time spent or in patient satisfaction (Madjar, 2004).

There is a wealth of literature suggesting that nurses lack knowledge about pain management (Clarke et al, 1996; McCaffery and Ferrell, 1997; Twycross, 2002; Madjar, 2004). To manage pain effectively, nurses need to understand the mechanisms that initiate and maintain pain. Management of pain by nurses should be based on current knowledge of pain physiology as well as understanding the context and the psychological, social, cultural and cognitive aspects that contribute to the pain experience (Clarke et al, 1996; Twycross, 2002).

The concepts introduced in this chapter reflect the principles, objectives and content of the pain curriculum for basic nursing education proposed by the International Association for the Study of Pain (IASP), particularly with regard to the physiological dimension of pain (IASP Subcommittee on Taxonomy, 1994).

While pain is much more than a physiological sensation, effective pain management depends in part on nurses having knowledge of the physiological mechanisms involved in the pain experience. This chapter and the next focusses on understanding pain: this chapter introduces the key concepts in contemporary pain physiology and explores the mechanisms that contribute to pain; chapter 7 enhances nurses' knowledge by exploring the biological basis of pain interventions that contribute to pain management.

Experience of pain

The pain experience varies for different individuals as a result of a multitude of factors and circumstances that are difficult to characterize. Different types of pain can be experienced; some pain is protective and acts as an early warning to alert the individual that tissue damage is occurring or about to occur. This sort of pain prevents further damage during healing and repair (Woolf, 1995). However, pain often outlives its warning role and becomes persistent and debilitating (Julius and Basbaum, 2001). Pain can be experienced when there is no evidence of tissue damage and phantom pains can be felt in a missing limb (Haigh and Blake, 2001). Any useful definition of pain has to encompass all these different pain manifestations.

The IASP defines pain as:

'... *an unpleasant sensory and emotional experience associated with actual or potential tissue damage or described in terms of such damage*' (IASP Subcommittee on Taxonomy, 1979).

The experience of pain is not a straightforward response to an unpleasant sensation. The perception and response to pain are dependent on many factors (*Table 6.1*). Pain also has a cognitive component, as the person experiencing pain will consider its meaning, significance and effect on his or her wellbeing (Casey, 1996).

Table 6.1: Factors that affect perception and response to pain

- The individual's emotional state
- Memories
- Genetic makeup
- Personality
- Motor activity and sensory inputs
- The cultural, environmental and socio-economic context

From Holdcroft and Power (2003)

The processing of pain information is complex, but follows a similar neural pathway as other types of sensory information; the incoming stimuli are changed into nerve impulses that are relayed along nerve fibres to the spinal cord and then to brain centres. Pain results from activation of specialized pain receptors, or nociceptors, in somatic or visceral tissues and the transmission of nerve impulses; this is called nociceptive pain and can be described as somatic or visceral (*Table 6.2*).

The pain system can be altered by injury, disease and genetic factors and, like other sensory systems, this can lead to disturbed functioning. Neuropathic pain is pain that follows injury to the nervous system itself and includes a range of neuropathies caused by different types of nerve damage (Dworkin, 2002; Sommer, 2003). Neuropathic pain is complex and has the potential to be severe and persistent (Woolf, 1995). In an intact nervous system the components that enable pain stimuli to be perceived as pain include nociceptors, sensory neurones, ascending tracts in the spinal cord and pain centres in the brain.

This chapter addresses the different steps involved in the pathway of nociceptive pain and introduces the gate control theory of pain developed by Melzack and Wall (1965).

Table 6.2: Causes of somatic and visceral pain

Somatic pain. This results from injury of:

- Skin and mucosa
- Muscle
- Bone
- Tendons
- Ligaments and joints
- Arteries

Visceral pain. This results from stimulation of nociceptors in internal organs

(e.g. stomach, kidney, gall bladder, intestines and bladder) as a result of tissue damage, such as:

- Distension
- Inflammation
- Obstruction
- Infection
- Ischaemia

From McCaffery et al (2003); Al-Chaer and Traub (2002)

Pain stimuli, nociceptors and nociception

Nociception encapsulates the molecular mechanisms whereby pain stimuli are detected and converted into nerve impulses. Stimuli that elicit pain are called noxious stimuli and include physical (mechanical or thermal) and chemical effects (McHugh and McHugh, 2000). Physical stimuli, such as a burn or physical blow, produce immediate pain, but a variety of chemicals released as a result of tissue damage can then also cause further pain (Cross, 1994; McHugh and McHugh, 2000). Types of tissue damage that cause pain include a deficiency of blood (ischaemia) and subsequent deficiency of oxygen (hypoxia); ulceration, infection, nerve damage and inflammation. In all cases, pain-stimulating chemicals will accumulate and trigger the cycle of events that cause pain.

Nociceptors are special free nerve endings, sometimes referred to as bare nerve endings at the distal end of pain-sensing neurones. They are found in the skin, muscles, joint capsules, visceral organs and arterial walls (Barasi, 1991; Bromm and Lorenz, 1998). Two broad types of nociceptor have been identified (Barasi, 1991; Cross, 1994; Julius and Basbaum, 2001): high-threshold mechanoceptors respond to intense mechanical stimulation; while polymodal nociceptors respond to noxious mechanical, thermal and chemical effects (Barasi, 1991). This categorization of pain stimuli and nociceptors is complex and evolving as new insights emerge from molecular studies (Julius and Basbaum, 2001).

The nociceptors themselves contain a multitude of specialized protein receptors located in the membrane. In response to noxious stimuli, the receptor proteins change shape to form pores or channels that allow ions to enter leading to electrical impulses in the pain-sensing neurones. There are two main groups of receptor channels: one group is responsible for detecting noxious stimuli, and includes transient receptor potential channels and acid-sensing channels; the other group of receptor channels is responsible for setting the threshold at which nociceptors generate electrical impulses (Stephan, 2005).

Nociceptors respond to noxious thermal and mechanical stimuli and a variety of inflammatory mediators released during tissue injury. These chemical mediators include peptides such as bradykinin, lipids including prostaglandins, neurotransmitters such as substance P, serotonin and adenosine triphosphate and neurotrophins, such as nerve growth factor (Cross, 1994; Julius and Basbaum, 2001).

The events that occur in nociceptors, which convert pain stimuli into nerve impulses, are not yet fully understood, but are thought to include a number of steps (Barasi, 1991; Monafo, 1995). Nociceptors are located next to mast cells and small blood vessels; the three components function together in response to injury with the inflammatory process (McHugh and McHugh, 2000; Julius and Basbaum, 2001) (*Figure 6.1*).

Mast cells release histamine in response to painful stimuli and this results in a range of neurochemicals including substance P (a neuropeptide) and glutamate (an amino acid) being released

Figure 6.1: Nociceptors in the skin situated next to a mast cell and capillary loop. Mast cells release their histamine in response to pain stimuli; the histamine in turn stimulates the nociceptors to secrete neurochemicals including substance P. A cascade of chemicals ultimately leads to activation of nociceptors, and action potentials are generated in the pain fibres and conducted to the spinal cord

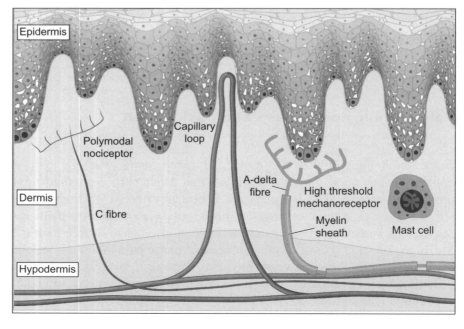

from the nociceptor ending (McHugh and McHugh, 2000; Julius and Basbaum, 2001). These neurochemicals stimulate mast cells further, and the resulting cascade of chemicals ultimately activates protein receptors in the nociceptor membrane, causing ion channels to open. Positively charged ions such as sodium or calcium flow into the nociceptor, lowering the voltage across the membrane. If the membrane voltage is sufficiently lowered, electrical impulses or action potentials will be generated and transmitted along nerve fibres towards the spinal cord (McHugh and McHugh, 2000). Nociceptors respond in proportion to the intensity of the stimulus; the greater the stimulus, the larger the voltage change and greater the number of impulses generated (Wood et al, 2005).

Transmission of pain impulses to spinal cord

There are two types of fibres for conducting pain nerve impulses: the relatively small-diameter A-delta fibres; and the even smaller C fibres (*Table 6.3*).

These sensory fibres carry the pain information from the nociceptors to the dorsal horn in the spinal cord (Monafo, 1995; Julius and Basbaum, 2001). Of the two types, A-delta fibres have a slightly larger diameter and are myelinated; both these attributes enable this type of fibre to carry pain impulses more quickly. They carry nerve impulses at a speed of about 5–25 m/s (Clancy and McVicar, 1998) and are sometimes referred to as 'fast fibres'. These fibres connect to the high-threshold mechanoreceptors. The C fibres are smaller-diameter, unmyelinated fibres, which therefore have a slower conduction velocity of about 1–2m/s (Barasi, 1991; Monafo, 1995). These fibres are often referred to as 'slow fibres' and they connect to the polymodal nociceptor (Julius and Basbaum, 2001).

Sometimes a distinction between 'first' and 'second' pain is made. First pain is the pricking or sharp pain associated with A-delta fibres, and the second or burning, dull, aching, poorly localized pain is associated with C fibres (Jackson, 1995; McHugh and McHugh, 2000; Julius and Basbaum, 2001). However, there is some debate about the physiological basis of these classifications (Barasi, 1991).

There are other types of sensory nerve fibres that are not usually associated with carrying pain information: the A-alpha and A-beta fibres (Julius and Basbaum, 2001; Wood et al, 2005). These

Table 6.3: Characteristics of the A-delta and C pain fibres

Fibre type	Diameter	Myelination	Conduction velocity (m/s)	Type of pain	Nociceptor at distal end
A-delta fibres	Large	Myelinated	5–25	'First' pain	High-threshold mechano-receptor
C fibres	Small	Unmyelinated	1–2	'Second' pain	Polymodal receptor

fibres conduct impulses more quickly than pain fibres and can modulate the transmission of pain information in the spinal cord.

Spinal cord processing of pain signals

A-delta and C fibres carry pain impulses to the spinal cord. Traditionally, sensory nerve fibres are thought to exclusively enter the dorsal (posterior) roots; however, some afferents carrying pain information do enter the ventral (anterior) roots (Cross, 1994). Nevertheless, most fibres carrying pain signals terminate in the dorsal horn of the spinal cord and then ascend or descend one or two segments in a thin tract of small axons capping the dorsal horn, known as Lissauer's tract. This branches off at different levels forming synapses with neurones in the grey matter of the dorsal horn (Cross, 1994).

The pain fibres entering the dorsal horn are first-order neurones and they synapse with second-order nociceptive neurones that crossover in the spinal cord and transmit the pain signals to the brain. There are two main groups of these second-order neurones:

- 'Nociceptive-specific' neurones (NS), which are only stimulated by noxious input
- 'Wide dynamic range' (WDR) neurones, which respond to gentle input from A-beta fibres as well as pain input from A-delta and C fibres (Cross,1994; Bromm and Lorenz, 1998).

The grey matter in the spinal cord is highly organized into a number of layers, or laminae: A-delta fibres terminate in laminae I, V and X, and C fibres end in laminae I–V (Cross, 1994). Afferent fibres terminating in the superficial laminae of the dorsal horn are small and tend to respond only to pain; whereas neurones in the deeper laminae respond to noxious and non-noxious input (Barasi, 1991). The location in the grey matter of the dorsal horn where the majority of C and A-delta fibres terminate is called the substantia gelatinosa (Dickenson, 1995). The substantia gelatinosa comprises lamina II and III and represents a system on each side of the spinal cord of densely interconnecting neurones that can modulate pain information (Melzack and Wall, 1965; Melzack, 1973). Within the spinal cord, each sensory or afferent fibre is likely to synapse with many small interneurones located in different regions (or laminae) of the spinal cord (Barasi, 1991).

Spinal transmission of pain information to the brain

Axons of both second-order neurones (WDR and NS neurones) crossover in the spinal cord into the white matter and rise up the spinal cord in a number of ascending pathways. The two major ascending pathways, the spinothalamic tract and spinoreticular tract, carry pain information to the brain in the anterolateral quadrant (Cross, 1994). Depending on which of the above pain pathways is being described, the second-order neurones synapse with third-order neurones in the thalamus or reticular formation (Barasi, 1991). The pain fibres of the spinoreticular tract ascend from the dorsal horn to the reticular formation in the brain stem, and third-order neurones project the pain information to the cerebral cortex (Barasi, 1991).

In the spinothalamic tract, the first-order neurones, the A-delta fibres and C fibres, synapse with the second-order neurones in the dorsal horn of the spinal cord. These crossover to the other side of

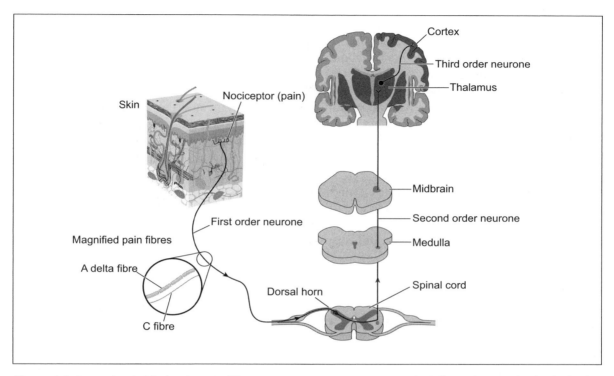

Figure 6.2: Lateral spinothalamic tract. Three sensory neurones carry pain information to the brain in this pathway

the spinal cord and ascend the spinal cord. The nociceptive spinothalamic fibres have two regions of the thalamus as their destination: the lateral nuclei and the medial nuclei. Axons that terminate in the thalamus synapse with third-order neurones, some project to the frontal cortex and others to the somatosensory cortex (Cross, 1994). Neurones projecting to topographically organized regions in the somatosensory cortex enable the pain to be localized (Barasi, 1991; Cross, 1994) (*Figure 6.2*).

Processing in the brain

Noxious information does not become pain until the brain adds meaning to the input arriving in the pain pathways. Many parts of the brain are involved in the experience of pain, and the classical view is that the specialized area of the cortex (the somatosensory cortex alluded to above) is responsible for interpreting pain from the many other signals representing touch, pressure, cold and heat that arrive there (Craig, 2005). This view is challenged by new ideas emerging from brain-mapping techniques and other experimental studies, suggesting that there may be specific pain centres in the brain (Craig, 2005).

An understanding of the role of the brain in the pain experience can be illuminated by recognizing that the sensation of pain is considered to have two components: the sensory-discriminative and affective-motivational components (Treede et al, 1999). The sensory-discriminative component gives information about the location, modality or intensity of stimuli, while the affective-motivational component relates to the emotional responses to the pain, including anxiety, fear, distress and the urge to respond (Ohara et al, 2005). The areas of the cortex that are involved in the processing of painful stimuli are thought to include the primary and secondary somatosensory cortices, the insula and the anterior cingulate cortex (Treede et al, 1999; Schnitzler and Ploner, 2000). The ability to locate and describe a painful stimulus arises in the primary somatosensory cortex, and the unpleasant and aversive features of pain relate to other cortical areas (Ohara et al, 2005).

Before reaching the cerebral cortex, pain information is relayed through a number of other brain areas, including the reticular formation and thalamus (Almeida et al, 2004). The reticular formation is a cluster of neurones in the brain stem that receives inputs via the spinoreticular tract; fibres from the reticular formation then radiate to other areas of the brain. The reticular formation has a role in the affective-motivational aspects of pain and is also thought to activate brain-stem areas involved in descending inhibitory pathways (Almeida et al, 2004). The reticular formation is thought to be partly responsible for integrating the autonomic responses observed when someone is suffering pain, such as sweating, changes in heart rate, blood pressure and respiratory rate, and which play an important part in the assessment of pain (Barasi, 1991; Carr and Mann, 2000).

The thalamus is of central importance to the sensation of pain. The projection of fibres carrying pain information to the hypothalamus also suggests a role for the hypothalamus in the autonomic changes associated with pain that is supported by imaging studies (Petrovic et al, 2004). The emotional aspects of pain are encoded in the limbic system (Blackburn-Munro and Blackburn-Munro, 2003).

Information about pain perception appears to be integrated in the anterior cingulate cortex. Pain alerts the individual to tissue damage, helps to evaluate how serious the danger might be and then helps learning to occur so that it can be remembered and avoided in the future. This region of the brain appears to play a unique role in collating all these pieces of information together (Motluk, 1999) and is involved in the perception of suffering and emotional response (Cross, 1994; Treede et al, 1999).

In addition to ascending pathways that carry pain to the brain, there are descending pathways that originate in the cortex, the thalamus and brain stem, which can influence the pain experience (Cross, 1994). The descending pathways, which modulate pain, are the basis for cognitive processes, such as past experience, and psychological processes, such as anxiety, which have significant impacts on the pain felt (Clancy and McVicar, 1998). The complexity of pain is highlighted by the role of descending pathways. Early studies on these pathways related to phenomena associated with acute stimuli, whereas more recent studies have focused on chronic pain conditions (Ren and Dubner, 2002). It now seems that the descending modulation of pain has two dimensions: inhibition and facilitation. The balance and timing between facilitation and inhibition is crucial, and shifts in this balance may contribute to chronic pain conditions (Ren and Dubner, 2002).

Gate control theory of pain

Melzack and Wall (1965) developed the gate control theory of pain, which explains how pain can be modulated in the spinal cord. They proposed the concept of a gating mechanism in the dorsal horn of the spinal cord through which pain information had to pass on its way to the brain (*Figure 6.3*).

The opening and closing of the gate to pain information can be influenced by a number of different factors and relates to the flow or suppression of pain information transmitted across synapses in the dorsal horn of the spinal cord (Clancy and McVicar, 1998).

Transmission of pain information from the body to the brain depends on the balance of activity in peripheral sensory neurones and modulation by descending inhibitory pathways (Clancy and McVicar, 1998). Nerve impulses from nociceptors and their sensory fibres (A-delta or C fibres) arrive in the dorsal horn. When information flows from A-delta or C pain fibres across the synapse to the second-order neurone via the secretion of excitatory neurotransmitters, the gate is said to be 'open'; the closing of the gate is achieved when this transmission is suppressed.

At the synapse between the pain fibres (A-delta or C fibres) and the second-order neurone are small interneurones (Barasi, 1991). Activity in these inhibitory neurones suppresses the flow of pain information to the brain by inhibiting the second-order neurones (McHugh and McHugh, 2000). These interneurones are stimulated by neurotransmitters secreted from larger diameter sensory neurones (A-beta fibres) carrying sensory information such as touch, pressure and temperature; this

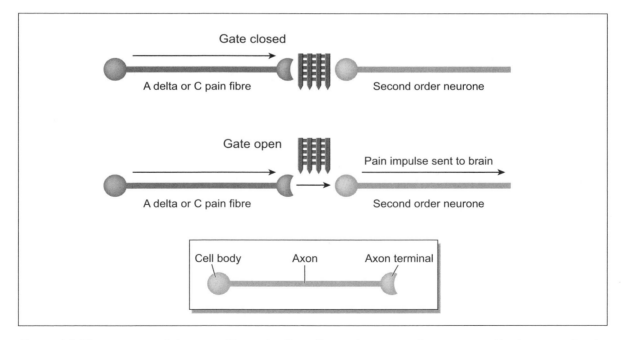

Figure 6.3: The concept of the gate. The pain fibre (first-order neurone) synapses with the second-order neurone in the dorsal horn of the spinal cord. These diagrams illustrate the concept of the gate that controls the flow of pain information to the brain. The arrows represent pain impulses

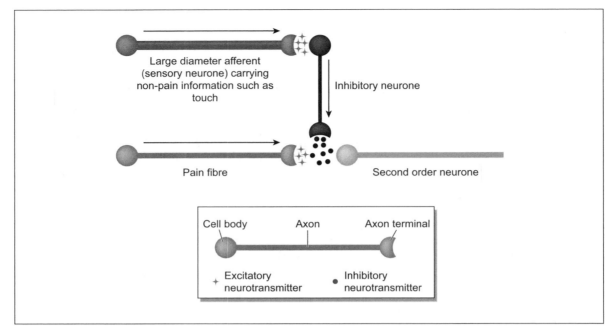

Figure 6.4: Gating mechanism. The gating mechanism in the dorsal horn of the spinal cord relies on a small inhibitory neurone, which when active suppresses the flow of pain information to the brain. Arrows represent nerve impulses

results in the suppression of upward transmission of pain information to the brain (Barasi, 1991) (*Figure 6.4*).

These non-pain sensory neurones secrete mainly excitatory amino acids and, in particular, glutamate (McHugh and McHugh, 2000). When the inhibitory interneurone is stimulated by these excitatory neurotransmitters it transmits nerve impulses, and at its synapse with the second-order neurone secretes inhibitory neurotransmitters that suppress the flow of pain information towards the brain.

In summary, activity in the large-diameter fibres tends to close the gate, while activity in the smaller pain fibres tends to facilitate transmission and opens the gate. The theory also suggests that it is the relative amount of activity in the two functionally distinct fibres that determines the pain intensity. As the activity in large-diameter fibres increases, less pain is perceived; while more activity in the small-diameter pain fibres means more pain is felt (Barasi, 1991).

The gate theory also proposes that information flowing down descending inhibitory pathways from higher brain centres closes the gate. The descending neurones, which arise in the brain, synapse with the inhibitory interneurones in the dorsal horn. As nerve impulses transmitted by descending neurones arrive at the synapse, they cause neurotransmitters, such as serotonin and noradrenaline, to be secreted (Cross, 1994; McHugh and McHugh, 2000). These neurotransmitters then excite the inhibitory neurone, which suppresses pain transmission in the second-order neurone to the brain (*Figure 6.5*). The inhibitory neurone secretes natural opioids (enkephalins, endorphins and dynorphins), and these peptides inhibit the second-order neurone (Barasi, 1991). The inhibitory interneurone can be excited either by the descending pathway or by sensory information arriving at the synapse in large-diameter sensory fibres. In both cases, the second-order neurone will be inhibited

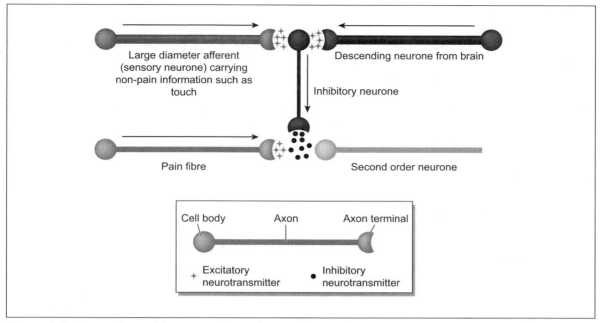

Figure 6.5: Descending inhibitory pathway. Descending pathways can also suppress the flow of pain information by stimulating the inhibitory neurone

by the natural opioids, sometimes described as endogenous opioids, secreted from the inhibitory neurone, and the flow of pain information up to the brain will be suppressed. This pain modulation by the body's own natural opioids may be described as endogenous opioid analgesia (Barasi, 1991).

There are a variety of ways in which these endogenous opioids can inhibit the flow of pain information. They prevent secretion of the neurotransmitter, substance P, from pain fibres and compete for substance P receptor-binding sites on the second-order neurone (Clancy and McVicar, 1998).

Sensitization

The neural pathways involved in the perception and modulation of pain are plastic, which means they can be modified in response to a range of stimuli, emotional as well as physical (Cross, 1994). Neurones that become used to carrying pain information can become sensitized. Changes to the sensitivity of both peripheral and central neurones are considered central to the concept of neuroplasticity. Neurones signalling tissue damage also secrete various chemicals leading to inflammation and sustained peripheral activity (Haigh and Blake, 2001). This leads to changes in sensitivity of neurones conducting pain information so that ordinary sensory information, such as pressure on an injured foot, becomes transformed into pain information (allodynia). This helps to explain why the pain someone feels may be out of proportion to the tissue damage (Youngson, 1992). The activity of excitatory amino acid receptors, particularly N-methyl-D-aspartate receptors on spinal neurones seems to be an intrinsic aspect of this plasticity (Haigh and Blake, 2001; Petrenko et al, 2003).

The phenomenon of sensitization illustrates that pain is an active process rather than just a relay of noxious information to the brain. Sensitization occurring in both the periphery and spinal cord reflects neuronal plasticity and leads to pain hypersensitivity (Woolf and Salter, 2000). The phenomenon of 'wind-up' is associated with C fibres that are responding to sustained pain stimuli; this causes a progressive increase (wind-up) in the response rate of the second-order neurones (McHugh and McHugh, 2000; Bolay and Moskowitz, 2002).

Hyperalgesia is an increased sensation to painful stimuli that may follow damage to soft-tissue-containing nociceptors.

Two types of hyperalgesia are described following cutaneous injury:

- Primary hyperalgesia occurring at the site of tissue damage is characterized by lowered pain thresholds and enhanced pain response to noxious stimuli
- Secondary hyperalgesia is pain felt in the surrounding undamaged areas in response to mechanical stimulation.

Primary hyperalgesia results from sensitization of peripheral receptors and central neurones; while secondary hyperalgesia appears to be caused by central sensitization alone (Treede et al, 1992).

Pain and homeostasis

Pain is clearly not just a sensory phenomenon. Injury and pain also disrupt homeostasis and, like changes in temperature, thirst or hunger, pain is a feeling producing an emotion that involves both a sensation and a behavioural drive (Craig, 2003). Pain disrupts homeostasis and elicits responses in neural, hormonal and behavioural activity, which are aimed at restoring homeostasis (Melzack, 1999). The gate control theory embraces the concept that the brain and spinal cord are essential components in pain perception as both engage in dynamic processes that can modulate pain. Acknowledging the role of the brain in pain processes is the basis for the neuromatrix model of pain (Melzack, 1999).

This model incorporates the concept of pain as a multidimensional experience evoked by a range of influences, including the role of the stress system, and recognizes the relationship between injury and disruption of homeostasis, stress and pain. The neuromatrix consists of a neural network of neurones and synapses in the brain that contribute to the sensory-discriminative, affective-motivational and evaluative-cognitive dimensions of the pain experience (Melzack, 1999). The neuromatrix is moulded by genetic and sensory influences and influenced by a variety of inputs, including those from the autonomic, endocrine and immune systems involved in mediating the stress response (Melzack, 1999). The mechanisms or programmes that are activated in response to injury are selected from a genetically determined range of programmes and reflect the magnitude of the injury (Melzack, 1999). The neuromatrix theory embraces many aspects of the gate control theory, but emphasizes that the perception of pain results from a range of influences, including past experience, cultural factors, emotional state, sensory inputs and modulation by opioids, and the endocrine, immune and autonomic nervous systems. This plethora of inputs is mediated by the networks that transform the neuromatrix into the pain experience.

Conclusions

Pain is a complex multidimensional experience. Pain stimuli trigger nociceptors to fire off impulses along nerve fibres to the spinal cord. A-delta fibres and C fibres carry pain information to the dorsal horn in the spinal cord. Here the relative activity of large-diameter afferents carrying sensory information, such as touch or warmth, modulates the pain signals passing to the brain. The 'gate' tends to close when the activity in the large-diameter afferents is greater than the activity in the pain fibres. When the activity in the small-diameter pain fibres is greater, the 'gate' opens and more pain is felt. Descending pathways from the brain also exert effects on the gating mechanism in the spinal cord, which explains how a variety of factors can influence the pain experience. Neural networks in the brain create a neuromatrix that integrates multiple influences or inputs to evoke the pain experience.

References

Almeida TF, Roizenblatt S, Tufik S (2004) Afferent pain pathways: a neuroanatomical review. *Brain Res* **1000**(1–2): 40–56

Barasi S (1991) The physiology of pain. *Surg Nurse* **4**(5): 14–20

Blackburn-Munro G, Blackburn-Munro R (2003) Pain in the brain: are hormones to blame? *Trends Endocrinol Metab* **14**(1): 20–7

Bolay H, Moskowitz MA (2002) Mechanisms of pain modulation in chronic syndromes. *Neurology* **59**(5 Suppl 2): S2–S7

Bromm B, Lorenz J (1998) Neurophysiological evaluation of pain. *Electroencephalogr Clin Neurophysiol* **107**(4): 227–53

Carr ECJ, Mann EM (2000) *Pain: Creative Approaches to Effective Management*. Palgrave Macmillan, Basingstoke

Casey K (1996) Match and mismatch: identifying the neuronal determinants of pain. *Ann Intern Med* **124**(11): 995–8

Clancy J, McVicar A (1998) Homeostasis: the key concept to physiological control: neurophysiology of pain. *Br J Theatre Nurs* **7**(10): 19–27

Clarke E, French B, Bilodeau M, Capasso V, Edwards A, Empoliti J (1996) Pain management knowledge, attitudes and clinical practice: impact of nurses' characteristics and education. *J Pain Symptom Manage* **11**(1): 18–31

Craig AD (2003) A new view of pain as a homeostatic emotion. *Trends Neurosci* **26**(9): 303–7

Craig AD (2005) *Mapping Pain in the Brain*. The Wellcome Trust, London (http://www.wellcome.ac.uk/en/pain/microsite/science2.html) (last accessed 8 August 2005)

Cross SA (1994) Pathophysiology of pain. *Mayo Clin Proc* **69**: 375–83

Dickenson AH (1995) Central acute pain mechanisms. *Ann Med* **27**(2): 223–7

Drayer RA, Henderson J, Reidenberg M (1999) Barriers to better pain control in hospitalised patients. *J Pain Symptom Manage* **17**(6): 434–40

Dworkin RH (2002) An overview of neuropathic pain: syndromes, symptoms, signs and several mechanisms. *Clin J Pain* **18**(6): 343–9

Fricker J (2003) *Pain in Europe: A Report*. Pain in Europe (http://www.painineurope.com/user_site/index.cfm?item_id=4405413) (last accessed 8 August 2005)

Haigh RC, Blake DR (2001) Understanding pain. *Clin Med* **1**(1): 44–8

Hasselstrom J, Liu-Palmgren J, Rasjo-Wrååk G (2002) Prevalence of pain in general practice. *Eur J Pain* **6**(5): 375–85

Holdcroft A, Power I (2003) Management of pain. *Br Med J* **326**(7390): 635–9

International Association for the Study of Pain Subcommittee on Taxonomy (1979) Pain terms: a list with definitions and notes on usage. *Pain* **6**(3): 247–52

International Association for the Study of Pain Subcommittee on Taxonomy (1994) Pain curriculum for basic nursing education. *J Pharm Care Symp Contr* **2**(2): 63–70

Jackson J (1995) Acute pain: its physiology and the pharmacology of analgesia. *Nurs Times* **91**(16): 27–8

Julius D, Basbaum AL (2001) Molecular mechanisms of nociception. *Nature* **413**(6852): 203–10

Latham J, Davis BD (1994) The socioeconomic impact of chronic pain. *Disabil Rehabil* **16**(1): 39–44

Madjar I (2004) Of pain, nursing and professional leadership: some personal reflections (editorial). *J Nurs Manag* **12**(3): 151–2

McCaffery M, Ferrell BR (1997) Nurses' knowledge of pain assessment and management: how much progress have we made? *J Pain Symptom Manage* **14**(3): 175–88

McHugh G, Thoms G (2001) Living with chronic pain: the patient's perspective. *Nurs Stand* **15**(52): 33–7

McHugh JM, McHugh WB (2000) Pain: neuroanatomy, chemical mediators and clinical implications. *AACN Clin Issues* **11**(2): 168–78

Melzack R (1973) *The Puzzle of Pain*. Penguin, Harmondsworth

Melzack R (1999) From the gate to the neuromatrix. *Pain* **6**(Suppl): S121–6

Melzack R, Wall PD (1965) Pain mechanisms: a new theory. *Science* **150**(699): 971–9

Monafo WW (1995) Physiology of pain. *J Burn Care Rehabil* **16**(3): 345–7

Motluk A (1999) Ouch! That hurt. *New Sci* **162**(2185): 17

Ohara PT, Vit JP, Jasmin L (2005) Cortical modulation of pain. *Cell Mol Life Sci* **62**(1): 44–52

Petrenko AB, Yamakura T, Baba H, Shimoji K (2003) The role of N-methyl-D-aspartate (NMDA) receptors in pain: a review. *Anesth Analg* **97**(4): 1108–16

Petrovic P, Petersson KM, Hansson P, Ingvar M (2004) Brainstem involvement in the initial response to pain. *Neuroimage* **22**(2): 995–1005

Ren K, Dubner R (2002) Descending modulation in persistent pain: an update. *Pain* **100**(1–2): 1–6

Rigge M (1990) Which? Way to health. *Pain* **Apr**: 66–8

Schnitzler A, Ploner M (2000) Neurophysiology and functional neuroanatomy of pain perception. *J Clin Neurophysiol* **17**(6): 592–603

Smith BH, Elliott AM, Chambers WA, Smith WC, Hannaford PC, Penny K (2001) The impact of chronic pain in the community. *Fam Pract* **18**(3): 292–9

Sommer C (2003) Painful neuropathies. *Curr Opin Neurol* **16**(5): 623–8

Stannard C, Johnson M (2003) Chronic pain management: can we do better? *Curr Med Res Opin* **19**(8): 703–6

Stephan MM (2005) Signals from the frontline. *The Scientist* Suppl March **28**: 20–3

Treede R, Meyer RA, Raja SN, Campbell JN (1992) Peripheral and central mechanisms of cutaneous hyperalgesia. *Prog Neurobiol* **38**(4): 397–421

Treede R, Kenshalo DR, Gracely RH, Jones AKP (1999) The cortical representation of pain. *Pain* **79**(2–3): 105–11

Twycross A (2002) Educating nurses about pain management: the way forward. *J Clin Nurs* **11**(6): 705–14

Whelan CT, Jin L, Meltzer D (2004) Pain and satisfaction with pain control in hospitalised medical patients: no such thing as low risk. *Arch Intern Med* **164**(2): 175–80

Wood JN, Beggs S, Drew LJ (2005) *Sensing Damage*. The Wellcome Trust, London (www.wellcome.ac.uk/en/pain/microsite/science1.html) (last accessed 8 August 2005)

Woolf CJ (1995) How to hit pain before it hurts you. *MRC News* **67**: 17–21

Woolf CJ, Salter MW (2000) Neuronal plasticity: increasing the gain in pain. *Science* **288**(5472): 1765–8

Yates P, Dewar A, Edwards H et al (1998) The prevalence and perception of pain amongst hospital in-patients. *J Clin Nurs* **7**(6): 521–30

Youngson R (1992) Pathways to pain control. *New Sci* **133**(1813): 30–3

Chapter 7

Understanding pain: Pain management

Helen Godfrey

Pain is a common experience for patients in hospitals (Whelan et al, 2004) and in the community setting (Smith et al, 2001). Despite a range of treatment approaches, pain remains a significant problem (Hader and Guy, 2004). Effective management of early pain is important, as this can influence the subsequent pain experience (Carr and Goudas, 1999). Successful pain relief can also reduce complications, including depression, anxiety and poor sleeping, and can shorten recovery time and length of hospital stay (Hader and Guy, 2004; Lellan, 2004). The control of pain is inevitably intricate, as pain is a complicated, active process. Additionally, pain is a multidimensional experience shaped by a variety of influences (Melzack, 1999). Although much is known about pain and how to control it, there are still many patients who suffer pain following surgery (Watt-Watson et al, 2001), and many whose chronic pain is not effectively managed (Stannard and Johnson, 2003).

Nurses play an important role in assessing and managing pain (Lellan, 2004; Madjar, 2004). Effective pain management is a major challenge (Barnason et al, 1998), and nurses' lack of knowledge about pain management is well documented (Clarke et al, 1996; McCaffery and Ferrell, 1997; Twycross, 2002; Madjar, 2004). To effectively manage pain and to select the appropriate approaches to alleviate pain, an understanding of the physiological basis of pain and pain interventions is required, together with an accurate assessment of the pain the individual is experiencing.

The last chapter explored the key concepts in contemporary pain physiology, while this chapter enhances nurses' knowledge by exploring the biological basis of pain interventions that contribute to pain management.

Pain assessment

Effective pain assessment is a prerequisite for choosing the most appropriate pain interventions to alleviate pain. Pain assessment is a complex issue, which has physiological, emotional, cognitive and social dimensions (Manias and Bucknall, 2002). Pain is a subjective experience and, since there are no precise objective measures, nurses should ask about pain, and the patient's self-report should be the primary source of assessment (Lynch, 2001; Martelli et al, 2004).

The assessment should include a description of the pain: its location, duration, frequency, intensity, aggravating and relieving factors, and the patient's cognitive response to pain. In addition the assessment should inquire about pain-related interference with activities and any pain-associated distress (Martelli et al, 2004). Two components to pain assessment can be considered: screening, which identifies the existence of pain at an initial assessment; and intensive assessment, which is the clinical evaluation of pain (Alcenius, 2004). Assessment of pain should be carried out frequently to identify changes in the intensity, quality and location of pain and to ascertain the effectiveness and side effects of pain management interventions (Lynch, 2001; Hader and Guy, 2004).

The use of a formal assessment tool can reduce the difficulty of assessing pain (Briggs, 1995; Carr, 1997; Lynch, 2001). However, selecting an appropriate tool from the range of pain assessment tools is difficult. The criteria for choosing a pain assessment tool include that it must be reliable and valid for the particular patient (Bird, 2003). Pain assessment tools usually incorporate numerical or verbal rating scales that record the intensity of pain and consequences on a range of activities of daily living and quality of life together with a range of other pain characteristics, such as location, description, onset, episodes and the effects of interventions (Lynch, 2001).

Since the effective assessment of pain is fundamental for successful pain control, this, in addition to routine monitoring of blood pressure, temperature, pulse and respiratory rate, is advocated, and pain is considered to be the fifth vital sign (Lynch, 2001; Hader and Guy, 2004). Although autonomic responses, such as changes in heart rate, blood pressure and respiratory rate, may be associated with the pain experience and should form part of the pain assessment (Briggs, 1995; Carr and Mann, 2000), as already emphasized, the patient's report of pain is the most reliable indicator of pain (McCaffery and Ferrell, 1997; Lynch, 2001).

Multimodal approach to managing pain

Pain management approaches develop from pain assessment and are aimed at removing the cause of pain, where possible, while achieving optimal comfort and function with minimal side effects from the interventions used (Lynch, 2001). The pain management system should use a multimodal approach that includes pharmacological and non-pharmacological interventions (Hader and Guy, 2004). A multimodal approach targets interventions at different points in the pain pathway, and knowledge of the neurones and neurochemicals involved in pain, and the psychosocial mechanisms that maintain pain, forms the basis of effective pain control (Holdcroft and Power, 2003).

Non-pharmacological interventions

There are a variety of non-pharmacological approaches to managing pain (*Table 7.1*), including physiotherapy, heat pads or ice packs, massage, relaxation and distraction therapies, hypnotherapy, transcutaneous electrical nerve stimulation (TENS) and acupuncture (Carr and Mann, 2000; Lynch, 2001).

Table 7.1: Non-pharmacological interventions to managing pain

---

- Physiotherapy for positioning and maintenance of function

- Heat pads or ice packs to reduce muscle aches, stiffness and oedema

- Massage for relaxation

- Relaxation and distraction therapies

- Hypnotherapy

- Transcutaneous electrical nerve stimulation (TENS)

- Acupuncture

From Carr and Mann (2000); Lynch (2001)

Complementary therapies for pain may be used to alleviate pain directly by inducing analgesia, or by acting indirectly to alleviate some of the comorbid symptoms such as nausea, vomiting, anxiety or depressed mood and by improving sleep (Chwistek, 2005).

In an American study of community-dwelling older adults (*n*=77), 84% of respondents reported use of at least one complementary therapy for pain, and most participants reported that the therapies were helpful in relieving pain (Kemp et al, 2004). There is evidence of increasing use of complementary therapies in the UK. A Scottish study comparing use of therapies between 1993–1999 suggests an increased use of complementary therapies for relief of pain from headaches and musculoskeletal problems (Emslie et al, 2002). Although there is evidence in the form of primary studies to suggest that non-pharmacological nursing interventions are effective in the management of pain, a meta-analysis of 49 of these studies failed to detect a difference between the treatment and control groups, emphasizing the need for randomized, controlled trials (RCTs) to test these interventions (Sindhu, 1996).

Acupuncture has been used in traditional Chinese medicine for thousands of years for the alleviation of pain (Lundeberg and Stener-Victorin, 2002; Goddard et al, 2005). Although acupuncture is now an accepted pain-relieving modality in most countries and is frequently used as a complement to other treatments (Lundeberg and Stener-Victorin, 2002), its efficacy in alleviating pain is controversial (Ernst, 2004). It is proposed that acupuncture may relieve pain in a number of ways, including the release of endogenous opioids, such as endorphins, which bind to opioid receptors (Lundeberg and Stener-Victorin, 2002). However, the notion of acupuncture-mediated endogenous opiate analgesia is contentious (Szmelskyj, 1998).

TENS is a non-invasive therapy used for pain relief in a variety of pain syndromes but, despite its frequent use, the evidence from RCTs for treatment of chronic pain remains inconclusive (Carroll et al, 2000). The possible mechanisms by which TENS produces pain relief are reviewed by Sluka and Walsh (2003) and include stimulation of large-diameter afferents (A-beta fibres), which inhibits pain impulse transmission in the dorsal horn as proposed by the gate control theory introduced in the last chapter. TENS is also thought to induce descending inhibition and to elicit the release of endogenous opioids (Sluka and Walsh, 2003). The stimulation of A-beta fibres may also underlie the pain relief afforded by massage (Lundeberg and Stener-Victorin, 2002). Massage is thought to stimulate large-diameter A-beta fibres, which will close the 'gate' and inhibit pain information conducted in A-delta and C fibres from reaching the brain. A systematic review indicates that massage might be beneficial for patients with chronic, non-specific, low-back pain, especially if combined with exercise and education (Furlan et al, 2002).

Heat therapy and cold therapy are other common forms of cutaneous stimulation that have been used to alleviate pain (Carr and Mann, 2000). In a study of 50 post-cardiac surgery patients, ice therapy before, during and after chest tube removal did not significantly reduce pain in the experimental group (Sauls, 2002). Both heat and cold treatments are commonly recommended in the treatment of low-back pain (Car and Sheikh, 2003), although a systematic review has yet to be published (French et al, 2004).

A number of interventions are based on the premise that changes in brain activity can be used to influence the experience of pain. Hypnosis and relaxation are commonly used as therapies in the treatment of acute and chronic pain, and there does seem to be some evidence for their effectiveness based on a review of RCTs by Kessler et al (2003). The neurophysiological mechanisms underlying analgesia mediated by hypnosis have yet to be elucidated.

In an experimental study of 20 healthy subjects, hypnosis significantly reduced subjective pain, and the findings also suggest that hypnosis modulated both the affective and sensory-discriminative components of pain (Sandrini et al, 2000). The authors suggest that hypnosis uses the descending inhibitory pathways for the control of pain.

In a more recent study (Faymonville et al, 2003) using positron emission tomography (PET), the anti-nociceptive effects of hypnosis were linked to increased activity in the anterior cingulate cortex and its functional connectivity to other regions in a neural network of cortical and subcortical regions. The anterior cingulate cortex is suggested to have a key role in modulating the processing of noxious stimuli within this large neural network in the hypnosis-related alteration of pain perception (Faymonville et al, 2003).

Another psychological approach used to control pain is cognitive–behavioural therapy (CBT). CBT is often used as an adjunct treatment to help patients with chronic illnesses to better manage their pain, and there is some evidence that CBT is effective for certain chronic conditions, such as rheumatoid arthritis, osteoarthritis, chronic fatigue syndrome and irritable bowel syndrome (Bradley et al, 2003). CBT addresses the psychological and emotional components of pain and can help an individual control his or her pain and anxiety (Garcia and Altman, 1997).

Pharmacological approaches

The use of drugs is an important component of pain management. Pharmacological interventions include opioid and non-opioid analgesia and adjuvant drugs (MacPherson, 2000; Lynch, 2001; Briggs, 2003; Miller, 2004). Adjuvants are drugs that are not usually analgesic themselves, but in combination with analgesic drugs may enhance the analgesic effect. Although opioids continue to be an integral component of pain management strategies, prominence is also given to adjuvant drugs and anti-inflammatory agents that can enhance pain control and decrease the use of opioids (MacPherson, 2000).

The World Health Organization analgesic ladder

The World Health Organization (WHO) analgesic ladder was introduced to improve pain control in patients with cancer pain (WHO, 1986), although it also provides a framework for other types of pain management as well (Garcia and Altman, 1997; Lynch, 2001). The WHO ladder embraces the combination of opioid, non-opioid and adjuvant medications, and emphasizes a systematic approach that stresses the use of analgesics in a sequential order according to the patient's response. There are three steps in the 'ladder', and they are only ascended when pain persists (*Figure 7.1*).

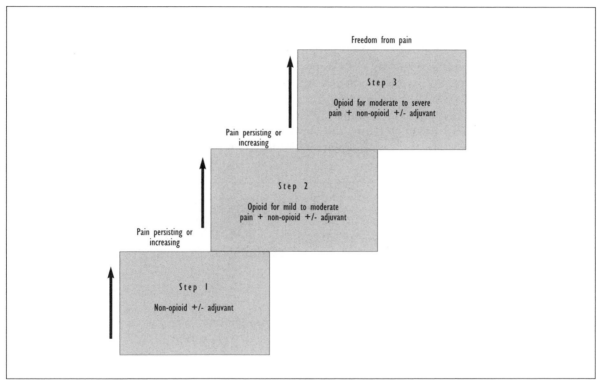

Figure 7.1: World Health Organization analgesic ladder (WHO, 1986)

The first step is to use non-opioid drugs, such as paracetamol (acetaminophen), or non-steroidal anti-inflammatory drugs (NSAIDs), such as ibuprofen, with or without adjuvants for mild pain. If the pain persists, the second step is to introduce weak opioids, such as codeine, with or without adjuvants. The third step of the ladder is ascended when pain continues, and strong opioids such as morphine are introduced with or without non-opioid and adjuvant analgesia (Garcia and Altman, 1997; Briggs, 2003; Miller, 2004). For patients who are still experiencing pain after this three-step approach, a fourth step may be necessary, which involves administration of intraspinal agents via epidural or intrathecal routes (Kedlaya et al, 2003). As well as stepping up the ladder, stepping down the ladder may be appropriate for some patients, for example as healing occurs (National Prescribing Centre, 2000).

Non-opioid agents

Non-opioid analgesia comprises paracetamol and NSAIDs, which include salicylates, such as aspirin. Paracetamol is one of the most commonly used over-the-counter drugs, and within its therapeutic range it has few side effects (Schug et al, 2003). Paracetamol is mainly metabolized by the liver and should be avoided in patients with liver dysfunction or those at risk of liver toxicity, such as those with a high alcohol intake (Schug et al, 2003; Miller, 2004). The mechanism for the analgesic effects of paracetamol remains unclear; however, it is thought to inhibit prostaglandin synthesis in the periphery (MacPherson, 2000). Other mechanisms might also operate, including the inhibition of prostaglandin synthesis in the central nervous system (CNS) (Garcia and Altman, 1997; Graham and Scott, 2005).

The mechanism of action for NSAIDS is the inhibition of cyclo-oxygenase (COX), an enzyme involved in prostaglandin synthesis. Since prostaglandins are involved in the activation and sensitization of nociceptors, a reduction in prostaglandin synthesis will tend to alleviate pain (Garcia and Altman, 1997).

There is a limit or 'ceiling' to their analgesic efficacy beyond which increasing the dose will have no effect (Lynch, 2001). Prostaglandins and thromboxanes are products of a pathway in which membrane phospholipids are converted into arachidonic acid (Gilron et al, 2003). COX exists in two forms, COX-1 and COX-2. The COX-1 enzyme is important in the synthesis of prostaglandins involved in gut and kidney function and platelet activation. The COX-2 enzyme produces prostaglandins that are involved in inflammation and pain (Jordan and White, 2001; Gilron et al, 2003; Miller, 2004) (*Figure 7.2*).

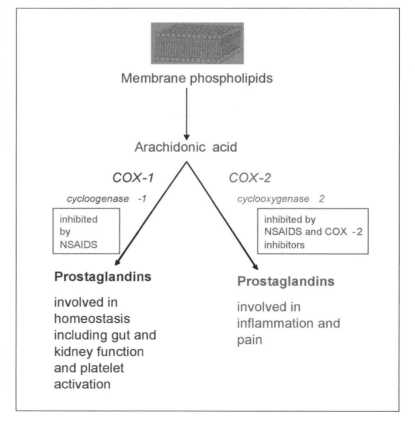

Figure 7.2: The role of cyclo-oxygenase in prostaglandin synthesis. NSAIDS=non-steroidal anti-inflammatory drugs

Most NSAIDs are non-selective and have some effect on both COX-1 and COX-2 (Gilron et al, 2003). The inhibition of both forms of the COX enzyme accounts for the adverse effects of NSAIDs, which include renal dysfunction, gastrointestinal ulceration and bleeding, and inhibition of platelet aggregation (Garcia and Altman, 1997; Gilron et al, 2003; Miller, 2004). NSAIDs have been developed that selectively inhibit COX-2; these COX-2 inhibitors have analgesic efficacy with fewer side effects (MacPherson, 2000; Gilron et al, 2003; Miller, 2004).

However, there is evidence that COX-2 inhibitors are associated with increased risk of adverse cardiovascular events (Jones, 2005), which has prompted manufacturer action and updated advice on their use (National Prescribing Centre, 2005).

Salicylates, such as aspirin, also exert their analgesia via inhibition of cyclo-oxygenase-mediated prostaglandin synthesis. Aspirin binds to both COX-1 and COX-2, interfering with enzyme activity and thus inhibiting prostaglandin synthesis (Vane and Botting, 2003). The adverse effects of salicylates include gastrointestinal upset, ulceration and bleeding, platelet dysfunction and allergic reactions (Garcia and Altman, 1997). In addition, aspirin is related to Reye's syndrome in children under 16 years of age (McGovern et al, 2001; Miller, 2004).

Opioids

Opioids are the main class of analgesics used in the management of moderate to severe pain (Garcia and Altman, 1997). Opioids are widely used in the management of somatic and visceral pain (Lynch, 2001) and cancer pain (Harrison, 2001). There are weak opioids, such as dihydrocodeine and codeine, which are used in step 2 of the WHO ladder, and strong opioids, such as morphine and pethidine, which are used in step 3 (Lynch, 2001; Miller, 2004).

Opioids produce analgesia by binding to specific opioid receptors inside and outside the CNS (Garcia and Altman, 1997) (*Figure 7.3*).

Opioid drugs (exogenous opioids) mimic the effects of naturally occurring opioids, the endorphins and enkephalins.

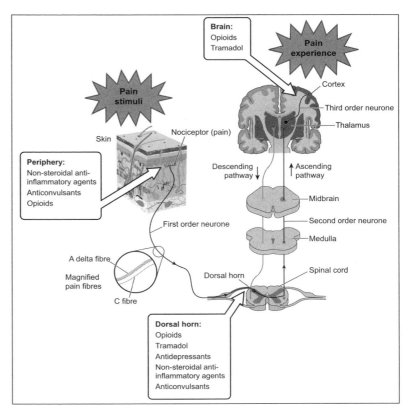

Figure 7.3: The pain pathway showing key sites for particular pharmacological interventions

Opioid receptors are usually stimulated by endogenous opioids. The last chapter described how endogenous opioids are secreted by inhibitory neurones in the dorsal horn of the spinal cord. Endogenous opioids interact with opioid receptors, suppressing substance P-mediated neurotransmission across the synapse. This inhibits the flow of pain information up to the brain and alleviates pain (Barasi, 1991; Clancy and McVicar, 1998).

Opioid receptors are found in low concentrations throughout the CNS, with the exception of the hypothalamus (Garcia and Altman, 1997). Opioids modulate pain via the gating mechanism in the spinal cord, although there is evidence that opioids may also have peripheral effects as opioid receptors are located on peripheral terminals of sensory neurones (Stein et al, 1995).

There are several different types and sub-types of opioid receptor. The three types of receptor associated with analgesia are: mu (μ), kappa (k) and delta (∂), with analgesia being most commonly related to mu receptors (Garcia and Altman, 1997; Schug et al, 2003). Opioid analgesics can be divided into agonists, such as morphine and fentanyl that express full receptor activation to mu receptors, and partial agonists, such as buprenorphine that, while possessing affinity for mu receptors, only elicits a partial response with reduced effects (Garcia and Altman, 1997; Schug et al, 2003; Johnson et al, 2005). There are also antagonists, such as naloxone, which bind to opioid receptors but lack analgesic effects (Garcia and Altman, 1997; Schug et al, 2003). The characteristics of the different groups of opioid drugs dictate their suitability for control of certain types of pain, but not others. For example, because pure agonists have a broad range of clinically effective doses they can be used by patients who require increasing doses of opioids (Garcia and Altman, 1997).

Opioid doses are given incrementally until pain is effectively controlled or unwanted side effects occur; this is called titration and is the adjustment of medication to achieve optimal analgesia. When these drugs are given at regular intervals, large fluctuations in blood levels are avoided, breakthrough pain is minimized and side effects are less likely (Lynch, 2001). The most common side effects of opioid drugs are nausea and vomiting, constipation and depressed breathing. Most side effects can be minimized if there is effective titration of the dose (Miller, 2004). Although respiratory depression is associated with greatest morbidity, nausea and constipation often distress the patient most (MacPherson, 2000). When opioid medication needs to change, perhaps because the side effects become unacceptable or pain control is inadequate, one opioid regimen may be changed for another, and in these circumstances equi-analgesia conversion charts may be used to determine the dose of the substituted opioid (MacPherson, 2000; Lynch, 2001).

Opioids have the advantage of being available in a variety of formulations and can be administered via traditional oral, intravenous and intramuscular routes together with other routes, which continue to be investigated, including transdermal, intranasal, inhalational, intrathecal and epidural routes (MacPherson, 2000; Lynch, 2001). The oral route for opioid administration is preferable because it is convenient, non-invasive and cost-effective (Garcia and Altman, 1997).

Some patients experience breakthrough or episodic pain. A number of mechanisms may lead to transient episodes of uncontrolled pain, including end-of-dose failure during initial titration or inadequate pain management; this pain can be managed by various classes of drugs delivered via a number of routes (Mercadante et al, 2002). The short-acting medication needed to manage breakthrough pain could include patient-controlled analgesia (Davis et al, 2005). Self-regulation of analgesic administration is an important method of pain control. Patient-controlled analgesia (PCA), in which drugs are administered via an electronically-controlled pump, is accepted as an important method of providing pain relief and is a developing field (Lehmann, 2005). Of two meta-analyses of trials comparing opioid administration in post-operative settings, one indicates that PCA improves analgesia and that patients prefer PCA (Walder et al, 2001); and another suggests that patients experience less pain with PCA compared with intramuscular opioids, although epidural analgesia appeared to be more effective than PCA (Dolin et al, 2002).

Tramadol is a centrally-acting analgesic which, although chemically unrelated to opioids (Garcia and Altman, 1997), is included here because it appears to have both opioid and non-opioid properties (Raffa, 1996; Miller, 2004). Tramadol seems to exert its analgesic effects in two ways: by binding to mu receptors and by inhibiting re-uptake of serotonin and noradrenaline (Raffa, 1996; Garcia and Altman, 1997; Miller, 2004). Both these neurotransmitters are involved in descending inhibitory pathways, which modulate pain in the spinal cord gating mechanism (*Figure 7.3*). The descending neurones synapse with the inhibitory interneurones in the dorsal horn and secrete serotonin and noradrenaline (Cross, 1994; McHugh and McHugh, 2000). These neurotransmitters then excite the inhibitory neurone, thereby suppressing pain transmission to the brain. By inhibiting reuptake of these neurotransmitters, tramadol enables serotonin and noradrenaline to remain in the synapse and stimulate the inhibitory neurone, thereby easing pain.

Adjuvant agents

Adjuvant analgesics are a variety of drugs with a primary indication other than pain (Lussier et al, 2004). Adjuvant agents include antidepressants, anticonvulsants, muscle relaxants, corticosteroids and local anaesthetics (Garcia and Altman, 1997; Lussier et al, 2004). Adjuvant medications enhance pain control and reduce opioid use (MacPherson, 2000).

Tricyclic antidepressants are considered to be useful in many painful disorders, including low back pain, fibromyalgia, post-herpetic neuralgia and neuropathic pain (Garcia and Altman, 1997). The analgesic effect of antidepressants is thought to be independent of their antidepressive effect because lower doses are effective and there is a more rapid onset of action (Garcia and Altman, 1997; MacPherson, 2000). The mechanism of action seems to involve inhibition of serotonin and noradrenaline re-uptake. Re-uptake inhibition would enhance pain modulation by the descending inhibitory pathways, and lead to analgesic effects by preventing the transmission of pain impulses across the synapse between the first- and second-order neurones in the dorsal horn (*Figure 7.3*) (Garcia and Altman, 1997; MacPherson, 2000).

Anticonvulsants are used widely in the treatment of neuropathic pain (Lynch, 2001). Damaged nerves may become more excitable and produce spontaneous bursts of action potentials (Garcia and Altman, 1997) by blocking sodium ion channels; this accounts for their analgesic effects (MacPherson, 2000).

Systemic local anaesthetics such as lidocaine have also been shown to be effective in neuropathic pain (Kalso et al, 1998; Lussier et al, 2004). The mechanism of action remains unclear but probably involves the blockage of sodium ion channels and reduction of spontaneous neuronal activity (Garcia and Altman, 1997; Kalso et al, 1998).

Several other drugs with different pharmacological profiles are under investigation for their role in therapeutic pain modulation, including cannabinoids (MacPherson, 2000). Endogenous cannabinoid mechanisms exist that are distinct from those involving the endogenous opioids. Cannabinoid receptors are mainly found in the CNS, although peripheral neurones also possess them

(Iversen and Chapman, 2002). A key problem in the use of cannabinoids is to alleviate pain without inducing psychoactive effects. A novel cannabinoid with this characteristic, along with anti-inflammatory and analgesic effects, is being investigated (Burstein et al, 2004).

Conclusions

Individuals continue to suffer pain despite the wide range of interventions available. Nurses can play a crucial role in pain management by using a range of strategies and interventions. To make an effective contribution to the alleviation of pain, nurses need to be knowledgeable about pain mechanisms and understand the physiological basis for the non-pharmacological approaches used. They should also appreciate the different points along the pain pathway that are potential targets for pain modulation. In addition, nurses need to be familiar with the means by which non-opioid and opioid analgesia exert their effects, and understand how adjuvant drugs intervene in the pain pathway. This knowledge and understanding will allow nurses to appreciate the significance of a multimodal approach in the control of pain and enable them to play a more informed role in pain management.

References

Alcenius M (2004) Successfully meet pain assessment standards. *Nurs Manage* **35**(3): 12

Barasi S (1991) The physiology of pain. *Surg Nurse* **4**(5):14–20

Barnason S, Merboth M, Pozehl B, Tietjen MJ (1998) Utilizing an outcomes approach to improve pain management by nurse: a pilot study. *Clin Nurse Spec* **12**(1): 28–36

Bird J (2003) Selection of pain measurement tools. *Nurs Stand* **18**(13): 33–9

Bradley LA, Mckendree-Smith NL, Cianfrini LR (2003) Cognitive–behavioral therapy interventions for pain associated with chronic illnesses. *Seminars Pain Med* **1**(2): 44–54

Briggs M (1995) Principles of acute pain assessment. *Nurs Stand* **9**(19): 23–7

Briggs E (2003) The nursing management of pain in older people. *Nurs Stand* **17**(18): 47–53

Burstein SH, Karst M, Schneider U, Zurier RB (2004) Ajulemic acid: a novel cannabinoid produces analgesia without a 'high'. *Life Sci* **75:** 1513–22

Car J, Sheikh A (2003) Acute low back pain. *Br Med J* **327**(7414): 541

Carr CJ (1997) Evaluating the use of a pain assessment tool and care plan: a pilot study. *J Adv Nurs* **26**(6): 1073–9

Carr DB, Goudas LC (1999) Acute pain. *Lancet North Am Ed* **353:** 2051–8

Carr ECJ, Mann EM (2000) *Pain: Creative Approaches to Effective Management*. Palgrave Macmillan, Basingstoke

Carroll D, Moore RA, McQuay HJ, Fairman F, Tramèr M, Leijon G (2000) Transcutaneous electrical nerve stimulation (TENS) for chronic pain. *Cochrane Database Syst Rev* **Issue 4**

Clancy J, McVicar A (1998) Homeostasis — the key concept to physiological control: neurophysiology of pain. *Br J Theatre Nurs* **7**(10): 19–27

Clarke EB, French B, Bilodeau ML, Capasso VC, Edwards A, Empoliti J (1996) Pain management knowledge, attitudes and clinical practice: the impact of nurses' characteristics and education. *J Pain Symptom Manage* **11**(1): 18–31

Chwistek M (2005) Integrative, evidence-based approach to the use of complementary therapies for cancer pain. *J Pain* **6**(3 Suppl 1): S53

Cross SA (1994) Pathophysiology of pain. *Mayo Clin Proc* **69:** 375–83

Davis M, Walsh D, Lagman R, LeGrand S (2005) Controversies in pharmacotherapy of pain management. *Lancet Oncol* **6:** 696–704

Dolin SJ, Cashman JN, Bland JM (2002) Effectiveness of acute postoperative pain management: 1. Evidence from published data. *Br J Anaesth* **89:** 409–23

Emslie MJ, Campbell MK, Walker KA (2002) Changes in public awareness of, attitudes to, and use of, complementary therapy in North East Scotland: surveys in 1993 and 1999. *Complement Ther Med* **10**(3): 148–53

Ernst E (2004) Acupuncture: who is missing the point? *Pain* **109**(3): 203–4

Faymonville ME, Roediger L, Del Fiore G et al (2003) Increased cerebral functional connectivity underlying the antinociceptive effects of hypnosis. *Brain Res Cogn Brain Res* **17:** 255–62

French SD, Cameron M, Clarke RB, Esterman AJ, Reggars J, Walker B (2004) Superficial heat or cold for low-back pain. *Cochrane Database Syst Rev* **Issue 2**

Furlan AD, Brosseau L, Imamura M, Irvin E (2002) Massage for low-back pain. *Cochrane Database Syst Rev* **Issue 2**

Garcia J, Altman RD (1997) Chronic pain states: pathophysiology and medical therapy. *Semin Arthritis Rheum* **27**(1): 1–16

Gilron I, Milne B, Hong M (2003) Cyclooxygenase-2 inhibitors in postoperative pain management: current evidence and future directions. *Anesthesiology* **99**(5): 1198–208

Goddard G, Shen Y, Steele B, Springer N (2005) A controlled trial of placebo versus real acupuncture. *J Pain* **6**(4): 237–42

Graham GG, Scott KF (2005) Mechanism of action of paracetamol. *Am J Ther* **12**(1): 46–55.

Hader C, Guy J (2004) Your hand in pain management. *Nurs Manage* **35**(11): 21–7

Harrison P (2001) Update on pain management for advanced genitourinary cancer. *J Urol* **165**(1): 1849–58

Holdcroft A, Power I (2003) Management of pain. *Br Med J* **326:** 635–9

Iversen L, Chapman V (2002) Cannabinoids: a real prospect for pain relief? *Curr Opin Pharmacol* **2:** 50–5

Johnson RE, Fudala PJ, Payne R (2005) Buprenorphine: considerations for pain management. *J Pain Symptom Manage* **29**(3): 297–326

Jones S (2005) Relative thromboembolic risks associated with COX-2 inhibitors. *Ann Pharmacother* **39**(7–8): 1249–59

Jordan S, White J (2001) Non-steroidal anti-inflammatory drugs: clinical issues. *Nurs Stand* **15**(23): 45–52

Kalso E, Tramèr MR, McQuay HJ, Moore RA (1998) Systemic local-anaesthetic-type drugs in chronic pain: a systematic review. *Eur J Pain* **2:** 3–14

Kedlaya D, Reynolds L, Waldman S (2003) Epidural and intrathecal analgesia for cancer pain. *Best Pract Res Clin Anaesthesiol* **16**(4): 651–65

Kemp C, Ersek M, Turner J (2004) Use and perceived effectiveness of traditional and complementary therapies for the management of chronic pain in community-dwelling elders. *J Pain* **5**(3 Suppl 1): S43

Kessler RS, Patterson DR, Dane J (2003) Hypnosis and relaxation with pain patients: evidence for effectiveness. *Semin Pain Med* **1**(2): 67–78

Lehmann K (2005) Recent developments in patient-controlled analgesia. *J Pain Symptom Manage* **29**(5)Suppl 1: S72–89

Lellan K (2004) Postoperative pain: strategy for improving patient experiences. *J Adv Nurs* **46**(2): 179–85

Lundeberg T, Stener-Victorin E (2002) Is there a physiological basis for the use of acupuncture in pain? *Int Congr Ser* **1238:** 3–10

Lussier D, Huskey AG, Portenoy RK (2004) Adjuvant analgesics in cancer pain management. *Oncologist* **9:** 571–91

Lynch M (2001) Pain as the fifth vital sign. *J Intraven Nurs* **24**(2): 85–94

MacPherson RD (2000) The pharmacological basis of contemporary pain management. *Pharmacol Ther* **88:** 163–85

Madjar I (2004) Editorial. Of pain, nursing and professional leadership: some personal reflections. *J Nurs Manag* **12**(3): 151–2

Manias E, Bucknall T (2002) Observation of pain assessment and management: the complexities of clinical practice. *J Clin Nurs* **11**(6): 724–33

Martelli M, Zasler N, Bender MC, Nicholson K (2004) Psychological, neuropsychological and medical considerations in assessment and management of pain. *J Head Trauma Rehabil* **19**(1): 10–28

McCaffery M, Ferrell BR (1997) Nurses' knowledge of pain assessment and management: how much progress have we made? *J Pain Symptom Manage* **14**(3): 175–88

McGovern MC, Glasgow JF, Stewart MC (2001). Reye's syndrome and aspirin: lest we forget. *Br Med J* **322**(7302): 1591–2

McHugh JM, McHugh WB (2000) Pain: neuroanatomy, chemical mediators, and clinical implications. *AACN Clin Issues* **11**(2): 168–78

Melzack R (1999) From the gate to the neuromatrix. *Pain* **6**(Suppl): S121–6

Mercadante S, Radbruch L, Caraceni A et al (2002) Episodic (breakthrough) pain. Consensus conference of an expert working group of the European Association for Palliative Care. *Cancer* **94**(3): 832–9

Miller E (2004) The World Health Organization analgesic ladder. *J Midwifery Womens Health* **49**(6): 542–5

National Prescribing Centre (2000) The use of oral analgesics in primary care. *MeReC Bulletin* **11**(1): 1–4

National Prescribing Centre (2005) Further advice on Cox-II selective inhibitors. *MeReC Extra* **16**

Raffa RB (1996) A novel approach to the pharmacology of analgesics. *Am J Med* **101**(suppl 1A): 40S–46S

Sandrini G, Milanov I, Malaguti S, Nigrelli MP, Moglia A, Nappi G (2000) Effects of hypnosis on diffuse noxious inhibitory controls. *Physiol Behav* **69**(3): 295–300

Sauls J (2002) The use of ice for pain associated with chest removal. *Pain Manag Nurs* **3**(2): 44–52

Schug SA, Garrett WR, Gillespie G (2003) Opioid and non-opioid analgesics. *Best Pract Res Clin Anaesthesiol* **17**(1): 91–110

Sindhu F (1996) Are non-pharmacological nursing interventions for the management of pain effective? A meta-analysis. *J Adv Nurs* **24**(6): 1152–9

Sluka KA, Walsh D (2003) Transcutaneous electrical nerve stimulation: basic science mechanisms and clinical effectiveness. *J Pain* **4**(3): 109–21

Smith BH, Elliott AM, Chambers WA, Smith WC, Hannaford PC, Penny K (2001) The impact of chronic pain in the community. *Fam Pract* **18**(3): 292–9

Stannard C, Johnson M (2003) Chronic pain management: can we do better? *Curr Med Res Opin* **19**(8): 703–6

Stein C, Schafer M, Hassan AH (1995) Peripheral opioid receptors. *Ann Med* **27**(2): 219–21

Szmelskyj A (1998) Do complementary therapies stimulate the body's natural painkilling medications? A literature review. *Complement Ther Med* **6**: 36–41

Twycross A (2002) Educating nurses about pain management: the way forward. *J Clin Nurs* **11**(6): 705–14

Vane JR, Botting RM (2003) The mechanism of action of aspirin. *Thromb Res* **110**(5–6): 255–8

Walder B, Schafer M, Henzi I, Tramèr MR (2001) Efficacy and safety of patient-controlled opioid analgesia for acute postoperative pain. A quantitative systematic review. *Acta Anaesthesiol Scand* **45**: 795–804

Watt-Watson J, Stevens B, Garfinkel P, Streiner D, Gallop R (2001) Relationship between nurses' pain knowledge and pain management outcomes for their postoperative cardiac patients. *J Adv Nurs* **36**(4): 535–45

Whelan CT, Jin L, Meltzer D (2004) Pain and satisfaction with pain control in hospitalized medical patients: no such thing as low risk. *Arch Intern Med* **164**(2): 175–80

World Health Organization (1986) *Cancer Pain Relief*. WHO, Geneva

Chapter 8

An overview of meningitis: Signs, symptoms, treatment and support

Ian Peate

Meningitis can be defined as inflammation of the meninges, the lining of the brain (Public Health Laboratory Service (PHLS), 2002) (*Figure 8.1*). Meningitis can be acute or chronic, infective or non-infective (Conlon and Snydman, 2004). According to the PHLS (2002), there are many infective agents that have been shown to cause meningitis, including viruses, bacteria, fungi and parasites.

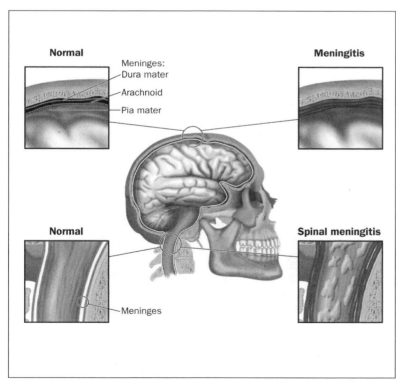

Figure 8.1: Diagrammatic representation depicting inflammation of the meninges in meningitis in the brain

Meningococcal disease can kill a healthy individual of any age within hours of the appearance of the first symptoms (Meningitis Research Foundation (MRF), 2002a). It is, therefore, important that the nurse is aware of what to look for in order to make an early diagnosis. The disease is rare but, despite this and because of the grave character of the illness, it is important for healthcare professionals to have an understanding of it. Prompt diagnosis and immediate treatment will reduce the mortality rate from meningococcal septicaemia (National Meningitis Trust (NMT), 2000). Meningitis is more common during the winter period and often follows epidemics of influenza (Long et al, 1995).

In the UK and Ireland all clinically diagnosed cases of meningitis and meningococcal septicaemia have to be notified to the local public health doctor: the public health doctor accountable in England, Wales and Northern Ireland is the consultant in communicable disease control; in Scotland it is the consultant in public health medicine; and in the Republic of Ireland the area medical officer and the authority in public health carries out this role (NMT, 2000). It is the responsibility of the public health doctor to determine what is to be done about every suspected case and to advise schools and employers, as well as ensuring that those who are at increased risk of infection are approached (McCormack, 1993).

Epidemiology

There has been a growth in the number of cases of meningococcal disease in Britain (NMT, 2000). However, with the introduction of the immediate use of benzyl penicillin, the survival rates in bacterial meningitis have improved (Strang and Pugh, 1992). *Figure 8.2* shows that the bulk of meningococcal infections are present in infants who are below 5 years of age, with a peak in incidence noticed in those children under 1 year of age (PHLS, 2000). It also demonstrates that a secondary peak occurs in those aged between 15–20 years of age (PHLS, 2000).

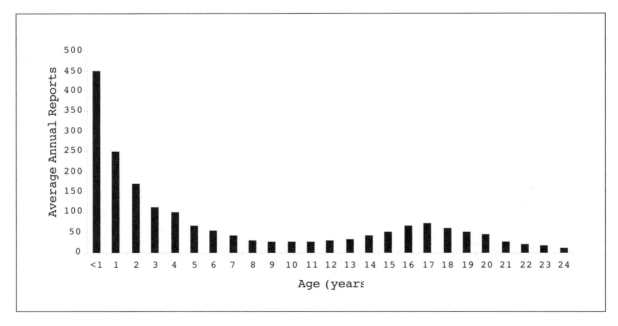

Figure 8.2: Average annual laboratory reports of meningococcal disease by age (years). England and Wales 1996–2000 (Source: www.hpa.org.uk/infections/topics_az/meningo/backgr.htm. Accessed 31.3.2006)

Acute bacterial meningitis

This form of meningitis should be seen as a medical emergency as the disease can quickly progress and a devastating chain of events may occur that may lead to death or disability (MRF, 2002b). The signs and symptoms of acute bacterial meningitis can develop over a few days and may have a rapid onset and fulminant course within a few hours (MRF, 2002a). The patient may have an accompanying septicaemia as one of the most common symptoms (Kumar and Clark, 1996).

Viral (aseptic) meningitis

The terms viral meningitis and aseptic meningitis are often used interchangeably. Viral meningitis is comparatively common in the UK; it is often benign and complications are rare (Boss, 1998). In some cases, the findings with viral meningitis are consistent with bacterial meningitis (Boss, 1998). Viral meningitis can take over 2–3 days to evolve (Roos, 1996).

Chronic meningitis

When signs and symptoms of meningeal inflammation have been present for a month or more, then the condition can be defined as chronic. Chronic meningitis is generally rare in the UK and the principal infective cause of the condition is the tuberculous bacterium (PHLS, 2002).

The rest of this chapter focuses on bacterial meningitis.

Meningococcal disease

Meningococcal disease has two main clinical presentations — meningitis and septicaemia — that often occur together. Patients with meningococcal septicaemia have a higher mortality rate than patients with meningococcal meningitis (MRF, 2002a). It is important to note that the presenting symptoms of a patient with meningococcal septicaemia are very different to those of a patient with meningococcal meningitis (MRF, 2002a).

There are various bacterial sero-groups (strains) that can cause meningococcal disease, such as B, C or W135. If laboratory tests detect any of these sero-groups then they are deemed 'laboratory confirmed'. However, in some cases laboratory tests do not confirm the presence of the bacterial groups — these are known as 'not confirmed'. In these cases the patient will have definite symptoms of meningococcal disease, so a diagnosis will be made on the patient's clinical symptoms and not laboratory test confirmation (NMT, 2000). There may be no positive detection of meningococcus in the patient's blood if he/she has already been treated for meningitis with antibiotic therapy at an earlier stage. Diagnosis can be made by lumbar puncture, but caution must be taken if there are signs of raised intracranial pressure and a risk of cerebral herniation (MRF, 2004). Even after the administration of antibiotics, a lumbar puncture may be valuable (NMT, 2000).

The most common strain of meningitis in the UK is group B, which accounts for approximately two-thirds of all cases reported. Group C accounts for one-third of all cases and group A strains are rare (Department of Health et al, 1996). Vaccinations are available that are effective against groups A and C strains, but there is no vaccine available against the group B strain (NMT, 1997). In sero-group B genome, a specific vaccine is unlikely to be widely available in the near future (Heyderman et al, 2003). In the meantime, however, the most effective and safest vaccine against meningitis is knowledge (Peate, 1999).

Diagnosis of meningococcal disease

Early detection of meningococcal disease can be problematic as during the prodromal stage of the disease (earliest phase of a developing disease) the patient may present with non-specific signs and symptoms (NMT, 2000). Often it is difficult to distinguish between illnesses such as influenza and other viral illnesses. *Figure 8.4* illustrates the progression of symptoms and signs of meningococcal disease.

The order in which the symptoms occur can differ and, indeed, some of the symptoms described may even be absent (NMT, 2000). In addition, babies may also display the symptoms listed in *Table 8.1* (MRF, 2002b).

Clinical examination

The majority of patients with meningococcal septicaemia will have a rash (MRF, 2002b). The rash is the most important sign for the nurse to recognize. In cases of meningitis the rash may not be so clear or pronounced and in certain cases it may even be absent (MRF, 2004).

During the early stages of the disease the rash may be blanching and maculopapular (lesions with a flat base surrounding papules — small elevations of the skin — in the centre); however, in the majority of cases the rash becomes a non-blanching red or brownish-coloured petechial (minute haemorrhagic spots of pinpoint to pinhead size) rash (*Figure 8.5*) or purpura (haemorrhage into the skin, varying in onset and duration) (*Figure 8.6*) (MRF, 2002a). If a glass tumbler is pressed firmly against the petechial or purpura rash and this does not blanch but remains visible through the glass tumbler (*Figure 8.7*), and if this non-blanching rash is present in a febrile or unwell patient, this would represent a medical emergency (MRF, 2002a). Examination of the whole skin is strongly recommended, as isolated pinprick spots may appear where the rash is predominantly maculopapular (MRF, 2002a). The nurse should ensure that there is good light source available, searching the entire body for small petechiae — this is particularly important when a child is in a febrile state with no obvious cause (MRF, 2002a).

A non-blanching rash and a rapidly evolving petchial or purpuric rash should be dealt with as an emergency. In rapidly evolving rashes, the prognosis is very poor (MRF, 2002a).

Nurses must be aware of what to look for in dark-skinned patients, in whom the rash may be more difficult to see. In this case, the nurse should examine the soles of the patient's feet, palms of the hand and conjunctiva or palate (MRF, 2002a).

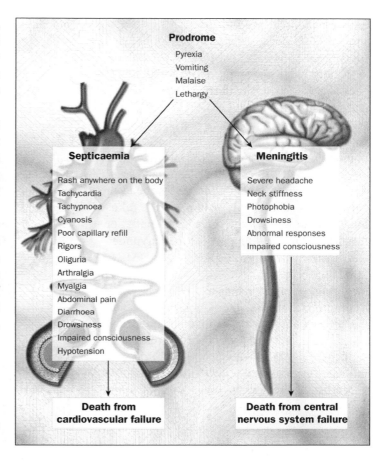

Figure 8.4: Development of symptoms and signs of meningococcal disease

Table 8.1: Symptoms of meningococcal disease in babies

- Tense fontanelle
- Pale or mottled skin or cyanosis
- Poor feeding
- Irritability, particularly when being handled
- High-pitched or moaning cry
- Abnormal tone — increased or decreased
- Abnormal posturing
- Vacant look/stare
- Poor response or lethargy

From MRF (2002b)

Shock

A patient who develops a life-threatening septicaemia will have a tachycardia, tachypnoea, an irregular respiratory pattern and there will be evidence of vasoconstriction — cold feet and/or hands and poor capillary refill (MRF, 2002b). Pressing on the big toenail, a fingernail, the forehead or the sternum for 5 seconds enables assessment of capillary refill. This is done in order to cause blanching and then the time it takes for capillaries to refill is noted. Capillary refill that takes over 2 seconds on the forehead or sternum is abnormal; when refill takes longer than 4 seconds on the toenails or fingernails in conjunction with tachypnoea and tachycardia it indicates shock (MRF, 2002a). Hypotension in adults is an important parameter that has to be assessed by the nurse. It may denote a shocked state, and although it may not indicate meningitis it may be related to life-threatening septicaemia (MRF, 2002a). In children it indicates critical illness (MRF, 2002a). *Table 8.2* indicates the normal values of vital signs.

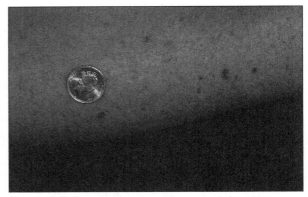

Figure 8.5: Petechial haemorrhages on the arm

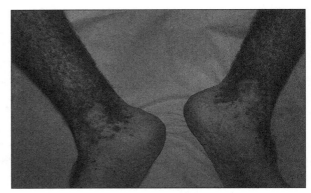

Figure 8.6: Purpuric rash on the lower limbs

Conscious level

The patient's level of consciousness must be assessed, and can be done by checking the mnemonic AVPU (alert, voice, pain, unresponsive; MRF, 2002a) and asking the following questions:

- Alert?
- Responds to voice?
- Responds to pain?
- Unresponsive?

In children the nurse must be extra vigilant; even those children who are in a serious state of shock may be attentive and talkative (MRF, 2002a). Drowsiness and/or impaired consciousness in children is a

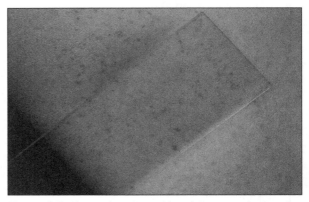

Figure 8.7: Example of non-blanching petechial rash

disturbing finding that carries with it a very poor prognosis; therefore, urgent action needs to be taken (MRF, 2002a).

Table 8.2: Normal values of vital signs

Age (years)	Heart rate per minute	Respiratory rate per minute	Systolic blood pressure (mmHg)
<1	110–160	30–40	70–90
1–2	100–150	25–35	80–95
2–5	80–120	20–25	90–110
5–12	80–120	20–25	90–100
>12	60–100	15–20	100–120

From Advanced Paediatric Life Support Group (2001)

Neck stiffness

While neck stiffness suggests meningitis, it is absent in septicaemia (MRF, 2002b). Assessment of neck stiffness can be achieved in two ways: by checking if the patient can kiss his or her knees; or by determining the effort of passive flexion in a relaxed patient (NMT, 2000). Nurses should be aware when attempting to assess young children for neck stiffness that it is unusual for the child to present with this symptom in meningitis (MRF, 2004). Neck stiffness and photophobia are unusual signs in early meningitis in young children (NMT, 2000). Approximately one-third of adult patients do not complain of neck stiffness in meningitis (MRF, 2002c).

Transmission

People are the only source of meningococci. Transmission is from the upper respiratory tract, through close and prolonged or direct contact — coughing, sneezing and intimate kissing (NMT, 2000). Prophylactic antibiotic and in some cases a vaccine are often offered to those in close contact with the infected person, such as immediate family members or household contacts. This will be coordinated by the public health team. If two or more cases occur within 4 weeks, for example in a childcare facility, antibiotics may be offered to all children and staff as advised by the public health doctor (NMT, 2004).

The consultant in communicable disease control (or the consultant in public health medicine) is responsible for ensuring that patient contacts, i.e. those who have had intimate or household contact with the patient, have been traced. All cases of meningococcal meningitis and septicaemia in the UK must be notified to the local health authority or the health board's consultant in communicable disease control or consultant in public health medicine (MRF, 2002a).

Treatment

If meningococcal infection is suspected, the best way to reduce mortality is to administer parenteral benzyl penicillin immediately (MRF, 2002a). Consequent dose, times and type of antibiotic need to be modified after full investigation and a detailed examination have taken place (Allen and Lueck, 2002).

The following intravenous doses are suggested in the British National Formulary (British Medical Association/Royal Pharmaceutical Society of Great Britain, 2004):

- Infant — 300 mg
- Child (1–9 years) — 600 mg
- Child (aged over 9 years) and adult — 1200 mg.

Parenteral antibiotics should be administered as soon as possible after a diagnosis has been made. In some instances the intravenous route may not be accessible, for example if the patient is in a severe state of shock with peripheral shutdown. If an intraosseous needle is available then the antibiotic can be given intraosseously (MRF, 2002a). If neither of the above routes can be accessed then the medication should be given intramuscularly. It is important to note that the intramuscular injection should be given as proximal as possible into a part of the body that is adequately perfused — a cold part of the limb should not be injected as the uptake of the medication will be variable if at all (MRF, 2002a).

Most cases of suspected meningococcal infections are seen in the primary care setting in the GP surgery. When this is the situation, the primary care setting will usually give advanced warning to a secondary care setting, such as an accident and emergency (A&E) department, an intensive care unit or paramedics, of the impending admission and whether antibiotics have been given. This is significant as the administration of antibiotics will affect subsequent microbiological investigations (MRF, 2002a).

Hospital management of suspected cases of bacterial meningitis or meningococcal disease should consist of the procedure shown in *Table 8.3* (MRF, 2002a).

The patient will be dependent on the nurse to ensure that all of his or her activities of living are assessed and that appropriate nursing intervention takes place to make sure that the patient is comfortable (Roper et al, 1996). Some patients may have a previous allergic reaction to benzyl penicillin. Only if there is an immediate (known) allergic anaphylactic reaction, i.e. severe dyspnoea, collapse and generalized itchy rash, should other antibiotics be considered. When the patient is at risk of developing an immediate allergic reaction where other antibiotics are available, a third-generation cephalosporin can be used (PHLS, 2001). If the patient has a history of immediate allergic reaction to benzyl penicillin and cephalosporins, chloramphenicol can be used (PHLS, 2001).

Prognosis and complications

Patients with meningococcal disease will encounter many potential problems, such as (MRF, 2002a):

- Headache
- Tiredness

Table 8.3: Hospital management of suspected cases of bacterial meningitis or meningococcal disease

- Prompt diagnosis
- Administration of antibiotics
- Early transfer to an intensive care unit
- Immediate resuscitation and maintenance of an airway (sometimes requiring mechanical ventilation)
- Correction of hypovolaemia with colloid replacement
- Maintenance of blood pressure with the use of inotropes
- Correction of electrolyte imbalance and acid—base disturbances
- Control of raised intracranial pressure

From MRF (2002a)

- Chronic fatigue
- Depression.

Deaths are not common in meningococcal disease. There are three main types of clinical presentation that are associated with a fatal outcome (NMT, 2000):

- Presence of shock
- Extensive and rapidly progressing skin rash
- Reduced level of consciousness.

In the majority of cases that result in death, the length of the illness subsequent to presentation is brief and the patient has septicaemia as opposed to meningitis (NMT, 2000). Those patients who are comatose, unrousable or non-responsive have a poor prognosis (NMT, 2000).

Seizures can occur in bacterial meningitis and have the potential to continue after the acute phase of the illness has abated (NMT, 2000). Ataxia (inability to coordinate muscle activity) can ensue as a pre-existing sign or a complication. Cranial palsies (eye and facial movements) may occur and the third, fourth, sixth and seventh cranial nerves may be affected (NMT, 2000). The auditory system may also be affected. Approximately 10% of cases of sensorineural deafness in children are caused by meningitis (Barton et al, 1962). Some patients with hearing loss in the acute phase of the illness return to normal hearing later. It is important, therefore, for nurses to ensure that patients who have bacterial meningitis have their hearing assessed by an audiologist (Fortnum, 1992).

Where a patient experiences raised intracranial pressure, neuronal damage may be caused to the visual cortex and/or the posterior visual pathways, which may result in cortical blindness (NMT, 2000). Partial obliteration of the cortex may proceed to partial loss of visual performance, where vision may remain for particular stimuli but not necessarily for others (NMT, 2000).

In certain circumstances it may be necessary to amputate limbs and/or digits after complications related to septicaemia such as gangrene (NMT, 2000). When amputation is to be considered, a full assessment of the patient is needed and a multidisciplinary approach is advocated to include the nurse, doctor, prosthetetist and occupational therapist. Prostheses can be either functional or cosmetic.

Purpura fulminans may result in the patient requiring large areas of skin grafting. This is a red, purplish severe lesion of the skin that appears suddenly — it is caused by seepage of blood from skin blood vessels (Epstein et al, 1997). The aim of skin grafting is to enhance healing time, protect underlying structures and reduce the risk of infection.

Depression may ensue during the acute phase and even after this phase has passed (NMT, 2000). Experienced nurses with counselling skills can help alleviate some of the symptoms associated with depression.

Long-term rehabilitation

Most people with bacterial meningitis will lead a normal life after the illness. Short-term difficulties may include (NMT, 2000):
- Difficulty in concentrating
- Problems with reading
- Intellectual impairment.

After the acute phase of the illness, it may take some months for the patient to improve depending on his or her situation, and the nurse needs to assess each patient individually. However, according to the NMT (2000), there may be some patients who will be left with multiple disabilities, such as:

- Severe intellectual deficits or disabilities
- Cerebral palsy
- Epilepsy
- Hydrocephalus
- Sensorineural deafness.

For these patients their complex needs must be considered when nurses are assessing and planning a long-term rehabilitation programme. Accepted management strategies will include a multidisciplinary approach in order to provide appropriate diagnosis and to devise suitable care plans.

Patient support

The effects of meningitis can be devastating for the patient, his or her family and the community. The nurse is ideally suited to provide information and support to all concerned. Referral to the appropriate agency is vital if the support is to have an impact on quality of life. The first referral may be to a national charity such as the NMT who can offer information based on the development of services over many years.

Emotional support provided to the bereaved by the nurse can help to overcome the devastation so often felt by loved ones, and the nurse must be aware of his or her limitations in these skills and be prepared to refer to experienced counsellors. The rate in which the disease may develop and the speed with which death can occur as a result usually shocks families. Often just talking over worries with patients and their families can help — the problem may not go away but it can help if a nurse takes time to listen. Financial help may be required to help pay for specialist care and specialist equipment needed by the patient and the family.

Nurses should be aware that there are a number of benefits available to patients, such as: income support; housing benefit; disability living allowance; and attendance allowance. Nurses can encourage patients and their families to claim financial help, as some people may not be aware of the benefits available.

Conclusion

The aim of this chapter is to raise awareness of meningitis and its symptoms, and to encourage nurses to provide practical support to patients and families. Often nurses in GP practices or A&E departments are the first people that patients may turn to for advice. Meningococcal disease can kill a healthy individual of any age within hours of the manifestations of the first symptoms. It is an uncommon disease but it is important because of its serious nature. A prompt diagnosis depends on the nurse's knowledge of the disease and the pertinent signs and symptoms. It is vital that benzyl penicillin is administered promptly if meningococcal disease is assumed, and the patient must be transferred to hospital as soon as possible. This is a medical emergency.

One in seven people with bacterial meningitis is left with a permanent disability, with loss of hearing being the most common (NMT, 2000). Other complications are epilepsy, sensorineural deafness and cortical blindness (NMT, 2000). Amputation and skin grafting may also be required. It is advocated that a multidisciplinary approach is used in order to assess and plan appropriate services in the acute phase and in the long term.

Nurses are ideally placed to support the patient, his or her family and the community. It is important that nurses recognize their limitations and make appropriate referrals where necesssary.

The author would like to thank Mrs Frances Cohen for her help and support.

References

Advanced Paediatric Life Support Group (2001) *Advanced Paediatric Life Support*. BMJ Publications, London

Allen CMC, Lueck CJ (2002) Neurological disease. In: Haslett C, Chilvers ER, Boon NA, Colledge NR, eds. *Davidson's Principles and Practice of Medicine*. 19th edn. Churchill Livingstone, Edinburgh: 1103–209

Barton ME, Court SD, Walker W (1962) Causes of severe deafness in school children in Northumberland and Durham. *Br Med J* **1:** 351–5

Boss BJ (1998) Alterations of neurological function. In: McCance KL, Huether SE, eds. *Pathophysiology: The Biological Basis for Disease in Adults*. 3rd edn. Mosby, St Louis: 510–73

British Medical Association/Royal Pharmaceutical Society of Great Britain (2004) *British National Formulary 47*. BMA/RPSGB, London

Conlon CP, Snydman DR (2004) *Infectious Diseases*. Mosby, London

Department of Heath, Welsh Office, Scottish Office Department of Health, Department of Health and Social Security (Northern Ireland) (1996) *1996 Immunisation Against Infectious Diseases*. HMSO, London

Epstein O, Perkin GD, de Bono DP, Cookson J, Solomons N, Robins A (1997) *Clinical Examination*. 2nd edn. Mosby, London

Fortnum HM (1992) Hearing impairment after bacterial meningitis: a review. *Arch Dis Child* **67:** 1128–33

Heyderman RS, Lambert HP, O'Sullivan I, Short JM, Taylor BL, Wall RA (2003) Early management of suspected bacterial meningitis and meningococcal septicaemia in adults. *J Infect* **46:** 75–7

Kumar P, Clark M (1996) *Clinical Medicine*. Saunders, London

Long BC, Phipps WJ, Cassmeyer VL (1995) *Adult Nursing: A Nursing Process Approach*. Mosby, London

McCormack A (1993) The notification of infectious diseases in England and Wales. *CDR Review* **3**(3): R19–25

Meningitis Research Foundation (2002a) *Meningococcal Meningitis and Septicaemia: Guidance Notes*. 3rd edn. MRF, Bristol

Meningitis Research Foundation (2002b) *Early Recognition of Meningitis and Septicaemia*. MRF, Bristol

Meningitis Research Foundation (2002c) *Meningococcal Meningitis and Septicaemia: Physical Signs in Children with Meningococcal Disease*. 3rd edn. MRF, Bristol

Meningitis Research Foundation (2004) *Lessons from Research for Doctors in Training*. MRF, Bristol

National Meningtis Trust (1997) *About Meningitis*. NMT, London

National Meningtis Trust (2000) *Meningitis Resource Pack*. NMT, London

National Meningtis Trust (2004) *Understanding Meningitis: A Guide for Early Years Professionals*. NMT, London

Peate I (1999) Meningitis: causes, symptoms and signs and nursing management. *Br J Nurs* **8:** 1290–8

Public Health Laboratory Service (2000) *Laboratory-Confirmed* Neisseria Meningitidis. *England and Wales by Age Group 1989–2001 (Mid Year Totals)*. Meningococcal Reference Unit, PHLS, London

Public Health Laboratory Service (2001) Pre-admission benzyl penicillin for suspected meningococcal disease: other antibiotics not needed in the GP bag. *Commun Dis Rep Wkly* **11**(7): news

Public Health Laboratory Service (2002) *Investigation of Cerebrospinal Fluid*. PHLS, London

Roper N, Logan WW, Tierney A (1996) *The Elements of Nursing*. 4th edn. Churchill Livingstone, Edinburgh

Roos KL (1996) *Meningitis*. Arnold, London

Strang JR, Pugh EJ (1992) Meningococcal infections: reducing the case fatality rate by giving penicillin before admission to hospital. *Br Med J* **305:** 141–3

Useful information

Meningitis Trust
www.meningitis-trust.org
Helpline: 0845 6000 800

Meningitis Research Foundation
www.meningitis.org
Helpline: 080 8800 3344

Department for Work and Pensions
List of benefits available:
www.dss.gov.uk/lifeevent/benefits
Benefits enquiry freephone: 0800 882 200

Cruse Bereavement Care
www.crusebereavementcare.org.uk
Helpline: 0870 167 1677

Disabled Living Foundation
www.dlf.org.uk
Helpline: 0845 130 9177

Chapter 9

Traumatic injuries to the head and spine: Mechanisms of injury

Anne McLeod

When a person sustains a head or spinal injury (or both), the goal of treatment is to stabilize him or her and to prevent further injury from occurring. Thus, staff managing the patient need to have an understanding of the different types of injuries that can occur and the specific complications that can result from that injury. This chapter reviews different intracerebral and spinal insults that can occur, and the underlying mechanisms of injury.

Causes

The primary causes of head and spinal injuries include road traffic accidents (RTAs), falls, assaults, sports injuries and accidents occurring at work or in the home. Head injuries sustained during a RTA are the most common cause of head trauma in young males, with alcohol frequently involved (Lindsay et al, 1998; Greaves et al, 2001). Although these only constitute about 25% of head injuries, they are potentially the most life-threatening, causing about 60% of deaths from traumatic head injury (Lindsay et al, 1998). Spinal injuries involve similar causes but are associated with a lower mortality rate. However, these injuries can lead to tetraplegia or paraplegia, with potentially no real prospect of full, functional recovery.

Mechanisms of injury

Every traumatic injury has a unique set of characteristics, features and consequences for the patient, but the patterns of injury will depend on the mechanisms that have been involved in the injury (Greaves et al, 2001). It is always essential to gain information from those at the scene of the accident, so that a full appreciation of the situation can be acquired. This will allow for the recognition of important clues as to what injuries are likely, allowing these to be identified or excluded. Some mechanisms of injury are highly predictive of serious injury and include, for example, a fall of more than 6 feet or 1.83 metres, and ejection from a vehicle or bike (Greaves et al, 2001) (*Table 9.1*).

Mechanisms of injury can be divided into four types (*Table 9.2*). These may occur in isolation or in combination and, indeed, some injuries may have an element of all four. As well as the type of injury that has been sustained, the surface area of tissue damage and length of time that force has been applied also need to be taken into consideration.

Table 9.2: Four mechanisms of injury

- Blunt
- Penetrating
- Thermal
- Blast

From Greaves et al (2001)

Table 9.1: Mechanisms predictive of serious injury

- Fall of >6 feet
- Pedestrian or cyclist hit by car
- Death of other occupant in same vehicle
- Ejection from vehicle/bike
- Major vehicular deformity or significant intrusion into passenger space
- Extrication time >20 minutes
- Vehicular roll-over
- Penetrating injury to head or torso
- All shotgun wounds

From Greaves et al (2001)

Blunt injury

In blunt trauma, the energy transfer is over a large area and is the most common form of traumatic injury in the UK (Greaves et al, 2001). Blunt injury can be subdivided by either the forces that caused the injury or by the type of incident (*Table 9.3*); again, often in blunt injury the forces that created it can be found in combination rather than in isolation.

The most common force found in blunt trauma involves direct impact or tissue compression and creates injury through direct pressure. This may cause only superficial tissue damage but can also cause deeper tissue injury as the energy from the impact is transmitted inwards (Greaves et al, 2001). Therefore, a blunt injury to the head could cause a scalp haematoma with possibly also a laceration. However, a more

Table 9.3: Subclassification of blunt trauma

Forces

Direct impact/compression
Shear
Rotation

Incident type

Road traffic accident	Vehicle occupants
	Vehicle vs vehicle
	Vehicle vs stationary object
	Motorcyclists/bicyclists
	Pedestrians
Fall	
Assault with blunt object	

From Greaves et al (2001)

forceful injury could cause a skull fracture, contusions and possibly an intracerebral haematoma. An injury like that may be seen after an assault with a weapon, such as a baseball bat (Hickey, 2002).

Blunt injury can also involve shearing forces. This occurs when tissue planes and organs move relative to each other (Greaves et al, 2001), tearing connective tissues and blood vessels. Acceleration and deceleration forces can lead to the shearing of tissues, and this type of injury is commonly seen in RTAs and high falls (Greaves et al, 2001).

Similarly, rotation can lead to the tearing of connective tissues and blood vessels. This can occur after the twisting of a body part relative to adjacent parts. Rotational forces can lead to spiral and oblique fractures, ligament damage and dislocations (Greaves et al, 2001). This may be seen in RTAs or after a fall from a height (Lindsay et al, 1998).

RTAs

Situations that may cause a blunt injury include RTAs, falls and assaults. In relation to RTAs, the direction and velocity of impact will give information as to the expected injuries. For example, front-impact RTAs can lead to head and neck injuries through impact on the steering wheel or windscreen, whereas side impact can cause the head to hit the side window or the neck to undergo compression injury on the side of the impact and a stretching injury on the other (Greaves et al, 2001).

Additionally, the nature of the impact is important to establish, for example whether the car hit another car or impacted onto a fixed stationary object such as a tree. If the RTA involved two cars, some of the force of the impact will have been dissipated into both cars; if a tree was hit, however, there will have been little movement or deformation of the tree and, therefore, most of the force of the impact will have been transmitted into the car and the occupants (Greaves et al, 2001). If an occupant has been ejected from the vehicle during the accident, it can be assumed that they will have suffered severe injuries, as considerable force will have been required to propel them from the car and they would have hit the ground at considerable speed.

Motorcyclists involved in RTAs display similar patterns of injury, but their injuries tend to be worse because of the speeds involved as well as not having the protection that a car offers. The use of helmets has reduced the number of life-threatening head injuries, but those involved in motorcycle accidents may have serious chest/abdominal trauma, which can be life-threatening (Greaves et al, 2001).

Injuries sustained by pedestrians involved in RTAs will depend on the size of the person as well as the speed and size of the vehicle involved. Adults tend to be hit side on as they either do not see the vehicle or are moving to get out of the way. This means that adults tend to be hit in the legs and then be thrown upwards onto the windscreen and bonnet. At this stage, head and neck injuries may be sustained (Greaves et al, 2001). Children, however, tend to turn to face the car before impact, which means that the pattern of injury tends to be frontal. As a result of their size, children are likely to sustain a head or neck injury as their head will strike the bonnet of the car (Greaves et al, 2001).

Falls

Injuries sustained during a fall will depend on the distance fallen, the surface fallen onto and the position of the body on impact (Greaves et al, 2001). As well as leg and ankle injuries, if the person lands on their feet, they can sustain compression fractures of the vertebral column (Lindsay et al, 1998).

Head injuries

In the UK, approximately 1 million people each year sustain a head injury. Of these, around 90% will have a minor head injury, but the remaining 100 000 will need to be admitted to hospital (Greaves et al, 2001). Around 1% of those admitted will need to be referred to a specialist neurosurgical unit (Greaves et al, 2001). Ultimately, around 5000 people each year will die from a head injury, while 50% of deaths after trauma will have involved a head injury (Greaves et al, 2001). Therefore, the overall mortality from a head injury is around 9 per 100 000 of the population while, of those that survive, 63% of moderate and 85% of severe head injury patients will be disabled 1 year after an accident (Greaves et al, 2001). Therefore, the devastating effects of head injury are evident, and those managing the patient need to be competent in the care required. To enable this, there needs to be an understanding of different cerebral trauma conditions and their pathophysiological effect.

Whatever the cause, the injuries that occur in a head injury are divided into primary or immediate, and secondary or delayed injury.

Primary brain injury

The primary injury refers to damage that occurs at the time of the actual event. Therefore, for example in a deceleration injury, which is when the head hits an immobile object, the axons in the brain can rip and shear (Lindsay et al, 1998; Greaves et al, 2001). If the head is hit by a large object, the skull can shatter, driving small particles of bone into the brain. Also, this type of insult causes the brain to move inside the skull through acceleration forces. This then can lead to contusions of the brain that may be on the side of the injury and on the opposite aspect of the brain surface (contracoup). Acceleration and deceleration injuries can also occur together, such as seen when the body is violently shaken (Lindsay et al, 1998). However, once the injury has been sustained, nothing can be done to alter the impact of the initial injury (Hickey, 2002).

The impact damage that occurs can be divided into two types, which may coexist. First, there can be cortical contusion or bruising and lacerations to the surface of the brain. These may occur under or contracoup to the site of impact (Lindsay et al, 1998), but most commonly involve the frontal and temporal lobes. Therefore, they can be multiple and occur bilaterally. Contusions themselves do not contribute to a decreased level of consciousness, but this may occur when bleeding into the contusion, or oedema around the contusion, develops (Hickey, 2002).

Second, diffuse white matter injury can result from the injury. This usually occurs after a shearing injury in which the axons become disrupted and tear because of the deceleration forces through the brain (Lindsay et al, 1998).

Secondary brain damage

This may occur any time after the initial injury, and care strategies are aimed at controlling secondary brain damage. Impact damage is unavoidable, but secondary brain damage may be prevented (Hickey, 2002). Secondary brain damage can present in five different ways (*Table 9.4*), and can not only be life-threatening but also lead to neurological dysfunction that may be severely disabling (Hickey, 2002).

Intracranial haematoma

Table 9.4: Secondary brain damage

• Intracranial haematoma	Extradural Subdural Intracerebral
• Cerebral swelling	
• Cerebral ischaemia	
• Tentorial/tonsillar herniation	
• Infection	

From Lindsay et al (1998)

After a head injury, haematomas may form either outside of the lining of the brain or just inside it. The lining, or meninges, is composed of three layers:

- The tough outermost dura mater
- The arachnoid mater
- The innermost tissue or pia mater that covers the brain's surface (Tortora and Grabowski, 2002).

When the middle meningeal blood vessels are torn, a clot will form rapidly between the skull and the dura mater. This arterial bleed, or extradural haematoma, is a neurosurgical emergency because of the speed at which it collects, thereby significantly increasing intracranial pressure (ICP) over a short period (Hickey, 2002).

A subdural haematoma forms when the bridging veins that cross between the sagittal sinus and the surface of the brain rupture. This causes a collection of venous blood between the dura mater and the arachnoid mater that does not have an underlying contusion. However, a subdural collection can occasionally form over a contusion; in these situations necrotic brain tissue may be mixed with the clot, and because of this it can be known as a burst lobe (Lindsay et al, 1998).

Although a bleed into the subarachnoid space is usually spontaneous and caused by an aneurysm or collection of blood vessels called an arteriovenous malformation, a subarachnoid haemorrhage can also be caused by trauma (Hickey, 2002). Finally, a haematoma into the brain tissue itself, or intracerebral haematoma, can be caused by trauma (Lindsay et al, 1998) (*Figure 9.1*).

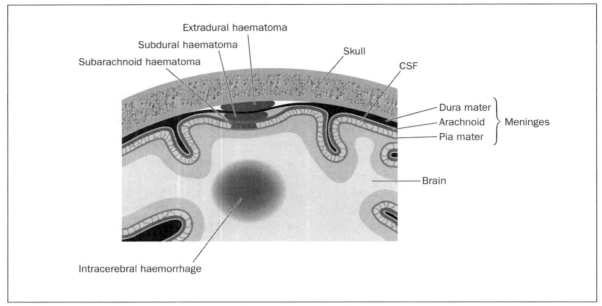

Figure 9.1: Location of intracranial bleeds. CSF=cerebrospinal fluid

Cerebral swelling

This can occur with or without intracranial haematoma. Although the exact pathogenesis of cerebral swelling in different injuries is unclear, it could result from either vascular engorgement or an increase in extracellular or intracellular fluid (Lindsay et al, 1998). Blood itself, when it is outside of blood vessels, acts as an irritant and causes an inflammatory reaction, which results in cerebral swelling (Hickey, 2002).

Additionally, the blood–brain barrier, which is formed by the plasma membranes of the brain capillaries and brain cells, may become disrupted. Normally, this is a highly selective barrier that only allows lipid-soluble substances and those that can use specific transport mechanisms to enter the brain (Vander et al, 2000). However, when it becomes disrupted after, for example, a head injury, there is an increase in the permeability of the blood–brain barrier allowing for the movement of plasma-like filtrate, which includes the large protein molecules found in blood, to leak into the extracellular space with the brain. This then can lead to cerebral oedema (Hickey, 2002).

Cerebral ischaemia

Cerebral ischaemia can occur after a head injury and, if not resolved, can develop into infarction (Hickey, 2002). This will worsen the prognosis of the patient. Generally, cerebral ischaemia results from either hypotension or hypoxia (Lindsay et al, 1998). Normally the brain can autoregulate, which is the ability to maintain a stable cerebral blood flow irrespective of changes in systemic blood pressure (Hudak et al, 1998). Therefore, if blood pressure increases, cerebral blood vessels will constrict and *vice versa* should systemic blood pressure drop. After a traumatic head injury, this ability to autoregulate occasionally becomes impaired (Lindsay et al, 1998) and cerebral blood flow becomes 'pressure passive', being directly influenced by systemic blood pressure. Therefore, ischaemia can occur if the patient is hypotensive (Hickey, 2002).

Ischaemia can also arise if the ICP is such that the cerebral blood vessels are compressed, thereby reducing cerebral blood flow (Lindsay et al, 1998). In these situations, the perfusion to the brain will be reduced. The brain is reliant on a continuous supply of oxygen and glucose for neuronal perfusion; if this supply does not meet neuronal metabolic requirements, ischaemia will occur. Cerebral perfusion pressure (CPP) is the difference between the systemic mean arterial pressure and the ICP, and is viewed as the blood pressure gradient across the brain. It is normally 80–100 mmHg (Hickey, 2002); it needs to be more than 60 mmHg for neuronal perfusion (Hickey, 2002). This is not the same as cerebral blood flow because CPP does not take cerebral vascular resistance into account; however, CPP does give an indication of global perfusion (Hickey, 2002).

Situations of increased cerebral metabolic rate can also lead to ischaemia. This may occur with an increase in temperature, which can occur if an infection is present or if there is damage to the central control of temperature, or the hypothalamus (Hudak et al, 1998). In this situation, normal thermoregulatory mechanisms will not be activated. Additionally, seizures may develop after a head injury. These also increase cerebral activity and, therefore, metabolic rate, which can cause ischaemia if cerebral perfusion is not maintained (Hickey, 2002).

If perfusion is not maintained, cellular mechanisms can become deranged (Oh, 1997). Ischaemia can rapidly lead to cellular energy failure and increased intracellular water. Energy failure occurs as the cells do not receive enough oxygen to undergo aerobic respiration and, therefore, the production of energy in the form of adenosine triphosphate (ATP) occurs anaerobically (Oh, 1997). Anaerobic respiration does not produce as much ATP as aerobic respiration, so energy-dependent processes fail. Therefore, the cell membrane channels that control intracellular and extracellular ion concentrations also fail as they require energy to maintain their activity (Oh, 1997). Thus, an influx of extracellular ions (sodium and calcium) and an efflux of potassium occurs.

The movement of sodium into the cells results in intracellular swelling as water tends to follow sodium (Oh, 1997). Additionally, a by-product of anaerobic respiration is lactate, which can then be used to form lactic acid (Vander et al, 2000). Acidotic conditions increase ICP because of cerebral vasodilation (Hickey, 2002). These consequences of ischaemia will actually worsen the ischaemia, as cerebral blood flow will be further reduced. Therefore, a worsening spiralling effect will result, which is potentially irreversible (Hudak et al, 1998).

Infection

A compound depressed skull fracture can lead to a tear in the tough dura mater, the outermost layer of the meninges. Similarly, a base of skull fracture can also result in a dural tear, which may be recognized if cerebrospinal fluid is seen to be dripping from the ears or the nose. Should this occur, there is a route of entry into the brain for bacteria. Therefore, meningitis and/or cerebral abscesses can develop (Lindsay et al, 1998).

Tentorial/tonsillar herniation

Brain damage can occur as a result of supratentorial or infratentorial herniation (Lindsay et al, 1998). This is the movement of brain tissue from one cerebral compartment into another through the dural fold that divides the brain into distinct compartments. Usually this movement is downwards towards the only place for escape, which is the foramen magnum at the base of the skull. Supratentorial herniation occurs when brain tissue moves through the tentorium that separates the cerebrum from the cerebellum (Lindsay et al, 1998). This is a result of increased pressure in the cerebrum and leads to pressure being exerted on the midbrain.

There are three main patterns of supratentorial herniation (Porth, 2003):

- Cingulate or subfalcial herniation is the displacement of the cingulate gyrus and hemisphere below the falx cerebri to the opposite side of the cerebrum (*Figure 9.2*)
- Central or transtentorial herniation involves the downward displacement of the cerebral hemispheres, basal ganglia, diencephalon and midbrain through the tentorium (see *Figure 9.2*)
- Uncal herniation is when a lateral mass pushes the brain centrally, thus forcing the medial aspect of the temporal lobe downwards (see *Figure 9.2*).

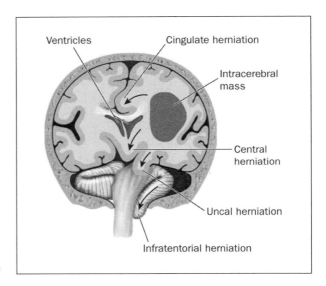

Figure 9.2: Cerebral herniation

Midline shift, which is evident on a computed tomography (CT) scan, occurs when pressure is mounting on one side and brain tissue is compressed away from the mass (Lindsay et al, 1998). On the CT scan this can be identified with the ventricle on the side of the mass becoming compressed and therefore collapsed, as well as the falx cerebri moving away from the mass. Finally, infratentorial herniation ('coning') occurs when the cerebellar tonsils are pushed through the foramen magnum, again by pressure. This will place pressure directly on the medulla oblongata and, therefore, brainstem dysfunction will ensue (Hickey, 2002).

Clinically, the different patterns of herniation are observed in different ways (Porth, 2003) (*Table 9.5*). Herniation is a life-threatening event, as direct pressure on the brainstem will lead to ischaemic damage and then infarction of the brainstem. The brainstem contains all the vital centres required for maintenance of life, such as the respiratory and vasomotor centres (Tortora and Grabowski, 2002). Additionally, the nuclei for the 12 cranial nerves are located in the brainstem; brainstem dysfunction can be demonstrated by abnormal cranial nerve function, such as reduced pupillary responses to light, reduced blink reflexes and reduced cough reflexes (Hickey, 2002). A late reflex seen with a marked increase in ICP is the central nervous system ischaemic response, which is initiated by ischaemia of the vasomotor centre in the brainstem (Porth, 2003).

Table 9.5: Different patterns of herniation — clinical signs

Central or transtentorial herniation	Initially the changes noted will be observed as a blurring of consciousness with bilaterally small pupils. The decrease in level of consciousness (LOC) is caused by pressure on the reticular-activating system (RAS), which has a key role in awareness. As the herniation continues, LOC continues to deteriorate with abnormal posturing viewed and an irregular respiratory pattern. When the midbrain becomes compressed, the pupils become fixed and midsized (about 5 mm)
Uncal herniation	This may initially be observed as ipsilateral (same side) dilation of the pupil as the oculomotor nerve on the side of the mass becomes compressed. Although LOC may be initially unimpaired as the RAS has not yet been affected, there can be a rapid deterioration. Motor function will become abnormal in conjunction with an altered respiratory pattern
Infratentorial herniation	The displacement of tissue that occurs in infratentorial herniation puts direct pressure on the brainstem. Therefore, medullary function becomes impaired leading to respiratory and cardiac arrest

In response to the ischaemia, the neurones in the vasomotor centre attempt to increase blood pressure in the brainstem to maintain perfusion and cerebral circulation. Therefore, the Cushing reflex is observed, which has a triad of signs (Porth, 2003):

- A marked increase in blood pressure
- A widened pulse pressure
- A reflex bradycardia.

If the raised ICP is not controlled and reduced (and the herniation reversed if possible), the consequence of herniation is brainstem death and is, therefore, a terminal event (Hickey, 2002).

Spinal injuries

Acute spinal injury predominately affects young men between the ages of 18–35 years (Greaves et al, 2001). The incidence within the UK is around 10–15 per million of population (Greaves et al, 2001). However, of these, 800 face permanent disability and paralysis, which has a major impact on them and their families — physically, financially and socially (Greaves et al, 2001). As with head trauma, RTAs as well as falls from heights account for the majority of people who sustain a spinal injury. However, sporting accidents, such as diving, horse riding and rugby, are also associated with spinal injuries. Additionally, penetrating injury, such as a stabbing, is as common as injuries sustained during sporting accidents (Greaves et al, 2001).

Anatomy and physiology

The vertebral column consists of 33 vertebrae, which surround and protect the spinal cord: there are 7 cervical, 12 thoracic and 5 lumbar vertebrae, along with 5 sacral and 4 coccygeal bones that are fused to form the sacrum and coccyx, respectively. The most flexible parts of the vertebral column are the cervical and lumbar areas, whereas the thoracic portion is relatively immobile because of the attachment of ribs (Tortora and Grabowski, 2002).

The stability of the vertebral column depends mainly on the ligaments and the intervertebral discs that are between the bodies of the vertebrae (*Figure 9.3*). The vertebral column has four ligaments that help maintain stability. The anterior longitudinal ligament is attached to the vertebral bodies and intravertebral discs, the posterior longitudinal ligament is attached to the posterior part of the vertebral body, the ligament flava connects laminae to adjacent vertebrae, and the supraspinous ligament links the spinous processes (Tortora and Grabowski, 2002). This pattern of attachment helps to prevent excessive flexion of the vertebral column (Tortora and Grabowski, 2002).

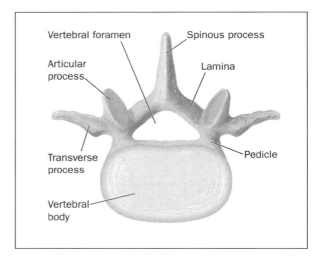

Figure 9.3: Diagram of typical vertebra

However, with this pattern there are three distinct columns of support: the anterior, middle and posterior. If two of these three columns are injured, the spine is unstable and movement may damage the spinal cord in the vertebral foramen (Greaves et al, 2001).

The spinal cord extends from the medulla oblongata, which forms the lowest portion of the brainstem, and usually terminates at the level of the first or second lumbar (L1–L2) vertebra (Tortora and Grabowski, 2002). At each verebral level, the anterior and dorsal nerve roots combine to form the spinal nerves as they exit from the spinal cord. The nerves that leave at each segment of the spinal cord innervate a specific body area (Hickey, 2002). By testing movement and sensation, it is possible to identify the lowest level of the spinal cord where damage has occurred; the area of skin that is specifically innervated by the nerves is called a dermatome (Lindsay et al, 1998) (*Figure 9.4*).

The spinal cord contains paired bundles of nerve fibres (or tracts), which carry ascending (or motor) information and descending (or sensory) information. The tracts have specific anatomical locations within the spinal cord, with the most important ones being the corticospinal and spinothalamic tracts, as well as the dorsal columns (Tortora and Grabowski, 2002) (*Figure 9.5*). Within the tracts, the most centrally located nerves innervate the more proximal areas of the body (such as the arms), whereas the more lateral nerves innervate the distal areas (such as the toes) (Tortora and Grabowski, 2002).

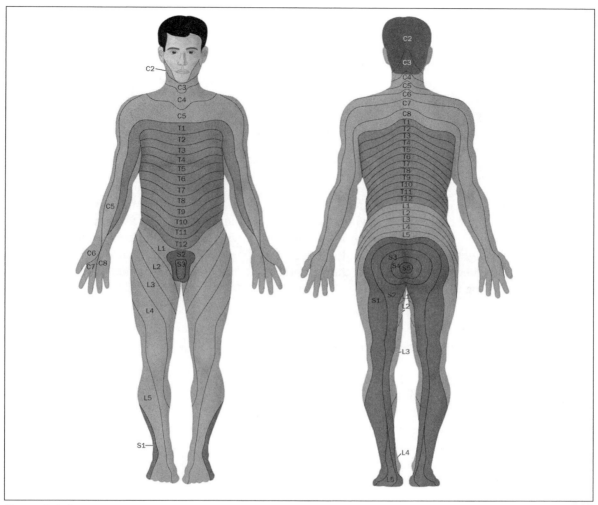

Figure 9.4: Dermatomes

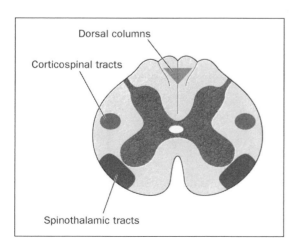

Corticospinal tracts

These are motor tracts and are found at the front of the spinal cord. Motor nerves cross over at the level of the medulla oblongata, which means that injury to the corticospinal tracts will result in functional loss on the same side as the injury (Hudak et al, 1998).

Figure 9.5: Cross-section of spinal cord

Dorsal columns

These tracts carry ascending sensory fibres and are at the back, or dorsum, of the spinal cord. These fibres transmit light touch, proprioception and vibration sense. Again, these fibres cross at the level of the medulla oblongata, so damage to the dorsal columns will be demonstrated as sensory alterations on the side of the injury (Hudak et al, 1998).

Spinothalamic tracts

These tracts are found in two places within the spinal cord and are associated with sensation. The lateral spinothalamic tracts transmit pain and temperature, whereas the anterior spinothalamic tract is associated with light touch (Hudak et al, 1998). These fibres enter and cross over the spinal cord before ascending; therefore, damage to the spinothalamic tracts will be demonstrated as sensory alterations on the opposite side of the injury (Hudak et al, 1998).

Pathophysiology of spinal injuries

There are five patterns of spinal injury that will damage the spinal cord in predictable ways (*Table 9.6*). Whatever the mechanism, around 14% of all spinal injuries will lead to spinal cord damage, with about 40% occurring in the cervical region, 35% in the thoracolumbar region, 10% in the thoracic region and only 3% in the lumbar region (Greaves et al, 2001). Generally, cervical spine injury is caused by extension or flexion movements, whereas compression with flexion or rotation is the main mechanism of injury in the thoracic and lumbar regions of the spinal column (Greaves et al, 2001).

Table 9.6: Patterns of spinal injury

- Flexion

- Flexion with rotation

- Extension

- Rotation

- Compression

From Greaves et al (2001)

Flexion

Flexion of the neck in, for example, a RTA, can cause damage to the anterior portion of the spinal cord in the cervical region of the vertebral column. Rapid deceleration in a flexed position, falls on the back of the head, diving and sports injuries may also cause flexion injuries (Greaves et al, 2001). This type of injury can be associated with fractures of the vertebrae and ligament damage (Greaves et al, 2001).

Flexion with rotation

A combination of hyperflexion and rotation is much more likely to cause significant injury to the cervical spine and thoracic region than any other mechanism. Around 50–80% of cervical spine injuries are caused by this mechanism, and this can occur after a RTA or direct trauma (Greaves et al, 2001). It is associated with damage to the posterior ligaments, which then can result in fractures of the vertebral bodies, lamina and transverse processes (Greaves et al, 2001).

Extension

Hyperextension injuries tend to occur in the cervical and lumbar regions of the vertebral column (Hudak et al, 1998). Hyperextension damages the anterior column but can also cause crushing of the posterior parts of the vertebrae. This may push bony fragments or the intervertebral disc into the vertebral foramen and so cause damage to the spinal cord (Lindsay et al, 1998).

Rotation

This rarely occurs in isolation and is usually associated with extension or flexion. If the ligaments are involved, an unstable spine can result (Greaves et al, 2001).

Compression

Wedge fractures within lumbar and thoracic vertebrae are a common result of compression damage, but are usually stable because the posterior ligaments remain intact (Greaves et al, 2001). However, a burst fracture can occur, when the force is such that the anterior and middle columns are damaged; movement of the posterior vertebral wall or the intervertebral disc could cause cord damage (Greaves et al, 2001). This may occur after either a fall from a height when the victim has landed on his or her feet, or an object has fallen onto his or her head (Lindsay et al, 1998).

Complete *vs* incomplete injury

If a spinal injury has been sustained, damage to the spinal cord needs to be assessed accurately (Hickey, 2002). This is usually ascertained by checking sensation and movements, using the sensory dermatones as a guide to what level of the spinal cord is injured (Lindsay et al, 1998). The lowest dermatone at which sensation is felt determines the level of the injury in relation to the spinal cord (Greaves et al, 2001).

A complete injury implies that motor and sensory function is lost below the level of the damage. In incomplete injury, some function is retained; however, the type of function is determined by the areas on the spinal cord that have been affected. There are four spinal cord syndromes, which are differentiated by the type of function that is retained.

Anterior cord syndrome

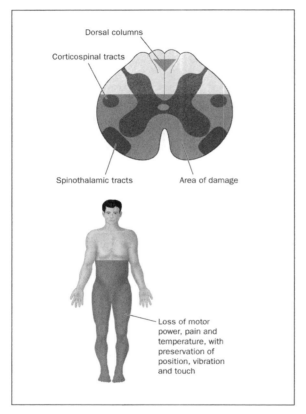

The damage sustained is at the front of the spinal cord (*Figure 9.6*). Thus the corticospinal tracts are affected, as are the spinothalamic tracts, but the dorsal columns are preserved. Therefore, patients will have variable motor function below the level of the injury with impairment of pain and temperature sensation. However, light touch, proprioception and vibration sense are retained (Hudak et al, 1998).

Figure 9.6: Anterior cord syndrome (left illustration)

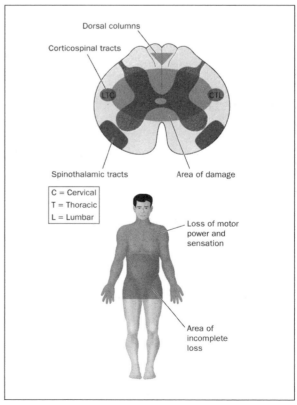

Central cord syndrome

In this situation, damage to the spinal cord is in its centre (*Figure 9.7*), usually through cervical hyperextension. Such patients will have arm weakness with some sensory changes. However, leg function is usually spared (Hudak et al, 1998).

Figure 9.7: Central cord syndrome

Posterior cord syndrome

This is unusual, but can occur after cervical hyperextension. Injury is at the back of the spinal cord, and the deficits observed result from a loss of the dorsal column functions. Therefore, light touch, proprioception and vibration sense are impaired (Hudak et al, 1998).

Lateral cord syndrome (Brown-Séquard syndrome)

A penetrating injury, such as that received during a stabbing, may cause damage to the spinal cord that only affects one side of the cord (*Figure 9.8*). Therefore, there is sensory and motor tract disruption on the affected side of the spinal cord. This can then give ipsilateral (same side) and contralateral (opposite side) deficits. Thus, below the level of the injury there is loss of motor function, proprioception, vibration sense and light touch on the side of the injury, with loss of pain and temperature sensation on the side opposite to the injury (Hudak et al, 1998).

It may be difficult to assess the patient's neurological function fully until any spinal shock resolves. Spinal shock can occur after severe spinal cord injury and is characterized by generalized flaccidity below the level of the injury (Grundy and Swain, 2002). Once this resolves, which may take up to several weeks, the patient's neurological deficits can be truly ascertained.

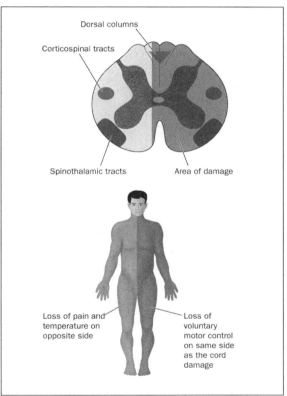

Figure 9.8: Brown-Séquard syndrome

Secondary injury

As with head injuries, the primary spinal insult can progress to develop secondary injuries. These are primarily caused by hypoxia, hypoperfusion and further mechanical injury to the spinal cord (Greaves et al, 2001). Secondary damage creates interstitial and intracellular oedema that may further reduce spinal perfusion and, hence, as with brain injury, a deteriorating spiral will be precipitated

(Hickey, 2002). As the oedema spreads and worsens, neurones are compressed and further neurological deterioration will be observed. With high thoracic and cervical injuries, this can lead to respiratory failure as the nerves innervating the diaphragm and intercostal muscles are not able to function normally (Lindsay et al, 1998).

Hypoxia

Hypoxia can result from head, upper airway and chest injuries, as well as from involvement of the respiratory nerves. The level of the spinal cord injury will determine the extent of the loss of respiratory muscle innervation (*Table 9.7*).

Hudak et al (1998) do not link C6 to a respiratory muscle dysfunction, but they do say that with C6 injury respiratory distress may occur because of ascending oedema and intestinal paralysis. Patients who have cervical spine injuries above C5 will nearly all require mechanical support to maintain their ventilatory requirements (Hickey, 2002). To reduce the risk of hypoxic-induced secondary damage, impairment to ventilation must be recognized immediately and the appropriate intervention instigated.

Table 9.7: Respiratory muscle innervation

Level of injury	Respiratory function
C1–4	Diaphragm and intercostal muscles paralysed C1, 2, 3 injuries will require permanent mechanical ventilation C4 injuries — patients may be able to breathe spontaneously for short periods
C5	Diaphragm may be impaired initially but spontaneous effort should return
C7	Diaphragm and accessory muscles can compensate for intercostal muscle impaired function

From Hudak et al (1998)

Hypoperfusion

Reduced regional blood flow, which is caused by capillary damage during the primary injury, will reduce oxygen and glucose delivery to the affected part of the spinal cord. Further hypoperfusion can occur because of reduced systemic blood pressure from, for example, hypovolaemic shock, or because of a loss of autoregulation (Greaves et al, 2001). As with head injuries, if spinal autoregulation is lost, spinal perfusion will reflect changes in systemic blood pressure (Greaves et al, 2001).

Mechanical damage

Further neurological damage can occur if the patient is mishandled and positioned incorrectly. Extreme caution should always be used when moving a patient with a suspected or known spinal injury, with care made to maintain alignment at all times (Hickey, 2002).

Management

Once the patient has been assessed and injuries identified, a decision needs to be made about whether the patient should be referred to a specialist centre. In relation to head injuries, there are clear guidelines on when to involve neurosurgeons (National Institute for Clinical Excellence, 2003); if there is significant spinal injury, specialist advice should be sought with a view to transfer to a specialist centre, be that neurosurgical or spinal.

Conclusion

In neurotrauma, there are a number of causative factors and influences that will determine the extent and type of injury sustained. Unfortunately, the primary injury that is sustained cannot be eradicated, but the secondary injury that ensues can be controlled by treating and managing the factors that create the cellular changes underlying the pathophysiology and consequences observed. It is these that must be the focus of care to ensure the best possible outcome for the patient and his or her family and loved ones.

The next chapter will explore the nursing considerations of patients with neurological traumatic injury.

References

Greaves I, Porter K, Ryan J (2001) *Trauma Care Manual*. Arnold, London

Grundy D, Swain A, eds (2002) *ABC of Spinal Cord Injury*. BMJ Publishing Group, London

Hickey JV (2002) *The Clinical Practice of Neuromedical and Neurosurgical Nursing*. 5th edn. Lippincott Williams and Wilkins, Philadelphia

Hudak CM, Gallo BM, Gonce Morton P (1998) *Critical Care Nursing: A Holistic Approach*. 7th edn. Lippincott, Philadelphia

Lindsay KW, Bone I, Callender R (1998) *Neurology and Neurosurgery Illustrated*. 3rd edn. Churchill Livingstone, London

National Institute for Clinical Excellence (2003) *Head Injury: Triage, Assessment, Investigation and Early Management of Head Injury in Infants, Children and Adults*. NICE, London

Oh TE (1997) *Intensive Care Manual*. 4th edn. Butterworth Heinemann, Oxford

Porth CM (2003) *Essentials of Pathophysiology: Concepts of Altered Health States*. Lippincott, Williams and Wilkins, Philadelphia

Tortora GJ, Grabowski NP (2002) *Principles of Anatomy and Physiology*. 10th edn. Harper Collins, London

Vander AJ, Sherman JH, Luciano DS (2000) *Human Physiology: The Mechanisms of Body Function*. 7th edn. McGraw-Hill, London

Chapter 10

Traumatic injuries to the head and spine: Nursing considerations

Anne McLeod

Each year, about 100 000 people are admitted to hospital after sustaining a head injury, while about 10–15 per million of population are admitted with a spinal injury (Greaves et al, 2001). These types of injuries can be devastating and the medical management and nursing care received by these patients is crucial to their future, as secondary injury needs to be treated and controlled. The last chapter reviewed the pathophysiology involved with neurological traumatic injury; the focus of this chapter is the management strategies that should be employed in the care of such patients. In view of cerebral trauma, this chapter also reviews more detailed pathophysiology of cerebral haemodynamics as this underpins nursing and medical management.

Head injuries

The care of patients who have sustained a severe head injury is generally focused on the management of the factors that are involved in the maintenance of cerebral blood flow (*Figure 10.1*). This then will ensure that the neurones continue to receive the oxygen and glucose they require for their metabolic function. If neurones become ischaemic (i.e. they do not receive enough oxygen and glucose), first reversible and then irreversible changes occur; this can happen after only 4–5 minutes (Oh, 1997). If this occurs, the outcome for the patient is worsened as the consequence of irreversible neuronal damage is a cerebral infarction. Additionally, secondary brain injury will be precipitated, as outlined in the last chapter.

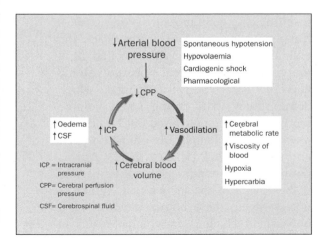

Figure 10.1: Factors that can cause cerebral ischaemia (Oh, 1997)

Intracranial pressure

Intracranial pressure (ICP) can be defined as the pressure exerted within the cerebral ventricles by the cerebrospinal fluid (CSF) (Hickey, 2002). It is also determined by brain tissue and cerebral blood volume within the cranium (Hickey, 2002). A normal ICP is 0–10 mmHg (Hickey, 2002) and is normally a fluctuating pressure, influenced by normal activities of living, such as sneezing. Such activities create a transient rise of pressure within the head, which is short-lived and has no lasting effect. However, in patients with a cerebral injury, a small rise could have devastating effects leading to herniation of brain tissue from one intracranial compartment to another (Vos, 1993; Lindsay et al, 1998), which can precede irreversible damage to the brainstem.

A raised ICP is more than 15 mmHg (Hickey, 2002) and intracranial hypertension is defined as an ICP of more than 20 mmHg (Hickey, 2002; Porth, 2003). However, if the ICP should become raised, certain compensatory mechanisms can be used in an effort to prevent herniation and therefore brainstem injury. The modified Monroe–Kellie doctrine states that within the rigid structure of the skull, there are three components that fill, to capacity, the vault in which they are contained (Hickey, 2002):

- Brain tissue (80%)
- Blood (10%)
- CSF (10%).

The doctrine states that should there be an increase in one of the compartments, there must be a reciprocal decrease in one of the other two compartments. This will have the net result of maintaining a normal ICP (Hickey, 2002). To achieve this, mechanisms such as increased absorption of CSF and the shunting of CSF to the spinal subarachnoid space occur (Hickey, 2002). The CSF is most able to accommodate an alteration in volume in response to an increase in ICP, whereas brain tissue is the least able to change in volume.

The ability to cope with an increase in ICP differs from person to person and is ultimately dependent on the compliance of the brain tissue (Porth, 2003). Compliance pertains to the brain's ability to cope with increased pressure but still maintain a stable ICP and represents the ratio of change in volume to the resulting change in pressure (Porth, 2003). Simply, it can be viewed as how 'slack' the cranial contents are. When plotted as a graph, a typical cerebral pressure/volume curve (*Figure 10.2*) is obtained, which demonstrates that, during small volume increases, ICP is not raised until a point is reached when changes in volume do elicit an increase in ICP (Hickey, 2002). At this point, cerebral compliance is altering and if the source of the increase in volume is not resolved, there comes a point when only small changes in volume result in

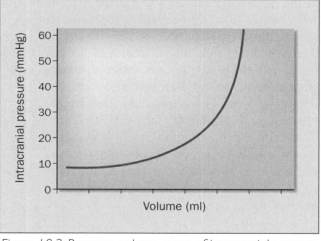

Figure 10.2: Pressure–volume curve of intracranial pressure

inappropriately large increases in ICP. Therefore, cerebral compliance is low and cerebral elastance (or stiffness) is high. At this point the likelihood of a positive outcome for the patient is slim (Hickey, 2002).

Cerebral blood flow

Intracranial hypertension leads to a decrease in cerebral blood flow (CBF) because blood flow is impeded as it attempts to flow through compressed blood vessels (Brinker et al, 1992). This can lead to a reduction in cerebral oxygen delivery (Cruz et al, 1993) and ultimately cerebral ischaemia can develop. Normal CBF is 50 ml/min/100 g of brain (or 750 ml/min in a 1500 g brain) (Hickey, 2002), and the brain has the ability to autoregulate the blood flow through it in order to maintain steady flow (Vander et al, 2000). This is usually in response to the cerebral perfusion pressure (CPP), or blood pressure gradient, across the brain. CPP is the difference between systemic mean arterial pressure (MAP) and the ICP, and is usually about 80–100 mmHg, with 60 mmHg being required for neuronal perfusion (Hickey, 2002).

Autoregulation is responsible for ensuring CBF is relatively stable, despite changes in systemic blood pressure (Vander et al, 2000). Thus, if the systemic blood pressure increases, the cerebral blood vessels will constrict; if the pressure should drop, the vessels will dilate. Autoregulation can only occur within a certain range of systemic mean arterial blood pressure (50–150 mmHg): outside this range, CBF becomes pressure-passive as it alters according to the MAP (Oh, 1997) (*Figure 10.3*), thus if the MAP decreases, so does the CBF.

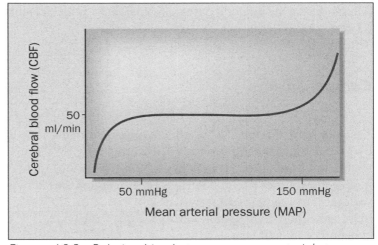

Figure 10.3: Relationship between mean arterial pressure and cerebral blood flow

There is no totally reliable method of measuring CBF. Transcranial Doppler can be used to measure the blood flow through the middle cerebral artery, and internal jugular bulb catheters can be used to measure the oxygen content of the blood leaving the brain (which will give an indication of oxygen extraction) (Oh, 1997).

ICP monitoring and calculation of CPP is the usual method for estimating cerebral perfusion (Hickey, 2002), but CPP does not take into account the cerebral vascular resistance that will alter CBF. When the influences on CBF are taken into consideration, the variables that can be manipulated in patient care can be identified. CBF can be calculated as shown on the next page (Muizelaar and Schroder, 1994).

$$CBF = K \frac{CPP \times d^4}{8 \times l \times v}$$

Where K=constant; l=length of blood vessels; d=diameter of blood vessels; v=blood viscosity; CPP=cerebral perfusion pressure

The CPP equation is CPP=MAP – ICP

The variables that can be manipulated are the MAP and ICP (and therefore the CPP), the diameter of the cerebral blood vessels and the blood viscosity. Of these, the blood vessel diameter has the most effect on CBF and therefore oxygen delivery to the brain (Muizelaar and Schroder, 1994).

Cerebral blood flow and respiratory gases

Alterations in respiratory gases can markedly affect cerebral blood vessels and, therefore, CBF (Hickey, 2002).

Carbon dioxide

Vascular smooth muscle is affected by hydrogen ion concentration, in that an increase in hydrogen ion concentration (and lowering of pH) causes the smooth muscle to relax, which results in vasodilation (Hudak et al, 1998). This will increase CBF and also ICP according to the modified Monroe–Kellie doctrine. Hydrogen ions are a byproduct of carbon dioxide metabolism so that any hypercarbia will increase the hydrogen ion concentration and can lead to cerebral vasodilation (Yoshihara et al, 1995). In view of this, carbon dioxide is viewed as one of the main influencing factors on CBF and ICP (*Figure 10.4*).

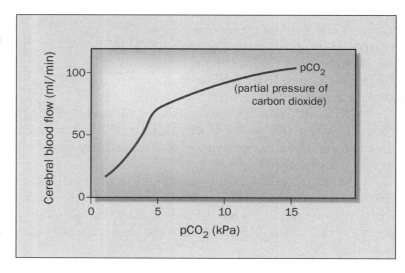

Figure 10.4: Carbon dioxide and cerebral blood flow

Oxygen

If the oxygen content of blood falls, the CBF increases in an effort to maintain cerebral oxygenation (*Figure 10.5*). This too will increase ICP (Price et al, 2003a).

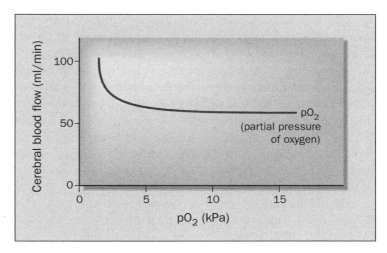

Figure 10.5: Oxygen and cerebral blood flow

Cerebral blood flow and pH alterations

Changes in the arterial pH affect CBF in a similar manner to carbon dioxide. Therefore, if the pH drops (i.e. the blood becomes more acidic), relaxation of the smooth muscle in the cerebral blood vessels occurs. This increases CBF and, therefore, potentially ICP (Hudak et al, 1998).

Care strategies

As the maintenance of CBF is the focus of care, then strategies that control the factors that influence CBF form the basis of patient management in conjunction with accurately observing for any deterioration.

Neurological

The patient's neurological status needs to be closely observed and any deterioration in level of consciousness promptly acted upon (Hickey, 2002).

The Glasgow Coma Scale is a commonly used tool for assessment of level of consciousness that assesses the patient's awareness of the environment and him/herself (Teasdale and Jennett, 1974). Three responses are assessed:

- Eye opening
- Verbal response
- Motor response.

The best score a patient can have is 15 out of 15; any score less than 8 is viewed as being unconscious and, therefore, the patient will need to be reviewed by an anaesthetist for possible intubation to ensure a patent airway is maintained (Hickey, 2002).

At the time of neurological assessment, pupillary response to light should also be documented. This gives information about the functioning of the third cranial nerve (oculomotor nerve), which arises from near the top of the brainstem. Dysfunction of the third cranial nerve, as indicated by dilated and/or a sluggish (or absent) response to light, implies that pressure is compressing the nerve (Hickey, 2002). Therefore, the brainstem is becoming compressed, and if that pressure is not relieved, ischaemic damage can occur. This may lead to brainstem death (Lindsay et al, 1998). As the cranial nerves do not cross over, dilation of one pupil indicates that pressure is building up on the same side as the dilated pupil (Hickey, 2002).

Should the patient's level of consciousness deteriorate abruptly, the osmotic diuretic mannitol may be prescribed. This does not enter the brain and so draws water out of the brain, helping to reduce ICP (Jastremski, 1998). However, when the blood–brain barrier is not intact, mannitol diffuses into the brain tissue and therefore takes water into the brain with it (Fisher, 1997). Mannitol can cause hypotension as well as electrolyte imbalances, such as hypokalaemia (Price et al, 2003a). If a patient has been given mannitol, it is also advisable to measure serum osmolality as this can give an indication of the patient's overall state of hydration and, therefore, whether further mannitol would be of use (Hickey, 2002).

Seizures may occur after a head injury; this can result from the brain injury itself or from hypoxia/hypotension (Price et al, 2003a). Seizures can worsen the secondary brain injury that develops after a severe head injury as cerebral hypoxia and ischaemia can be exacerbated (Adam and Osbourne, 1997). Seizures must be controlled with anticonvulsants, such as phenytoin, and therapeutic levels achieved (Price et al, 2003b).

Respiratory system

The control of respiratory gases is an essential part of acute head injury management because of the effect they have on CBF and, therefore, cerebral perfusion. Mechanical ventilation may be required to control the partial pressures of oxygen (pO_2) and carbon dioxide (pCO_2) (Hickey, 2002). If a patient is intubated and mechanically ventilated, admission to the intensive care setting is essential (Hillman and Bishop, 1996). Hypoxia should be avoided and a pO_2 within normal limits (11–13 kPa) should be the aim (Adam and Osbourne, 1997); pCO_2 needs to be carefully controlled, and if the patient is mechanically ventilated, a pCO_2 that is towards the low end of normal is generally the ideal. Therefore, a pCO_2 of 4.5–5 kPa and a normal pH (7.35–7.45) is required (Adam and Osbourne, 1997; Wright, 1999; Wong, 2000).

Endotracheal suctioning (ETS) can cause ICP to rise (Johnson, 1999), as well as causing transient hypoxia. Additionally, coughing can lead to sharp increases in ICP (Johnson, 1999). However, pulmonary secretions can lead to hypoxaemia and hypercarbia (increased pCO_2), which will also have a potentially deleterious effect on cerebral perfusion (Johnson, 1999). Therefore, the decision to perform ETS should always be based on individual patient indications.

Parsons and Shogan (1984) studied the effect of ETS and manual hyperinflation on patients who had a severe head injury. They found that ETS could be safely performed on this group of patients if their baseline ICP was <20 mmHg and their CPP was >50 mmHg. Even so, Prendergast

(1994) recommends that nurses limit suctioning to one or two suction passes, with each pass being for a maximum of 10 seconds. Preoxygenation with 100% oxygen and optimal sedation/analgesia can help to avoid the complications associated with suctioning (Hall, 1997).

Cardiovascular system

One of the components that influences CBF is the CPP. Therefore, the control of the MAP is an essential part of caring for the patient with a cerebral injury. The MAP should be sufficient to maintain a CPP of >70 mmHg (Hickey, 2002). This may require a MAP of 85–90 mmHg (Eisenhart, 1994; Young and Meredith, 1995). To enable this, it is likely that the patient will require adequate fluid resuscitation that can be guided by central venous pressure readings. If necessary, vasoactive drugs, such as noradrenaline or dobutamine, may be required to support pharmacologically the MAP (Oh, 1997).

The thickness, or viscosity, of blood is also a factor that influences CBF. The administration of colloid solutions may reduce the viscosity of the blood by haemodilution (Oh, 1997). The extent of this can be ascertained by measuring the haemocrit, normally about 45–50% (Oh, 1997). This can be reduced to 30–33% during colloid therapy without having a negative effect on oxygen delivery, which may be reduced during haemodilution (Muizelaar and Schroder, 1994).

Hydration and nutrition

Generally, patients with a severe head injury require about 80% of their normal fluid requirements in order to ensure adequate hydration but not to the point of precipitating cerebral oedema. Therefore, a fluid intake of about 100–125 ml/hr is advocated (Oh, 1997). Sodium chloride 0.9% is the intravenous fluid of choice to ensure extracellular electrolytes are replaced rather than causing cellular rehydration, as is seen with the use of dextrose-containing solutions (Hudak et al, 1998). The dextrose-containing solutions contain free water, which then can exacerbate cerebral oedema (Oh, 1997). Enteral nutrition, if the patient is unable to eat normally, should be commenced as soon as possible so that nutritional requirements are met. This is supported by the findings of a systematic review of nutrition after head injury in which early enteral nutrition was associated with better patient survival and outcome (Yanagawa et al, 2004). However, in any patient with head trauma an orogastric rather than a nasogastric tube should be used so that passage of the tube into the brain via a base of skull fracture is avoided (Greaves et al, 2001).

Blood glucose should be maintained within normal limits (Wong, 2000) as it is metabolized to carbon dioxide and water, and an excess of these could increase ICP as cerebral oedema will worsen (Woodrow, 2000). Additionally, normal electrolyte levels should be maintained, especially sodium. A slightly elevated sodium (for example 147 mmol/l) is acceptable, but hypernatraemia is associated with dehydration and sluggish CBF, whereas hyponatraemia is associated with overhydration and cerebral oedema — both of these situations should be avoided (Hickey, 2002).

Excretion

A normal urine output greater than 0.5 ml/kg/hr should be maintained as this demonstrates normal renal function (Oh, 1997). Patients with a traumatic head injury may develop neuroendocrine disorders as a consequence of the head injury. Therefore, diabetes insipidus (DI) may be observed, which can result from damage to the hypothalamus, which controls the pituitary gland (Hickey, 2002). Normally, the posterior lobe of the pituitary secretes antidiuretic hormone (ADH) in response to osmotic stimuli. However, in DI, ADH is not released and therefore large volumes of dilute urine are passed (*Table 10.1*).

If left untreated, the patient can become dehydrated rapidly, and sodium levels can become elevated. This can lead to sluggish CBF and a risk of ischaemia. DI is treated by administering desmopressin, which is an analogue of ADH, thereby promoting the reabsorption of water in the collecting duct of the renal tubules (Oh, 1997).

Constipation should be avoided as the increase in intra-abdominal pressure can increase ICP because the raised intra-abdominal pressure increases intrathoracic pressure, which in turn increases ICP (Hickey, 2002). Straining at a stool will also increase ICP (Hickey, 2002). Stool softeners should be administered to prevent constipation and to avoid the use of enemas, which may increase intra-abdominal pressure (and therefore ICP) (Hickey, 2002).

Table 10.1: Diabetes insipidus

- Urine output >3 ml/kg for 2 hours
- Hypotonic urine (specific gravity 1000–1005)
- Urine osmolality inappropriately low compared with serum osmolality

From Oh (1997)

Temperature regulation

Hyperthermia in patients with a severe head injury has been shown to increase the cerebral metabolic rate, thereby increasing the demands of the brain for oxygen and glucose (Hickey, 2002). This increases the cerebral blood volume and hence ICP (Johnson, 1999). Studies into the benefits of induced hypothermia have been inconclusive so this cannot be recommended, but active warming should be discouraged (Sutcliffe, 2001).

Hyperpyrexias should be controlled with antipyretic agents, such as paracetamol, which 'reset' the hypothalamus and thus induce normal physiological cooling (such as sweating) (Johnson, 1999) and passive cooling methods, such as tepid sponging, which can promote heat conduction in hyperthermia (Johnson, 1999). Price et al (2003b) compared various methods of cooling, such as paracetamol, ice packs and cooling blankets. Their findings were inconclusive, but they did conclude that paracetamol might be of use in managing hyperpyrexia in patients with an intact thermoregulatory response. One risk of cooling patients is that they may shiver — this should be avoided as it generates more heat and increases the metabolic rate, thereby potentially increasing ICP (Johnson, 1999).

Positioning and mobility

An essential component of ICP management is to promote cerebral venous drainage. Therefore, head and neck alignment should be maintained (Williams and Coyne, 1993), and it may be of benefit to elevate patients' heads by 30° (Hickey, 2002). This could decrease the patient's MAP and, therefore, CPP.

Increases in intra-abdominal pressure can also increase ICP, so it is recommended that patients' legs are not bent more than an angle of 90° at the hip when they are lying on their side (Hickey, 2002). Additionally, optimal sedation/analgesia during repositioning can prevent a rise in ICP (Hickey, 2002).

In view of passive movements, changes in ICP during passive limb exercises seem to be small (Price et al, 2003a). Studies have found no significant rise in ICP during limb movements (Koch et al, 1996; Brimioulle et al, 1997). However, it is unclear whether there is a cumulative effect if movements are performed at the same time as other activities, and it is unclear whether passive limb exercises have a therapeutic benefit (Halbertsma et al, 1999).

Communication and the environment

Communication and environmental stimuli have both been shown to alter ICP and may be a positive influence (Price et al, 2003a). Common stressors, such as excessive noise, painful procedures, unnecessary lighting and an unfamiliar environment, can all increase ICP (Chudley, 1994; Hall, 1997; Jastremski, 1998), but the impact of these can be minimized by nurses recognizing the negative effect and controlling these environmental factors, including pain. Relatives/loved ones can also influence ICP, with some evidence suggesting that they reduce ICP (Hendrickson, 1987; Allan, 1989; Chudley, 1994). However, in a small study (*n*=12), Treloar et al (1991) found that there was no statistical significance between familiar and unfamiliar voices on the ICP of comatose patients. Walleck (1983) found that stroking patients' cheeks reduced their ICP (25 out of 30 patients), but their ICP did not change when their hands were touched. This may indicate that patients, even when comatose, respond to a sense of comfort and reassurance.

Nursing interventions

The timing and frequency of nursing interventions have been shown to influence ICP (Hickey, 2002). There is no consensus as to whether nursing activities should be clustered together or spread over a period of time; however, there is agreement that response to nursing interventions should be assessed on an individual patient basis, with the aim of avoiding prolonged increases in ICP (Hickey, 2002).

Spinal injuries

The aim of care in the management of patients who have sustained a spinal injury is to control the development of secondary damage, to optimize stability of the spinal cord and to commence rehabilitation as soon as possible (Grundy and Swain, 2002). Much of the care required by the patient with a spinal injury is supportive in nature; therefore, complications need to be identified and managed accordingly (Hickey, 2002). If possible, the patient should be referred to a specialist spinal centre as early as possible for specialist nursing and multidisciplinary team input (Grundy and Swain, 2002). If the patient has to wait for a bed, the referring hospital should commence establishing the specialist centre's protocols and regimens, especially in relation to bowel and bladder management.

Immobilization

The cervical spine is the most mobile part of the spinal column, and immobilization of this area is essential for any patient who has been involved in, for example, a road traffic accident (Greaves et al, 2001). Immobilization of the cervical spine is crucial in any patient where a neck injury is suspected, to help prevent any further damage to the cervical spine through movement. Cervical spine immobilization can be achieved through the use of a rigid cervical collar, and sand bags can be placed on either side of the head (Chiles and Cooper, 1996). The thoracic spine has considerable intrinsic stability because of the rib cage and limited mobility of this area. However, the thoracolumbar junction (T11–L2) is a point of mobility and is the second most common site of spinal injury (Chiles and Cooper, 1996). Injuries to this area of the spinal column should be considered as being unstable, with patients at risk of further damage to the spinal cord.

Logrolling, which is turning the patient in complete alignment, helps to prevent further damage to the spinal cord, irrespective of what anatomical level is at risk,by helping to prevent flexion or extension of the spine (Grundy and Swain, 2002). It requires four people to perform the turn and usually a fifth to, for example, inspect the back/change sheets (*Table 10.2*; *Figure 10.6*).

Table 10.2: Positions in log rolling

1st person/ team leader	Maintains head–neck alignment Coordinates turn
2nd person	Holds the patient's shoulder with one hand and places the other on the patient's waist/pelvis
3rd person	Holds pelvis with one hand and places the other under the patient's opposite thigh
4th person	Places both arms under the patient's opposite lower leg and supports it during the turn
5th person	Examines/washes back/changes sheet

From Greaves et al (2001)

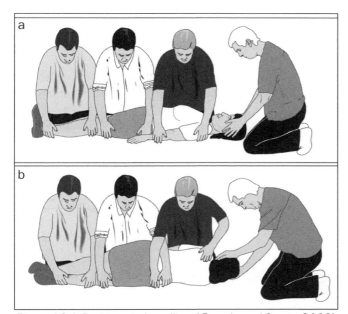

Figure 10.6: Positions in logrolling (Grundy and Swain, 2002)

The staff member who has responsibility to maintain the inline stabilization of the head and neck acts as the team leader and coordinates the roll. With logrolling, it is essential that clear instructions are given and everyone is aware of their role so that the logroll is performed smoothly and safely in a coordinated manoeuvre (Hickey, 2002).

Patients with an unstable spinal injury should be nursed on a specialized spinal bed (Hickey, 2002). If this is not available, a normal bed can be used but the mattress must be firm and not a pressure-relieving mattress that uses fluctuating pressure in air sacs. These mattresses can cause instability in the spinal cord because of differing pressures and support being placed through the spine (Zejdlik, 1992).

Stabilization of the spine can either be achieved through conservative management or surgical intervention (Grundy and Swain, 2002). Conservative management usually consists of bedrest for a period of time, enabling the vertebral column to heal.

Cervical spine

Patients with cervical spine injuries may initially need spinal traction to reduce any fractures or dislocations, to relieve pressure on the spinal cord and to splint the spine. This may require skull callipers and weights, which are gradually reduced. A neck roll should be placed under the neck to maintain normal lordosis, or curvature, of the spine (Grundy and Swain, 2002). Pressure ulcers on the patient's occipital region can develop, so this area needs to be cushioned when the patient is positioned. Skull traction will be needed for at least 6 weeks if surgery is not performed (Grundy and Swain, 2002). The decision about when to operate will depend on the available expertise and facilities, but this may be undertaken in the district general hospital rather than in a spinal injuries unit.

Neck stability is assessed with frequent X-rays, and at 6 weeks will show whether there is any bony union if fractures were sustained. Once stability has been achieved, the patient can gradually start to sit up with the use of a hard cervical collar, such as a Miami or Philadelphia collar. Patients with high cervical injuries may have postural hypotension when first mobilized, and this is owing to alterations in their autonomic nervous system function (Grundy and Swain, 2002). The use of anti-embolic stockings and an abdominal binder can help to prevent pooling of blood.

Halo traction, which is a form of skull traction, can be used as an alternative to skull callipers once any fractures or dislocations have been reduced. It provides stability and allows for earlier mobilization. It will need to be in place for approximately 12 weeks (Grundy and Swain, 2002).

Thoracic injuries

The thoracic spine is relatively stable because of the articulation with the ribcage. The majority of patients who have a thoracic spinal cord injury are managed conservatively by 6–8 weeks of bedrest (Grundy and Swain, 2002).

Thoracolumbar and lumbar injuries

Patients with a thoracolumbar injury are generally managed conservatively with 6–8 weeks' bedrest, after which mobilization can commence with the use of a spinal brace (Grundy and Swain, 2002). During the period of bedrest, normal spinal curvature needs to be maintained through placing a pillow under the lumbar spine (*Figure 10.7*).

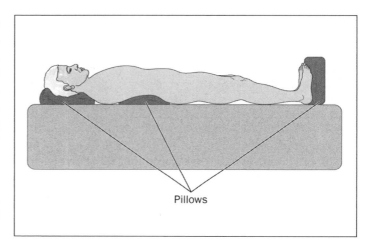

Pillows

Figure 10.7: Support for patients with a thoracolumbar spinal injury (Grundy and Swain, 2002)

Pharmacological treatment

Within 8 hours of the injury, high-dose methyl-prednisolone should be administered, which has been found to improve maximal motor function over the long term (Bracken et al, 1992). If this is not started within 8 hours, administering steroids over an extended period of 48 hours may be of benefit (Bracken et al, 1997). The regimen is:

- 30 mg/kg bolus over 15 minutes immediately
- 5.4 mg/kg/hr over 23 hours (commenced 45 minutes after initial bolus) (Greaves et al, 2001).

Respiratory system

Patients with a cervical spine injury involving C1–4 will require intubation and mechanical ventilation, as the nerve impulses to the respiratory muscles will be affected by the injury (Hudak et al, 1998). These patients should also have early tracheostomy placement, as it is likely that they will require mechanical ventilatory support permanently (Hudak et al, 1998). Patients who have a spinal injury at C5–7 may develop respiratory insufficiency as spinal oedema increases (Hudak et al, 1998). The requirement for mechanical ventilation in these patients can be assessed by measuring vital capacity, which is an indicator of respiratory muscle strength. Generally, this will deteriorate before arterial blood gas alterations, and a vital capacity of <15–20 ml/kg would normally indicate the need for mechanical ventilatory support (Greaves et al, 2001).

Complications associated with poor respiratory function, such as chest infections and lobar collapse, need to be avoided as they will worsen an already poor gas exchange (Hickey, 2002). Judicious chest care needs to be performed and chest infections treated. This will require close coordination of the multidisciplinary team and patient education regarding assisted coughing (Grundy and Swain, 2002). Assisted cough is when a nurse or carer supports the diaphragm during coughing in order to elicit a stronger cough. Additionally, clinical signs of a chest infection need to be assessed, including respiratory rate, oxygen saturations and chest auscultation.

Cardiovascular system

After a spinal injury, neurogenic shock can develop. Injuries at or above T6 are associated with loss of sympathetic autonomic outflow (Greaves et al, 2001). Therefore, vasomotor tone is reduced and sympathetic innervation of the heart can be reduced if the spinal injury is high enough. The reduction in vasomotor tone results in profound hypotension because of peripheral vasodilation, and the loss of sympathetic innervation to the heart leads to significant bradycardia (Hudak et al, 1998). The onset of neurogenic shock can be minutes or several hours after the injury occurred.

Management of neurogenic shock is aimed at re-establishing vasomotor tone until the shock resolves. This normally requires the use of vasopressors, such as noradrenaline (Oh, 1997). Bradycardias can be treated with, for example, isoprenaline (Hudak et al, 1998). Careful fluid management is required as pulmonary oedema could be precipitated if large volumes of fluids have been used once vasomotor tone returns (Oh, 1997).

Autonomic dysreflexia

This is a serious potential complication that all patients with an injury that is at T6 or above may experience. It is created by an abrupt and excessive discharge from the sympathetic nervous system, leading to hypertension, cardiac rhythm changes, severe headache and profuse sweating (Gardner and Kluger, 2004), as well as flushing or blotchiness of the skin above the level of the injury (Grundy and Swain, 2002). It can be caused by any stimulus arising from below the level of the injury, including constipation, a blocked urethral catheter, ingrowing toenails and pressure ulcers. Management of autonomic dysreflexia includes identification and removal of the cause, sitting the patient upright and administering vasodilators such as sublingual nifedipine and glyceryl trinitrate (Gardner and Kluger, 2004). As the patient will not be able to feel the stimulus (such as a distended bladder), patient and family education will need to be provided so that they recognize the symptoms of this potentially dangerous situation.

Neurological status

In complete spinal injury, assessment of level of sensation needs to be performed, as this will provide information as to the level of the spinal cord at which the injury has occurred. In incomplete injury, motor and sensory function need to be assessed in order to ascertain the level of injury and the type of injury that has been sustained (Hickey, 2002) (*Table 10.3*).

Table 10.3: Segmental values for dermatomes and myotomes

Segment	Dermatome	Myotomes
C5	Sensation over deltoid	Deltoid muscle
C6	Sensation over thumb	Wrist extensors
C7	Sensation over middle finger	Elbow extensors
C8	Sensation over little finger	Middle finger flexors
T1	Sensation over inner aspect of elbow	Little finger abduction
T4	Sensation around nipple	
T8	Sensation over xiphisternum	
T10	Sensation around umbilicus	
T12	Sensation around symphysis	
L1	Sensation in inguinal area	
L2	Sensation anterior upper thigh	Hip flexors
L3	Sensation anterior mid-thigh	Knee extensors
L4	Sensation on medial aspect leg	Ankle dorsiflexors
L5	Sensation between 1st and 2nd toes	Long toe extensors
S1	Sensation on lateral border of foot	Ankle plantar flexors
S3	Sensation over ischial tuberosity	
S4/5	Sensation around perineum	

Dermatome=sensory level; myotome=motor function
From Greaves et al (2001)

Ongoing assessment is important as function may return as oedema resolves, or if oedema ascends up the spinal cord then levels could change. This is especially important in the C5–7 level injuries, when ascending oedema could create respiratory difficulties (Oh, 1997).

Spinal shock can occur after a spinal cord injury and is viewed as the complete loss of all neurological function, including reflexes, rectal tone and autonomic control, below the level of the injury. However, it is unrelated to neurogenic shock or other forms of shock. The complete loss of function usually lasts for about 24–72 hours; however, despite the profound paralysis that occurs in this stage, compete recovery is possible. Until spinal shock resolves, complete and incomplete injury cannot be determined (Greaves et al, 2001).

Nutrition

After acute spinal cord injury, support may be required to maintain nutritional status. A nutritional risk assessment should be performed with the dietitian (Grundy and Swain, 2002). If necessary, nasogastric feeds should be commenced once bowel sounds are heard in all four quadrants of the abdomen. There is a risk of paralytic ileus after a spinal cord injury, which may be slow to resolve, so total parenteral nutrition may be required (Hickey, 2002). Initially, the nasogastric tube may need to be on free drainage to decompress the stomach, thereby avoiding respiratory compromise because of gastric distension (Chiles and Cooper, 1996). There is a potential risk of regurgitation and aspiration of enteral nutrition while on flat bedrest, which can be minimized with gently tilting the bed after agreement by medical staff. Once able, an oral diet should be encouraged. Feeding aides may be required depending on the level of the injury and motor function.

Bladder function

Bladder dysfunction may occur after a spinal injury. During the spinal shock phase, an indwelling catheter will be required to ensure bladder emptying. Once the spinal shock phase has resolved and the level of injury has been determined, bladder management depends on the level of injury.

In injury above L1, the patient may have a hyperreflexic (or spastic) bladder (*Figure 10.8*), and this occurs because the level of the injury is above the reflex voiding centre in the sacral portion of the spinal cord (Zejdlik, 1992). Both motor and sensory function are damaged, resulting in a loss of sensation to void and a loss of voluntary control over the voiding centre. Therefore, patients with hyperreflexic bladders are unaware of the normal sensation of fullness and cannot control voiding. When the bladder becomes full, the stretch receptors in the muscle wall of the bladder become stimulated and a simple reflex arc results, causing an uncontrolled contraction of the bladder (Zejdlik, 1992).

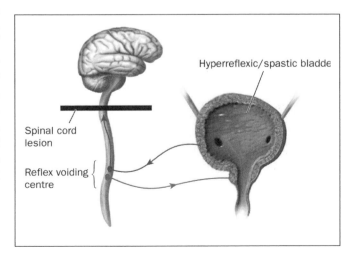

Figure 10.8: Hyperreflexic bladder (Zejdlik, 1992)

Where the injury is below L2 (*Figure 10.9*), the bladder is areflexic because the injury to the sacral portion of the spinal cord damages the voiding reflex centre itself (Zejdlik, 1992). The interruption in the sensory stimulation and motor reflex arcs at this spinal cord level breaks the communication pathways with the intact sensory and motor tracts above the level of the injury (Zejdlik, 1992). This results in diminished reflex activity and bladder tone. The patient will be unaware of the normal sensation of bladder fullness and is unable to initiate emptying of the bladder, and thus it becomes overdistended (Zejdlik, 1992).

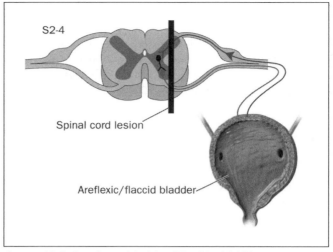

Figure 10.9: A reflexic bladder (Zejdlik, 1992)

Bladder management

Alteration in bladder control is probably one of the most disruptive problems a person with a spinal cord injury will face. The maintenance of bladder emptying is a major nursing responsibility, requiring a combination of knowledge, skill and patience in order to ensure individualized, tailormade programmes (Zejdlik, 1992). Assessment of voiding patterns must initially be undertaken. Any voluntary control of voiding must be observed for and documented, as well as any awareness that the patient has of sensation of fullness or spontaneous voiding. This may not be a simple lower abdominal sensation of pressure but, for example, the quadriplegic patient may perspire more when his/her bladder is full (Zejdlik, 1992). Bladder management also requires an assessment of functional ability, such as hand motor function, as well as patient cooperation. Successful implementation will require patient motivation, responsibility and receptiveness (Zejdlik, 1992).

An indwelling catheter is almost always necessary during at least the first 12 hours after injury, and it may be required for a longer period to monitor the seriously ill patient through the acute phase (Grundy and Swain, 2002). However, the method of choice, and the desired aim in patients with neurogenic bladder dysfunction, is intermittent catheterization (Zejdlik, 1992). The underlying principle is to empty the bladder at regular intervals with the use of a non-retaining urethral catheter, thereby avoiding overdistension and the complications associated with this, such as ascending infections, which can cause kidney damage (Hudak et al, 1998). If the patient has the motor abilities, intermittent self-catheterization can be taught.

In conjunction with intermittent catheterization, manual techniques to elicit bladder emptying can be used. Intermittent catheterization facilitates this by allowing filling and emptying of the bladder, thereby stimulating any existing spinal cord reflexes and also maintaining bladder tone (Zejdlik, 1992). Manual techniques are trigger voiding, straining to void and manual expression (or Credé manoeuvre).

Trigger voiding

After a trigger response, the detrusor muscle of the bladder contracts through a spasm or reflex, expelling urine and emptying the bladder. This can be useful as the reflex contractions that can occur when the bladder is full do not usually empty the bladder completely; therefore, by creating an additional trigger, the voiding contraction is augmented (Zejdlik, 1992). However, this technique can only be used if the reflex arcs to the sacral voiding centre are intact. Trigger stimuli include firmly tapping, stroking or pinching the abdomen and inner thigh (Zejdlik, 1992).

Straining to void

Using a Valsalva manoeuvre can help with bladder emptying. This technique requires strong abdominal muscles, and the level of injury needs to be below T6–12 as it is at these levels that the abdominal muscles are innervated. This technique can be useful in patients with an areflexic bladder (Zejdlik, 1992).

Manual expression (Credé manoeuvre)

This involves the application of external pressure over and around the bladder, aiming to increase the pressure within the bladder and, therefore, overcoming the resistance of the bladder neck and urinary sphincters. This technique is only used in a flaccid bladder and when voiding cystourethrography (which visualizes the voiding cycle through fluoroscopy) confirms the absence of ureterovesical reflex (Zejdlik, 1992). It should be used with caution as it can increase the risk of hernias and haemorrhoids, and if undertaken in patients with a hyperreflexic bladder can cause reflux, thereby increasing the risk of infection (Zejdlik, 1992).

Despite various techniques and management programmes, an unbalanced bladder with high residual volume may persist, leading to a constant, dribbling incontinence or an inability to completely empty the bladder (Zejdlik, 1992). These types of symptoms are caused by bladder and sphincter dysfunctions occurring at the same time and, for the patient with a spastic bladder, detrusor–sphincter dyssynergia can create major difficulties in bladder management. The detrusor muscle and the external urethral sphincter contract at the same time, leading to obstructed urine flow (Zejdlik, 1992). Anticholinergic drugs, such as oxybutynin, may be of help as these inhibit bladder contractility (Grundy and Swain, 2002). In some patients, surgical intervention, such as sphincterectomy, may be required to relieve the symptoms, especially in view of bladder neck obstruction (Grundy and Swain, 2002).

Bowel function

As with bladder function, independent bowel function after a spinal cord injury can be difficult, and bowel management must commence from the day of admission. During the spinal shock phase, stool softeners should be commenced and either daily or alternate day suppositories should be given (Zejdlik, 1992). An accurate bowel chart must be established to document clearly the effectiveness of the bowel regimen. Once spinal shock has resolved, then the level of the injury will influence bowel management.

Where the injury is above T12, the reflex defaecation centre, which is in the sacral portion of the spinal cord, is intact (Zejdlik, 1992). Reflex activity is uninhibited but ascending sensory signals are interrupted. Thus the patient is unable to feel the normal sensation or urge to defaecate. However, descending motor signals are also blocked and so normal control of the external anal sphincter activity is also blocked. Therefore, the patient has a spastic bowel with contraction of the anal sphincter (Zejdlik, 1992). If the injury is below L1, the reflex defaecation centre is directly damaged, leading to a flaccid bowel (Zejdlik, 1992). Even though intrinsic contractile responses remain, there are ineffective peristaltic actions because of the diminished spinal reflex. Also, the patient loses the normal sensation to defaecate and cannot voluntarily control the external anal sphincter (Zejdlik, 1992).

Bowel management

In the early days after spinal cord injury, it is a nursing responsibility to maintain bowel elimination, and an effective bowel-management programme should be established (Coggrave, 2004). However, loss of control over bowel function can be distressing and upsetting for the patient. Success of the programme will need patient cooperation, and the aim of the programme is to ensure a planned, predictable bowel movement (Zejdlik, 1992). This then should avoid both incontinence and constipation. The following strategies can be used to achieve this aim.

Diet

High-fibre foods, such as fruit and vegetables, should be encouraged, with additional fibre taken if necessary (Coggrave, 2004). High-fibre diets can contribute to abdominal distension because of fermentation of food, which may be uncomfortable.

Fluids

A fluid intake of 2000–3000 ml/day is necessary to keep stools soft (Zejdlik, 1992) and helps to avoid cramping constipation when high-fibre and/or stool softeners or bulking agents are used.

Exercise and activity

This should be within the patient's functional ability but, even when on bedrest, passive movements can help to prevent sluggish bowel activity, which can lead to constipation (Zejdlik, 1992). Once the patient is in a wheelchair, encouraging him or her to participate in dressing, feeding or pushing the wheelchair will also help to promote bowel function as well as rehabilitation.

Increasing abdominal pressure

Patients who have strong abdominal muscles can perform the Valsalva manoeuvre to evacuate their bowel. Leaning forward also increases intra-abdominal pressure and may help (Zejdlik, 1992).

Abdominal massage

This is thought to stimulate the colon to push faeces into the rectum. It can be used as an adjunct to other techniques to assist in bowel evacuation, such as suppositories, anorectal digital stimulation or manual evacuation (Coggrave, 2004).

Oral laxatives

These are not required for all spinal-injured patients and should not be viewed as an essential part of their bowel programme, even if required during the acute phase (Coggrave, 2004). Laxatives may have undesired side-effects, such as cramping, flatulence, loose stools and dehydration (Coggrave, 2004). If used, a response may not be seen until 24 hours later because of the reduced bowel activity (Zejdlik, 1992).

Stimulation techniques

These are used in the patient with a spastic bowel. In this situation, digital stimulation is required. However, initially a glycerine suppository can be administered; this may have the effect of lubrication and stimulation of reflex bowel activity. If no stool is evacuated after this, anorectal digital stimulation can be used, which encourages the anal sphincter to relax and thus the stool to be passed (Zejdlik, 1992).

Manual evacuation

A patient with a flaccid bowel will require manual evacuation to remove the stool, especially if other techniques, such as bearing down and leaning forward, have been unsuccessful (Coggrave, 2004). A suppository, such as bisacodyl, that will stimulate the colon to empty the stool into the rectum may be useful (Zejdlik, 1992).

Privacy is paramount throughout and, whenever possible, normal toileting facilities should be used as this will aid bearing down (Coggrave, 2004).

Pressure areas

Pressure ulcers are among the most common complications in patients with a spinal injury (Hickey, 2002). This patient group will be unable to relieve their pressure areas independently, and because of sensory abnormalities may not be able to feel pain in these areas. Therefore, meticulous pressure area care is a priority of therapy, and patient education around maintaining intact skin should commence as soon as possible. In this way, patients take a responsibility within their care. To help facilitate pressure area care, a turning clock can be used, which divides the day into 2-hour periods and indicates what position the patient should be in at any given time (Zejdlik, 1992). An electric spinal bed may be useful, particularly in heavy patients or those with multiple injuries (Grundy and Swain, 2002). This allows the patient to be turned at small increments such as 10–20° at a given time period. Careful alignment must be maintained at all times, and logrolling will still be required for examination of pressure areas and for bowel care.

Care of the joints

The joints must be passively moved through a full range of movement to prevent stiffness and contractures. This is essential, so that joints that may recover function remain functional, thereby enabling rehabilitation (Grundy and Swain, 2002). Splints for the hands are particularly important to maintain the hand in a functional position, while ankle splints can help to avoid foot drop and shortening of the Achilles tendon (Grundy and Swain, 2002). Once any recovery of limb function has occurred, participation in daily activities should be encouraged.

Psychosocial care

Patients with spinal injury will experience a number of emotional responses as they pass through the initial injury phase and commence rehabilitation (Hickey, 2002). Sensory deprivation is a major concern for these patients. They will not have normal sensory input from their body, which means that they have visual, auditory and tactile sensory deprivation (Hickey, 2002). Confinement to bed, which is usually kept flat or slightly sloping upwards, means that patients will not be able to see around them and will normally only have the ceiling within their visual range. Sound may be distorted by traction and the machinery around them. Therefore, the patient can feel isolated and socially deprived (Hickey, 2002).

Nursing interactions, such as providing bed mirrors and reading tables, may help to avoid the sensory deprivation these patients may experience. Additionally, the provision of a radio or television can be beneficial.

Patients' self-concept will have been altered and their social position threatened. They will be aware that they may never be able to function independently in the future, and if they are the main wage earner in the family they will be worried and concerned about finances (Zejdlik, 1992). If patients are young, they are likely to be anxious and worried about their development as a functional person within society as well as having their plans for their future development as an adult curtailed.

Therefore, many patients with a spinal injury will go through the steps of the grieving process in their path to accepting their injury:

- Denial
- Anger
- Bargaining
- Depression
- Acceptance (Kubler-Ross, 1969).

Nurses will be required to support them through this and provide information as required. The psychological rehabilitation of the patient is as important as the physical rehabilitation, as it is by accepting the change that has resulted from the injury that patients can take hold of their life and take responsibility for it themselves (Zejdlik, 1992).

Conclusion

The nurse caring for the patient with a traumatic neurological injury will face a challenge to ensure the best possible outcome for the patient. The aim of care is to minimize the impact of factors that can cause secondary injury and, therefore, prevent ischaemia from occurring. However, the impact of the primary injury cannot be removed and it is this, especially in spinal injuries, that will greatly influence the patient's future prospects. The care of this patient group requires insight and skill in the management of physiological systems, but the psychosocial aspects are as important, especially in the acceptance and future circumstances of both the patient and his or her family and loved ones.

References

Adam S, Osbourne S (1997) *Critical Care Nursing: Science and Practice*. Oxford Medical, Bath

Allan D (1989) Intracranial pressure monitoring: a study of nursing practice. *J Adv Nurs* **14:** 127–31

Bracken MB, Shepard MJ, Collins WF (1992) Methylprednisolone or naloxone treatment after acute spinal cord injury: 1-year follow-up data. Results of the second National Acute Spinal Cord Injury Study. *J Neurosurg* **76**(1): 23–31

Bracken MB, Shepard MJ, Holford TR (1997) Administration of methylprednisolone for 24 or 48 hours or tirilazad mesylate for 48 hours in the treatment of acute spinal cord injury. Results of the third National Acute Spinal Cord Injury randomized controlled trial. *JAMA* **277:** 1597–604

Brimioulle S, Moraine J, Norrenberg D, Kahn R (1997) Effects of positioning and exercise on intracranial pressure in a neurosurgical intensive care unit. *Phys Ther* **77:** 1682–9

Brinker T, Seifert V, Dietz V (1992) Cerebral blood flow and intracranial pressure during experimental subarachnoid haemorrhage. *Acta Neurochir (Wien)* **115**(1–2): 47–52

Chiles B, Cooper P (1996) Current concepts: acute spinal injury. *N Engl J Med* **334:** 514–20

Chudley S (1994) The effect of nursing activities on intracranial pressure. *Br J Nurs* **3:** 454–9

Coggrave M (2004) Effective bowel management for patients after spinal cord injury. *Nurs Times* **100**(20): 48–51

Cruz J, Raps EC, Hoffstead OJ, Jaggi JL, Gennarelli TA (1993) Cerebral oxygenation monitoring. *Crit Care Med* **21:** 1242–6

Eisenhart K (1994) New perspectives in the management of adults with severe head injury. *Crit Care Nurs Q* **17**(2): 1–12

Fisher M (1997) Paediatric traumatic brain injury. *Crit Care Nurs Q* **20**(1): 36–51

Gardner B, Kluger PJ (2004) Mini-symposium: spinal trauma (iv). The overall care of the spinal cord injured patient. *Curr Orthop* **18**(1): 33–48

Greaves I, Porter K, Ryan J (2001) *Trauma Care Manual*. Arnold, London

Grundy D, Swain A (2002) *ABC of Spinal Care Injury*. 4th edn. BMJ Books, London

Halbertsma J, Mulder I, Geken L, Eisma W (1999) Repeated passive stretching: acute effect on the passive muscle movement and extensibility of short hamstrings. *Arch Phys Med Rehabil* **80:** 407–14

Hall C (1997) Patient management in head injury care: a nursing perspective. *Intensive Crit Care Nurs* **13:** 329–37

Hendrickson S (1987) Intracranial pressure changes and family presence. *J Neurosci Nurs* **19:** 14–17

Hickey J (2002) *The Clinical Practice of Neurological and Neurosurgical Nursing*. 5th edn. Lippincott, Philadelphia

Hillman K, Bishop G (1996) *Clinical Intensive Care*. Cambridge University Press, Cambridge

Hudak CM, Gallo BM, Gonce Morton P (1998) *Critical Care Nursing: A Holistic Approach*. 7th edn. Lippincott, Philadelphia

Jastremski C (1998) Head injuries. *RN* **60**(12): 40–6

Johnson L (1999) Factors known to raise intracranial pressure and the associated implications for nursing management. *Nurs Crit Care* **4**(3): 117–20

Koch S, Fogarty S, Signorino C, Parmley L, Mehlhorn U (1996) Effects of passive range of motion on intracranial pressure in neurosurgical patients. *J Crit Care* **11**(4): 176–9

Kubler-Ross E (1969) *Death and Dying*. Macmillan, New York

Lindsay KW, Bone I, Callender R (1998) *Neurology and Neurosurgery Illustrated*. 3rd edn. Churchill Livingstone, London

Muizelaar JP, Schroder ML (1994) Overview of monitoring of cerebral blood flow and metabolism after head injury. *Can J Neurol Sci* **21**(2): S6–S11

Oh TE (1997) *Intensive Care Manual*. Butterworth Heinemann, Oxford

Parsons LC, Shogan JS (1984) The effects of endotracheal tube suctioning/ manual hyperinflation procedure on patients with severe closed head injuries. *Heart Lung* **13**: 372–80

Porth CM (2003) *Essentials of Pathophysiology: Concepts of Altered Health States*. Lippincott, Williams and Wilkins, Philadelphia

Prendergast V (1994) Current trends in research and treatment of intracranial hypertension. *Crit Care Nurs Q* **17**(1): 1–8

Price A, Collins TJ, Gallagher A (2003a) Nursing care of the acute head injury: a review of the evidence. *Nurs Crit Care* **8**: 126–33

Price T, McGloin S, Izzard J, Gilchrist M (2003b) Cooling strategies for patients with severe cerebral insult in ITU (part 2). *Nurs Crit Care* **8**: 37–45

Sutcliffe AJ (2001) Hypothermia (or not) for the management of head injury. *Care of the Critically Ill* **17**: 162–5

Teasdale G, Jennett B (1974) Assessment of coma and impaired consciousness. A practical scale. *Lancet* **2**: 81–4

Treloar D, Nalli B, Guin P, Gary R (1991) The effect of familiar and unfamiliar voices on ICP. *J Neurosci Nurs* **23**: 295–9

Vander AJ, Sherman JH, Luciano DS (2000) *Human Physiology: The Mechanisms of Body Function*. 7th edn. McGraw-Hill, London

Vos HR (1993) Making headway with intracranial hypertension. *Am J Nurs* **93**(2): 28–35, 37–9

Walleck C (1983) The effects of purposeful touch on ICP. *Heart Lung* **12**: 428–9

Williams A, Coyne S (1993) Effects of neck position on intracranial pressure. *Am J Crit Care* **2**(1): 68–71

Wong F (2000) Prevention of secondary brain injury. *Crit Care Nurs* **20**(5): 18–27

Woodrow P (2000) *Intensive Care Nursing: A Framework for Practice*. Routledge, London

Wright M (1999) Resuscitation of the multitrauma patient with a head injury. *AACN Clin Issues* **10**(1): 32–45

Yanagawa T, Bunn F, Roberts I, Wentz R, Pierro A (2004) Nutritional support for head-injured patients (Cochrane Review). In: *The Cochrane Library*, Issue 2. John Wiley and Sons, Chichester

Yoshihara M, Bandoh K, Marmarou A (1995) Cerebrovascular carbon dioxide reactivity assessed by intracranial pressure dynamics in severely head injured patients. *J Neurosurg* **82**: 386–93

Young JS, Meredith JW (1995) Does oxygen delivery-directed resuscitation worsen outcome of head injured patients with multisystem injuries? *Am Surg* **61**: 419–23

Zejdlik CP (1992) *Management of Spinal Cord Injury*. 2nd edn. Jones and Bartlett, Boston

Chapter 11

Multiprofessional follow up of patients after subarachnoid haemorrhage

Anne Jarvis, Louise Talbot

Approximately one in 10 000 people in Britain will experience subarachnoid haemorrhage (SAH) (Lindsay and Bone, 1997). It is a life-threatening illness and people are struck down by it suddenly and without warning. In SAH, bleeding occurs from the system of cerebral arteries called the Circle of Willis, which runs through the subarachnoid space (*Figure 11.1*). This space is normally filled with cerebrospinal fluid (CSF). Aneurysms form on the cerebral arteries, usually at the point where they branch off, and when they rupture this causes SAH (*Figure 11.2*). Seventy-five per cent of cases of SAH will be caused by an aneurysm of the cerebral circulation (Bonita and Thomson, 1985).

Little is known of the reason for aneurysm formation, although it is known that approximately 2% of the general population have cerebral aneurysms that never cause a problem during their lifetime (Fox, 1983). Aneurysm rupture is influenced by four factors:

- High cholesterol levels
- Hypertension
- Excess alcohol intake
- Smoking (Teunissen et al, 1996).

There are no particular groups that are more at risk of SAH; the risk of one in 10 000 applies to the general population regardless of background, race or other differences.

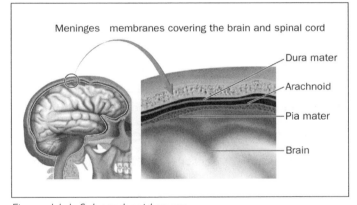

Figure 11.1: Subarachnoid space

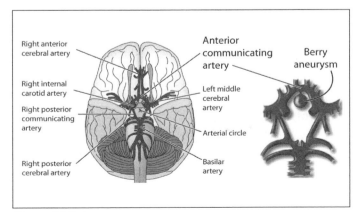

Figure 11.2: Aneurysm

This illness carries a high chance of mortality. Out of 100 people suffering SAH from a ruptured aneurysm, only around 25% would survive beyond 2 years if no treatment were sought (Lindsay and Bone, 1997). Consequently, a large proportion of patients in the acute stage of the illness are nursed in either intensive care or high-dependency environments. Neurosurgical nurses are required to observe patients closely for complications specific to SAH, such as re-bleed, delayed cerebral ischaemia and hydrocephalus (Rees et al, 2002).

It is estimated that only 7% (around 10 people discharged from the authors' specialist unit per year) of survivors suffer physical deficit (Stegan and Freckmann, 1991) whereas, disturbingly, around two-thirds of those sufferers classed as having made a good recovery actually experience a range of debilitating cognitive or emotional difficulties (Bindschaedler et al, 1997; Buchanan et al, 2000) such as fatigue, anxiety and even memory impairment. It seems that a good recovery is generally accepted to be one where the patient is deemed 'grade one' on the World Federation of Neurological Surgeons' Grading Scale at outcome/discharge (*Table 11.1*; World Federation of Neurological Surgeons Committee, 1988). Patients, even though physically recovered to grade one, can still report the difficulties summarized in *Table 11.2* that hinder return to daily life, work and social adjustment.

Table 11.1: World Federation of Neurological Surgeons' Grading Scale

Grade	GCS	Comments
I	15	+/- nerve palsy
II	13–14	
III	13–14	+motor/sensory/ speech deficit
IV	7–12	
V	3–6	

From World Federation of Neurological Surgeons Committee (1988); GCS=Glasgow Coma Score

Table 11.2: Possible resultant deficits following SAH

Physical	Cognitive	Emotional
Motor weakness or sensory deficits to limbs	Memory disturbance	Symptoms of panic
Cerebellum problems, e.g. ataxia, problems with coordination	Concentration difficulties	Anxiety symptoms
Speech problems	Planning/organizational difficulties	Depression symptoms
Cranial nerve palsy	Acquired reading difficulties	Unable to venture outside although physically able
Overwhelmed by fatigue, unable to resume activities	Memory problems leading to concerns about safety	Unable to be left alone owing to anxiety
Altered level of consciousness, e.g. disorientation	Unable to be left unsupervised owing to problems with memory	Lack of physical progress owing to non-physical factors

SAH=subarachnoid haemorrhage

At Hope Hospital in Salford, approximately 12 aneurysmal SAH patients per month are discharged to the specialist centre. In April 1998, a system was set up to help support the survivors of SAH. This involved contact with a specialist nurse before discharge home from the specialist centre. The follow-up programme brought together specialized neurosurgeons, interventional neuroradiologists, a specialist nurse and neuropsychologists to form a neurovascular team. The team's aim was to provide the patient with information, guidance and intervention according to his or her individual needs. It was hoped the system would provide much-needed consistency of information for the recovering haemorrhage patient together with a mode of early detection of problems that may be emotional or cognitive in nature, thereby preventing the development of longer-term incapacity brought about by deeply entrenched problems. Ultimately, it was hoped that the system would promote independence and a return to previous activities.

The system was put in place after a pilot project identified that there was a need for support following discharge that was unmet. This pilot project was not published, but examined anxiety and depression levels in SAH patients and the trend of these measures over a 12-month period following the haemorrhage.

The purpose of this chapter is to demonstrate patient need in those experiencing SAH within the first 12 months of discharge, and to describe the follow-up service that has been created at the Greater Manchester Neurosciences Centre (GMNC), which attempts to address the need.

Follow-up procedure

At Hope Hospital it was noted that follow up of patients after discharge was haphazard in nature. This meant that some patients were being followed up medically in outpatient clinic around 6 weeks following discharge from hospital, while others may face a wait of 6 months–1 year to be seen in clinic by their consultant.

The specialist nurse service aims to bridge the gap between inpatient stay and home, so contact is made with the patient before discharge and through the period at home before being seen in clinic. Contact is flexible, so it is very much led by patient progress. If there is distress and anxiety reported by the patient, contact is frequent; conversely, if the individual is happy with his or her progress and has no issues of concern, there would be minimal contact.

The flowchart (*Figure 11.3*) reflects the patient journey from discharge through follow up in terms of contact or support that they may expect. The main aims of this follow-up programme are outlined in *Table 11.3*.

An unpublished pilot project carried out at Hope Hospital and outlined above followed patients in recovery after SAH. This project allowed a nurse to support people after discharge from hospital and also examined how people fared regarding levels of anxiety, depression and distress, as monitored by the Hospital Anxiety and Depression Scale (HADS) questionnaire (Zigmond and Snaith, 1983) and the Impact of Events Scale (IOES) questionnaire (Horowitz et al, 1979); both of these scales are described in more detail later in this chapter.

The pilot project demonstrated that patients had a variety of invisible difficulties experienced once home that the present system did not cater for, such as fatigue, which in some cases were fairly debilitating. Also the project identified that levels of distress, depression and anxiety (as assessed by the measures outlined above) were abnormally high even at the 12-month stage. The present system as described in this chapter came about in response to this pilot project.

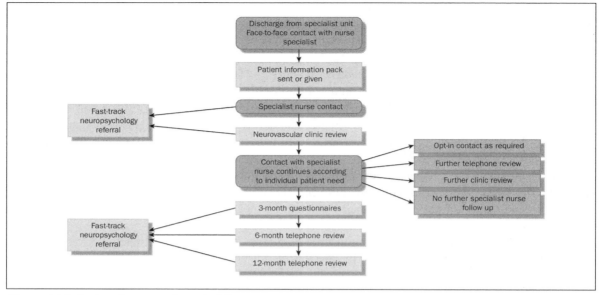

Figure 11.3: Patients' journey through follow up

Table 11.3: The main aims of the follow-up programme

- Standardize follow up for patients

- Empower the patient with information about the illness and his or her recovery

- Aid the patient to retrieve accurate information about his or her illness

- Minimize patient anxiety following discharge

- Identify nurse specialist as link back into specialist centre

- Identify those patients with psychological problems and refer as appropriate

Once the person is ready for discharge from the specialist neurosurgical unit following admission for SAH, face-to-face contact is made with the nurse specialist and an information pack is given to the patient. The information pack contains a booklet written for sufferers specifically about this illness, its aetiology and investigation, treatment options, and other written information containing useful contact numbers of various local bodies where support can be sought.

Once home, the person is then contacted 1–2 weeks later by the specialist nurse to talk through any issues that the person or close family members have. A home visit can be carried out following telephone contact if there are many issues or complex issues present at this stage. Six weeks later a clinic visit is arranged, when the person is able to discuss his or her progress with the doctor and the nurse jointly. Contact is tailored to individual patient need, and referral to the neuropsychologist is possible at any stage. This is done by reviewing the patient's progress against a set of behavioural criteria or indices, which are common problems that people may notice in recovery. If three or more of these difficulties are present, the patient can be referred via the fast-track system, which means that the neuropsychologist will see the patient within 1 month of referral. These indices can be seen in *Table 11.4*.

Table 11.4: Behavioural indices

- Anxiety/panic symptoms
- Depression symptoms
- Unable to be left unsupervised owing to anxiety
- Unable to venture outside although physically able
- Other emotional difficulties, e.g. irritability, guilt or anger
- Excessive fatigue
- Lack of physical progress owing to non-physical factors
- Memory difficulties leading to concerns over safety
- Unable to be left unsupervised owing to memory difficulties
- Planning/organizational difficulties
- Acquired reading difficulties
- Problems that prevent a return to work

The psychology department send out questionnaires to patients who are recovering at home at 3, 6 and 12 months following their discharge. If these measures are returned and the client scores are abnormally high, the assistant psychologist will contact the patient, which is equally an opportunity to review the patient's progress. The psychology assistant will also liaise with the nurse specialist when reviewing the patient at this stage. The assistant psychologist collects data regarding these outcome scores at certain stages of recovery for audit purposes.

On first contact with the nurse specialist, whether this is face to face or by telephone, patients are given the following minimum standard information in verbal and written form:

- What happens when SAH occurs
- What the management of the patient is that then follows
- A description of treatment options
- What to expect in terms of symptoms in recovery
- Advice regarding returning to activities including work and driving
- Information about professionals that a patient may come into contact with in recovery
- Frequently-asked questions and answers
- Information about medical follow up, such as check scans
- Information about the support group and helpline.

Description of measures used

It is well documented that survivors of SAH are at risk of problems with emotional and social adjustment as well as cognitive and physical impairment (Pritchard et al, 2001; Jarvis, 2002; Kirkness et al, 2002). A summary of such potential problems were outlined in *Table 11.2*.

In the earlier pilot study, a number of questionnaires were used to examine aspects of outcome such as social adjustment, health state and wellbeing.

It was found during this preliminary stage that the main indicators of patients experiencing emotional difficulties were the HADS and the IOES.

The HADS (Zigmond and Snaith, 1983) measures subjective and behavioural symptoms of anxiety and depression, with maximum scores of 21 for each of the anxiety and depression subscales. Scores of 11[+] fall within the clinical range and hence indicate referral to neuropsychological services. Within the revised IOES (Horowitz et al, 1979), participants are asked to indicate how often they have experienced various types of intrusive thoughts, such as flashbacks or nightmares, and how often they have engaged in avoidance behaviour during the past week. The maximum score on this questionnaire is 75. Within the follow-up design, participants who returned questionnaires with scores of 15[+] were thought to merit referral.

On receipt of completed IOES and HADS questionnaires, patients were telephoned to discuss any symptoms and, where appropriate, referral to neuropsychology. However, these questionnaires did not always reveal difficulties when they were present. Other problems became evident and were reported to the nurse specialist by patients, and subsequently these issues evolved into behavioural criteria or indices. This meant that patients were referred to neuropsychology if either these measures were found to have scored abnormally or patients reported as experiencing any of the behavioural criteria.

Currently, to monitor for altered mood states and post-traumatic stress symptoms, patients are sent questionnaires at 3 months post-discharge from the neurosciences centre (see *Figure 11.3*).

The characteristics of the group of patients that this chapter examines are outlined in *Table 11.5*; of these, 62 patients returned their 3-month questionnaires, and of those, seven did not have qualitative behavioural indices recorded. The most frequent reason for this is that it was not possible to contact the person by telephone to discuss his or her questionnaires. The patients in this group, whose questionnaire scores indicated a referral, were referred to the neuropsychologist and an appointment offered for a preliminary assessment. The behavioural indicators of psychological difficulties that were discussed during this informal telephone interview are shown in *Table 11.4*. Presence or absence was recorded on a tick-box basis. The severity was not recorded for audit purposes, but the details would be noted for the purposes of referral to neuropsychology.

Table 11.5: Characteristics of the client group

Characteristic	Number
Sex	
Female	72
Male	39
Treatment	
None	6
Surgery	57
Guglielmi detachable coil	48
Discharged to	
Home	60
District general hospital	35
Rehabilitation unit	16
Total	111

Patient profile

In a 1-year period, 111 surviving patients had experienced the system of follow up designed by the neurovascular team at Hope Hospital. Of these, 72 were female and 39 male. The mean age was 51.22 years.

All patients had experienced an acute SAH that was aneurysmal in nature. This means that an aneurysm of the cerebral circulation had developed and ruptured, causing the person to become acutely ill. Of the 111 patients, six had no treatment for their condition, 57 had surgical clipping of the aneurysm and 48 underwent endovascular coiling of the aneurysm (where the aneurysm is packed with platinum coils to prevent blood from entering it).

Following a stay within the specialist unit, 60 of the patients were then discharged directly home, 35 to a district general hospital and 16 to a rehabilitation unit. Please refer to *Table 11.5* for a summary of the client characteristics.

Table 11.6 shows information regarding referral to neuropsychology, together with the return rate for 3-month questionnaires. Patients who did not return questionnaires were sent out a second package with an accompanying letter explaining reasons for completion of the measures and encouraging them to comply. If the pack was not returned a second time, it was assumed that the individual had chosen to decline the offer of this type of follow up or ongoing monitoring, and this would be classed as missing data.

Table 11.6: Referrals to neuropsychologist

	Number	**Percentage**
Number of referrals into follow-up service	111	
Three-month questionnaire return rate	62	56
Number of patients referred to neuropsychology at 3 months	32	29 of total patients 52 of returned questionnaires
Number of patients referred at other times	8	7 of total
Percentage of patients referred into follow-up service referred to neuropsychology	40	36 of total

Findings

Information from the patients who returned questionnaires, and subsequent informal interviews with these patients, showed three trends:

- Questionnaire scores and/or behavioural indices that indicated a referral to neuropsychology, to which patients had consented
- Questionnaire scores and/or behavioural indices that indicated a referral to neuropsychology, but patients did not consent to such a referral
- Questionnaire scores and/or behavioural indices that did not indicate a referral to neuropsychology.

Table 11.7 summarizes the numbers of patients with abnormal scores at 3 months.

Table 11.7: Abnormal 3-month IOES/HADS scores

	Number	Percentage
Patients with IOES scores >15	23	37
Patients with HADS anxiety scores >11	22	35
Patients with HADS depression scores >11	14	23

IOES=Impact of Events Scale; HADS=Hospital Anxiety and Depression Scale

The information gathered via questionnaires showed that the patients who had scores indicative of a referral to neuropsychology tended to have high IOES scores yet subclinical anxiety and depression scores. *Table 11.8* demonstrates the prevalence rates of the various behaviours that indicate referral to neuropsychology.

Examples of the actual effect that the SAH had in real terms are illustrated in the following case studies.

Table 11.8: Behavioural problems reported by patients

Behavioural indices	Number	Percentage
Anxiety/panic symptoms	17	31
Depression symptoms	17	31
Unable to be left unsupervised owing to anxiety	5	9
Unable to venture outside although physically able	8	15
Other emotional difficulties	13	24
Excessive fatigue	17	31
Lack of physical progress owing to non-physical factors	6	11
Memory difficulties leading to concerns over safety	4	7
Unable to be left unsupervised owing to memory difficulties	5	9
Planning/organizational difficulties	5	9
Acquired reading difficulties	4	7
Problems that prevent a return to work	24	44

Of the 62 questionnaires returned, seven patient's behavioural indices were not recorded; therefore, the sample size for the above is *n*=55. Patients may experience more that one symptom

Case study one

A 26-year-old man suffered SAH and underwent surgical clipping of an anterior communicating artery aneurysm. He was reviewed in the clinic at the 6-week stage by the nurse specialist, when he reported vague anxiety symptoms including a fear of a recurrent SAH and panic symptoms that restricted his ability to return to work. His anxiety was preventing him from being able to be left alone.

Questionnaires were sent out to him at the 3-month stage and his IOES score (52/75) and HADS score (16/21) were both found to be abnormally high. The assistant psychologist then followed this up with a telephone call, when he identified problems of anxiety and panic symptoms and an extreme reluctance to stay in or go out alone (he would rather be accompanied by his children than be alone). He was traumatized by the experience of his illness and constantly worried about having another SAH. As a result, he misinterpreted common physical symptoms and had feelings of guilt. He had developed a fear of heights and panic attacks, which were preventing him from returning to work. He was also avoiding social situations.

He was referred to neuropsychology services on the basis of the emotional impact that his SAH experience had caused him. His first appointment was within 4 weeks of referral, and in all he was seen five times by the consultant neuropsychologist. When he was discharged, he was told he could access the system again any time by telephone if necessary.

In comparison, his scores at discharge were IOES 17/75 and HADS 1/21. He did require to be seen once more through the opt-in facility for purposes of reassurance, but following this intervention he was able to return to work, resume social activities and was able to go out or stay in alone without undue anxiety.

Case study two

A 36-year-old woman suffered SAH and underwent coiling treatment of a right-sided middle-cerebral artery aneurysm. She was reviewed by telephone at the 6-week stage, when she reported vague anxiety symptoms and physical limitations caused by a left-sided weakness or hemiparesis. Questionnaires (HADS and IOES) were sent to her at the 3-month stage. Her results were abnormally high (IOES 47/75 and HADS anxiety 16/21). At the same stage, the patient reported symptoms of anxiety, panic and depression. She was frequently tearful, lacking in motivation and emotionally passive. She was also reluctant to venture outside alone and there were problems that were preventing her from returning to work that included fatigue, low mood and cognitive difficulties.

Referral to the neuropsychology services was on the basis of her emotional difficulties; she had difficulty with labile mood and had poor motivation, which was preventing rehabilitation by physiotherapy and occupational therapy services. She recognized that she was over-dependent upon her partner and mother, and there was some disassociation between events and her emotions surrounding the SAH. Ultimately, her confidence was affected because of her perception of her cognitive and physical difficulties. She was reluctant to spend time alone, and was unable to return to work, social and physical activities. These behaviours were reinforced by her family members.

Her first appointment was within 2 weeks of referral, and she attended eleven times in total. On discharge from neuro-psychology services, her scores were much improved in comparison to referral scores: IOES 23/75 and HADS anxiety 8/21. She was also discharged with the ability to opt into the system again if she felt necessary. She did use this to gain reassurance by telephone, but no further appointment was necessary. She gained increased independence, increased social and physical activity and also made the decision to retire from work on the grounds of ill health.

Conclusions

Previous research has highlighted the need for structured support and treatment after SAH (Jarvis, 2002; Kirkness et al, 2002). The follow-up system devised at Hope Hospital provides this much-needed structured support and intervention via dedicated services from the SAH specialist nurse to provide information and advice, the interventional neuroradiologist and neurosurgeons for medical follow up, and fast-track access to neuropsychological interventions on the basis of individual patient need. As far as the authors are aware, the system at Hope Hospital was the first of its kind, with the Wessex Neurological Centre developing a similar system thereafter (Pritchard et al, 2001). Novel work in this area by nurse specialists has demonstrated that care of the SAH patient continues way beyond discharge because the needs of this group of patients are much longer term than the period of acute illness and hospitalization.

Collaborative work between the two centres (Greater Manchester Neuroscience Centre and the Wessex Neurological Centre) led by the SAH nurse specialists has recently resulted in the design and construction of a SAH web site aimed at providing patients and their loved ones with credible information about their illness and recovery. This can be viewed at www.srht.nhs.uk/SAH.

A service such as the one described is necessary in order to address those needs, and care must be holistic. That means that when the patient leaves hospital looking well, i.e. walking and talking, this is not necessarily a true indication of complete recovery. Care must be more than physical – it must also include emotional support following an illness such as SAH.

Patient need may be anticipated, the patient monitored beyond discharge from hospital and fast-tracked to the appropriate service. The service at Hope Hospital is user-friendly, it has easy access for patients who are at home following and recovering from this illness. They can opt into the service as necessary and also can avoid waiting lists in the case of fast-track referrals to neuropsychology.

As intervention is available on an opt-in basis, there is a risk that some patients will fail to access the necessary services, which means that the prevalence rates represented in this sample may be under-inclusive. Ideally, it would be possible for the specialist nurse to offer home visits to all patients in the first weeks following their discharge from hospital in order to engage patients in the follow-up procedure and to detect patients who are experiencing difficulties. Unfortunately, owing to the large number of patients entering and leaving the centre, it is not practical for this to be included in the process at this time with limited staff resources available.

The nurse specialist role described in this document has changed dramatically from when the role was first created and described (Wild, 2000). At that time, the post was funded by a local charity (Brain And Spinal Injury Charity; BASIC) and has subsequently been substantiated by the trust.

Although the main aims of the role remain, the role has been shaped and developed very much according to the nurse specialist model and its five distinct components:

- Educator
- Leader
- Researcher
- Practitioner
- Consultant (Finlay, 1998).

The follow-up procedure currently in place focuses on screening patients for emotional difficulties at 3 months post-discharge from hospital, with patients indicating cognitive difficulties on a self-report basis. The questionnaires are an ideal 'safety net' for the identification of those who may be suffering emotionally after discharge with delayed presentation of anxiety or depression symptoms.

Review of the service is vital in order to continue the development of it according to patient need, and this is assisted by the trust's protected time for clinical governance that can be used for this purpose. Flexibility of the system must also be maintained in order that change and development can be achieved.

There is no doubt that the service described in this chapter offers a valuable facility to clients. It is vital to help support and identify those people suffering from non-physical difficulties in the aftermath of SAH, which prevent them from returning to normal daily life. It is an example of best practice and goes some way to forming a component of an integrated care pathway for SAH patients.

References

Bindschaedler C, Assal G, De Tribolet N (1997) Cognitive sequelae following rupture of aneurysms of the anterior communicating artery and the anterior cerebral artery. *Rev Neurol* **153**(11): 669–78

Bonita R, Thomson S (1985) Subarachnoid haemorrhage: epidemiology, diagnosis, management and outcome. *Stroke* **16**: 591–4

Buchanan KM, Elias U, Goplen GB (2000) Differing perspectives on outcome after subarachnoid haemorrhage: the patient, the relative, the neurosurgeon. *Neurosurgery* **46**: 831–8

Finlay LD (1998) Susan Quaal: the global and local impact of a transformational leader. *J Cardiovasc Nurs* **12**(2): 88–93

Fox JL (1983) *Intracranial Aneurysms*. Springer Verlag, New York

Horowitz M, Wilner N, Alvarez W (1979) Impact of Event Scale: a measure of subjective stress. *Psychosom Med* **41**: 209–18

Jarvis A (2002) Recovering from subarachnoid haemorrhage: patients' perspective. *Br J Nurs* **11**(22): 1430–7

Kirkness CJ, Thompson JM, Ricker BA, Buzaitis A, Newell DW, Dikmen S, Mitchell PH (2002) The impact of aneurysmal subarachnoid haemorrhage on functional outcome. *J Neurosci Nurs* **34**(3): 134–41

Lindsay K, Bone I (1997) *Neurology and Neurosurgery Illustrated*. 3rd edn. Churchill Livingstone, Edinburgh

Pritchard C, Foulkes L, Lang DA, Neil-Dwyer G (2001) Psychosocial outcomes for patients and carers after aneurysmal subarachnoid haemorrhage. *Br J Neurosurg* **15**(6): 456–63

Rees G, Shah S, Hanley C, Brunker C (2002) Subarachnoid haemorrhage: a clinical overview. *Nurs Stand* **16**(42): 47–54

Stegen G, Freckmann N (1991) Outcome and rehabilitation after aneurysmal subarachnoid haemorrhage. *Zentralbl Neurochir* **52**: 37–9

Teunissen LL, Rinkel GJE, Algra A, Van Gijn J (1996) Risk factors for subarachnoid haemorrhage: a systematic review. *Stroke* **27:** 544–9

Wild A (2000) The role of the specialist nurse. *Nurs Times* **96**(4): 42–3

World Federation of Neurological Surgeons Committee (1988) Report of World Federation of Neurological Surgeons Committee on a Universal Subarachnoid Hemorrhage Grading Scale. *J Neurosurg* **68**(6): 985–6

Zigmond AS, Snaith RP (1983) The hospital anxiety and depression scale. *Acta Psychiatr Scand* **67:** 361–70

Chapter 12

A care plan approach to nurse-led extubation

Diana De

Since the publication of the Department of Health's (DoH's) document on *Comprehensive Critical Care* (DoH, 2000), critical care environments have been rapidly expanding outside the traditional confines of the intensive care unit (ICU). Additionally, with reduced working time initiatives (British Medical Association, 2000), physician responsibilities are shifting dramatically, resulting in more onus being placed on the shoulders of the nurse. This is even the case in high-care areas, such as critical care settings, where the author has witnessed nurses already implementing a number of expanded roles, such as arterial blood gas analysis, electrocardiogram implementation and cardiac output study measurements where a Swan-Ganz catheter has been placed to monitor a patient's fluid status more accurately.

Weaning patients from mechanical ventilation and extubating them was traditionally seen as a duty of medical staff. However, in many critical care settings this responsibility is being taken over by appropriately trained nurses, particularly in the cardiothoracic ICU setting. Advances in anaesthetic and cardiac surgical technique, which have led to a warmer and more haemodynamically stable patient, have enabled this procedure to become more accelerated (Gale and Curry, 1999). Jenkins (1997) found that early extubation not only improved patient care standards and physical and psychological patient recovery, but also reduced cost by increasing the throughput of patients. It also led to patients returning to independence much more quickly owing to less overall time in hospital.

However, evidence has shown that major differences in weaning practices exist between critical care environments at local, national and international level (Gale and Curry, 1999). Positive findings have shown that ICUs, which have an explicit weaning protocol or strategy and where nurses (or respiratory therapists) initiate the weaning process, will extubate patients much more quickly than physician-directed units (Esteban and Alia, 1998). With Scheinhorn et al (1994) estimating mortality rates from long-term mechanical ventilation as high as 30–40%, more rapid extubation can only be of benefit to a patient's recovery. The role nurses can play in decreasing the duration of intubation times is being deemed a successful part of rapid recovery programmes, which see the overall length of hospital stay by patients being shortened (Riddle et al, 1996).

Early extubation of patients after cardiac surgery is becoming much more widely accepted and is gaining ever-increasing interest as a means of improving patient care worldwide (Jenkins, 1997). The nurse's potential in this has already been recognized and highlighted in the DoH and Royal College of Nursing (RCN) (2003) document *Freedom to Practice: Dispelling the Myths*. As Anderson and O'Brien (1995) highlight, the development of this type of policy has also provided nurses with a new and challenging role in critical care.

The introduction of the nurse-led extubation procedure into high-dependency care environments has been slow, despite the publication of the Intensive Care Society's (2000) weaning guidelines. Lowe et al (2001) found that often nurses felt their ability to make decisions to progress weaning in some units was hampered by having to seek medical approval for each step taken to reduce ventilation.

This calls on the need for more uniformity of care between critical care environments. Therefore, this chapter aims to disseminate information to provide a guide/education tool for high-dependency ward nurses so that they too can be involved in the weaning process or even assist in the extubation procedure itself. It is based on compilation of evidence from a range of critical care journal literature between 1994 to the present, using the Cinahl database and the key words 'nurse-assisted extubation', 'nurse-led extubation' and 'nurse-led weaning'. Information has also been gathered from discussion with patients following extubation, ICU consultants, consultant anaesthetists and critical care nurses.

This chapter provides and supplements useful information on nurse-led extubation to any critical care area considering or promoting this expanded nursing role, using a care-plan approach (*Figures 12.1*, *12.2* and *12.3*). The format is intended to be used either as an actual care plan or as a template for writing new unit protocols. The proposed care should be used in conjunction with careful assessment and planning of an adult patient's suitability for nurse-assisted extubation, based on the extubation criteria being met and an anaesthetist being informed. This latter point is an important safety procedure that will be especially significant if initial intubation by an anaesthetist was difficult to implement (Anderson and O'Brien, 1995). This is often classed as a grade 3 intubation or above (see 'Glossary').

Mechanical ventilation is a method for using machines to help patients breathe when they are unable to breathe sufficiently on their own (American College of Chest Physicians, 2004). Please refer to the glossary for brief explanations of ventilatory terms.

Extubation criteria

Weaning is defined as the process of assisting patients to breathe spontaneously without mechanical ventilatory support (Knebel et al, 1998). Extubation is the removal of either the plastic endotracheal, nasopharyngeal or tracheostomy tube from the patient's airway. The decision to wean has long been based on a composite of objective data, professional experience and clinical judgment (Brooks, 1983). It is important to note that weaning and extubation are separate decisions (Sharar, 1995).

This chapter promotes the safety of the patient, first and foremost, and although promoting the role of the nurse, the actual decision to extubate a patient despite the existence of formal guidelines should be ideally based on the clinical judgment of a consultant anaesthetist (Oztekin and Weriman, 2001).

Preparation for the procedure	
ACTION	**RATIONALE**
Enteral feed should be stopped as soon as extubation has been considered. Aspirate the patient's naso/orogastric tube	To prevent risk of aspiration if the patient vomits during the procedure
Sedation should be stopped as soon as extubation has been considered. If a minimal amount is necessary, sedation scores (*Table 12.1*) need to be regularly monitored and reversal agents kept at hand	To enable the patient to be aware and able to obey commands (Howie, 1999) and to reduce anxiety
Collect equipment	To enhance preparation for the procedure
ǐ Suction circuit (functioning) ǐ Yanker suction catheter ǐ Suction catheters x 2 (appropriate size)	To remove unwanted secretions, prevent increased airway resistance (Robb, 1997) and maintain airway patency (McKelvie, 1998) and a reduction in gas exchange (Robb, 1997)
ǐ Wear eye protection	To maintain universal precautions (Pierce, 1995)
ǐ Scissors	To cut tapes/ties
ǐ 10ml syringe	To deflate cuff
ǐ Face mask	To optimize humidified oxygen delivery post-procedure
ǐ Elephant tubing (wide corrugated oxygen tubing)	
ǐ Set up bacterial filter and a humidified circuit☐	To reduce risk of pneumonia and airway mucosa drying (Ballard et al, 1992)
ǐ FIO$_2$ supply (100%/98%) (this needs prescribing)	To prevent hypoxia post-procedure
Prepare equipment for re-intubation, check ventilator and position emergency intubation trolley near patient's bed area	To ensure equipment is present, working and readily available if rapid re-intubation/ventilation is required
ǐ Correct size endotracheal tubes (same size and one size smaller)	To be prepared if rapid re-intubation is required. Assessment of the need for re-intubation is based on the deteriorating patient's condition, in relation to respiratory function, cardiovascular status and level of consciousness (Lowe et al, 2001)
ǐ Sterile scissors ǐ Lubricant ǐ 10ml syringe ǐ Working laryngoscope ǐ Forceps (Magills) ǐ Introducer	To ensure patient safety
ǐ Induction agents, e.g. Xylocaine, propofol, suxamethonium, atracurium besylate, atropine (trust/consultant variable)	To ensure anaesthetic agents are on hand if re-intubation is necessary and patient needs to be anaesethized/paralysed rapidly
Sit patient upright if safe so to do	This position will aid chest expansion, help the patient to cough effectively and minimize vomiting and subsequent aspiration. Knowledge about positioning patients with respiratory compromise in order to allow maximum gas exchange to occur, is of great importance in preventing hypoxic damage to tissues (Wheeler, 1997)
Explain clearly the whole procedure to patient	To inform patient of procedure and aid co-operation and communication (Arnold and Underman Boggs, 1999) To ensure patient understands his/her role and allay stress, fear and anxiety To provide encouragement and to allay stress, fear/and anxiety (Logan and Jenny, 1997)
Ensure patient is pain free by carrying out a pain assessment	To ensure breathing is not compromised by restricted movement or chest expansion due to pain
Suitable analgesia should be provided (without suppressing respiratory centres or level of consciousness). For example, fentanyl has a relatively non-sedative effect (McPherson et al, 1990)	To alleviate pain/discomfort from endotracheal suctioning (Sawyer, 1997; Todres et al, 2000) and to increase patient comfort
Provide the patient with 100% prescribed FIO$_2$ 3 minutes before planned extubation	To optimize oxygenation and prevent hypoxia (Grap et al, 1996)

Figure 12.1: Care plan showing the preparatory care necessary for extubation

During the procedure	
ACTION	**RATIONALE**
Nurse 1: suction oropharynx	To prevent secretions draining into chest when endotracheal tube (ETT) cuff is deflated
Nurse 2: silence ventilator alarms (if still attached)	To minimize noise and to reduce anxiety
Nurse 1: suction ETT using aseptic technique	To remove existing secretions and to clear chest
Nurse 2: re-attach O_2 source to ETT following suctioning procedure	To maximize oxygenation
Nurse 2: cut tapes and hold tube steady and inform patient to keep mouth open (if oral ETT) and that tube will soon be removed	To free ETT and reduce trauma caused by ETT movement and to prepare patient for removal
Nurse 1: suction ETT twice (on 2nd entry leaving the catheter in situ) and request nurse 2 to deflate cuff	To free ETT To remove remaining chest secretions and then remove ETT when the patient breathes out, suctioning all the way out of the airway and paying special attention to removing those secretions from oral/nasal cavity

Figure 12.2: Care plan showing the recommended procedure during the extubation

Following the procedure	
ACTION	**RATIONALE**
Nurse 2: apply face mask immediately with 100% prescribed FIO_2 for 3ñ5 minutes. Following this period nurse 1 should then reduce the amount of oxygen gradually back down to the level being administered to the patient before the extubation	To reduce risk of damage to airways by administering high-dose oxygen saturations greater than 96%
Encourage patient to cough and deep breath. Provide sputum pot and tissues	To clear any sputum, maintain the parient's airway patency and prevent pooling of secretions in the chest
Liaise with physiotherapists and other multidisciplinary staff to position patient optimally and encourage regular deep breathing	To teach and support patient how to breathe effectively and so allow for maximal air entry to the chest
Give patient constant support and reassurance	To encourage the patient to continue to breath spontaneously
Nurse 1: to check arterial blood gases 20 minutes (or sooner if the patient's condition dictates) following extubation and regularly thereafter alongside continuous oxygen saturation monitoring	To compare and contrast a series of observations and detailed results in order to identify signs of improvement or early deterioration (Howie, 1999)
Observe closely for signs of deterioration and document findings in nursing notes and inform physician if patient develops: ï dyspnoea ï flaring of the nostrils ï posture ï central cyanosis ï stridor ï aspiration ï cardiac/respiratory arrest ï dysphasia ï tachycardia ï excessive sweating ï new arrhythmias ï hypotension ï disorientation, irritability, negative facial expressions (Harris, 2001)	To monitor for signs of respiratory distress, hypoxaemia and hypercapnia. Classically, severe hypercapnia is characterized by a cherry red facial complexion (Lowe et al, 2001) To assess and examine the patient in respiratory difficulty and make an expert decision whether or not patient requires re-intubation To provide effective record keeping and recognize accountability (Nursing and Midwifery Council (NMC), 2002a)
Ongoing regular chest physiotherapy, postural drainage and pharyngeal suction should be implemented thereafter	To maintain and improve respiratory status (Lowe et al, 2001)

Figure 12.3: Care plan showing the recommended procedure following the extubation

Table 12.1: An example of a sedation scale — the Ramsay Sedation Scale*

1. Patient is anxious and agitated or restless, or both

2. Patient is cooperative, oriented, and tranquil

3. Patient responds to commands only

4. Patient exhibits brisk response to light glabellar tap or loud auditory stimulus

5. Patient exhibits a sluggish response to light glabellar tap or loud auditory stimulus

6. Patient exhibits no response

Table 12.1 refers to Table 2 cited in Figure 12.1 (second point under 'Action')

Guideline criteria for extubation are:

- Patient is awake and responsive to command (Logan and Jenny, 1997)
- Patient is able to maintain and be nursed in an upright position. Be aware of patients with conditions such as head injury or hypotension who cannot be nursed at 90° (McLean, 2001). These patients will need to be positioned as upright as their condition allows
- Patient has a respiratory function greater than 8 breaths per minute and a rate no greater than 30 breaths per minute (Cull and Inwood, 1999) on a spontaneous breathing mode such as continuous positive airway pressure (Davies, 1997), T piece (Gale and Curry, 1999) or a face mask over an endotracheal tube (ETT) (Anderson and O'Brien, 1995). A T piece is a simple, large bore, non-rebreathing circuit attached directly to an ETT or tracheostomy tube (Oh, 1997)
- Underlying disease has been resolved (Lowe et al, 2001)
- The patient has no clinical signs of haemorrhage, and blood pressure, pulse and cardiac output studies are all showing stability (Goldstone, 1993) and the patient has minimal inotropic support (Anderson and O'Brien, 1995)
- Cough, swallow and gag reflexes are present. This will indicate the patient's potential ability to maintain his or her airway following extubation and reduce the retention of any sputum that may later lead to respiratory failure (Howie, 1999)
- On chest auscultation breath sounds are equal and clear on both sides of the chest (Lowe et al, 2001)
- Chest X-ray review by a physician to check lung fields are clear (Lowe et al, 2001)
- Satisfactory recent arterial blood results, i.e. pH between 7.35–7.45 (Cull and Inwood, 1999), a PO_2 level greater than 10 kPa (Henry and Duffy, 1995) and a PCO_2 level less than 6 kPa (Davies, 1997)
- An O_2 saturation reading by pulse oximetry of 95% or above (Slutsky, 1993)
- Oxygen requirement (FIO_2) is 40% or less (Henry and Duffy, 1995).

Care plan aim

A care plan's written aim and outcomes should emerge from what the patient and nurse hope to achieve, and should be presented in terminology that is concise, realistic, measurable and clear (Moorhouse et al, 1997). The aim in this care plan is for the nurse to wean the ventilated patient safely through to extubation, with minimal intervention from a physician.

General patient outcomes

The general patient outcomes are that the patient/client breathes independently, unassisted by the ventilator, with maintenance of adequate spontaneous ventilation and gas exchange as indicated by arterial blood gases, oxygen saturations and respiratory rate within normal limits. Lungs should be fully expanded, and breath sounds on auscultation clear with absence of retractions (contraction of neck and shoulder muscles) and use of accessory muscles from the abdomen and neck for respiration effort.

Standard/benchmark

The standard is to ensure safe, quick and efficient removal of an ETT. ETTs are curved, hollow tubes made of polyvinylchloride and are designed for insertion via the nose or mouth into the trachea. An inflatable balloon/cuff provides a seal and keeps the tube in place within the trachea.

Patient safety/nurse priorities

The nurse's priorities are to promote adequate oxygenation of the brain and prevent hypoxia. Oxygen delivery can be supplemented by pre-oxygenating the patient before the procedure with 100% oxygen for 3 minutes (Grap et al, 1996). The nurse must also provide clear explanations of the proposed procedure to the patient in order to minimize discomfort. This will reduce anxiety/stress for both the patient and family (McIntyre, 1995).

Proposed care plan

The format for the care plan consists of and is based on the patient's diagnosis and relevant assessment data derived from information obtained during the history, physical examination, diagnostic studies, laboratory results and, equally important, visual observation. The care plan will be divided into three main sections — pre-extubation (see *Figure 12.1*), peri-extubation (see *Figure 12.2*), and post-extubation (see *Figure 12.3*) — and will apply to nasally or orally intubated adult patients. Goal statements and priorities have also been formulated to give direction to the nursing care and to improve quality, safety and effectiveness. This is a two-nurse procedure in order to ensure patient safety and improve efficiency (Pickles, 1999).

Conclusion

Nurses must remember that no two patients are ever the same. Although these patient outcomes have been stated in general terms in this care plan, practitioners are permitted to modify them by adding other considerations based on an individual patient's circumstances, needs or other specifics such as respiratory history, time spent mechanically ventilated, lung pathology (Lowe et al, 2001), anaesthetic drug sensitivities, chest infection, sputum consistency or previous extubation complications.

It is hoped that early nurse-led extubation practice will become more widespread, developed and practised throughout the UK in order to benefit quality of patient care and more effective use of resources by nurses spending less time caring for patients on mechanical life support machines. However, many factors will continue to influence patient care planning including resource management, staffing ratios, computerization, differentiation between and replacement by care pathways as well as ongoing financial constraints.

Patient care plans can ensure that critically ill patients receive efficient, effective, individualized quality care (Nursing and Midwifery Council (NMC), 2002a). Care plans can also help highlight evidence in documentation to promote the potential impact of innovative nursing and accountability on patient-focused care (NMC, 2002b). This will no doubt contribute to further improvements in UK national standards without compromising patient care, while also promoting a more autonomous role for the nurse.

References

American College of Chest Physicians (2004) *Mechanical Ventilation: Beyond the ICU*. American College of Chest Physicians, Illinois, US (http://www.chestnet.org/education/patient/guides/mech_vent/p1.php) (accessed 23 September 2004)

Anderson J, O'Brien M (1995) Challenges for the future: the nurse's role in weaning patients from mechanical ventilation. *Intensive Crit Care Nurs* 11(1): 2–5

Arnold E, Underman Boggs K (1999) *Interpersonal Relationships*. WB Saunders, Philadelphia: 445–75

Ballard K, Cheeseman W, Ripiner T, Wells S (1992) Humidification for ventilated patients. *Intensive Crit Care Nurs* 8(1): 2–9

British Medical Association (2000) *Junior Doctors' Comittee. Implications for Health and Safety of Junior Doctors' Working Arrangements*. BMA, London

Brooks C (1983) The adult way to wean from mechanical ventilation. *Crit Care Nurs* 3: 64–5

Cull C, Inwood H (1999) Extubation in intensive care unit: enhancing the nursing role. *Prof Nurse* 14(9): 618–21

Davies N (1997) Nurse-initiated extubation following cardiac surgery. *Intensive Crit Care Nurs* 13(2): 77–9

Department of Health (2000) *Comprehensive Critical Care: A Review of Adult Services*. DoH, London

Department of Health, Royal College of Nursing (2003) *Freedom to Practice: Dispelling the Myths*. DoH, London

Esteban A, Alia I (1998) Clinical management of weaning from mechanical ventilation. *Intensive Care Med* **24**: 999–1008

Gale C, Curry S (1999) Evidencing nurse-led accelerated extubation post-cardiac surgery. *Nurs Crit Care* **14**(4): 165–70

Goldstone JC (1993) Weaning from mechanical ventilation. *Br J Hosp Med* **50**: 345–7

Grap MJ, Glass C, Croley M, Parks T (1996) Endotracheal suctioning: ventilator versus manual delivery of hyperoxygenation breaths. *Am J Crit Care* **5**: 192–7

Harris J (2001) Weaning from mechanical ventilation: relating the literature to nursing practice. *Nurs Crit Care* **6**(5): 226–31

Henry L, Duffy J (1995) A cardiovascular intensive care nursing staff response to managed care: a change in practice. *Crit Care Nurs Q* **18**(3): 28–35

Hinds CJ (1996) *Intensive Care: A Concise Textbook*. 2nd edn. Saunders, London

Howie A (1999) Rapid shallow breathing as an indicator during weaning from ventilator support. *Nurs Crit Care* **4**(4): 171–8

Intensive Care Society (2000) *Intensive Care Society National Guidelines: When and How to Wean*. Intensive Care Society, London (available on http://www.ics.ac.uk/downloads/weaning.pdf) (last accessed 17 September)

Jenkins M (1997) Early extubation post-cardiac surgery: implications for nursing practice. *Nurs Crit Care* **2**(6): 276–8

Knebel A, Shekleton M, Burns S, Clochesy J, Hanneman S (1998) Weaning from mechanical ventilatory support: refinement of a model. *Am J Crit Care* **7**: 19–152

Logan J, Jenny J (1997) Qualitative analysis of patients' work during mechanical ventilation and weaning. *Heart Lung* **26**: 140–147

Lowe F, Fulbrook P, Aldridge H, Fox S, Gillard J, O'Neil J, Papps L (2001) Weaning from ventilation: a nurse-led protocol. *Crit Care Nurs Eur* **1**(4): 124–33

McIntryre NR (1995) Psychological factors in weaning from mechanical ventilatory support. *Respir Care* **40**: 277–81

McKelvie S (1998) Endotracheal suctioning. *Nurs Crit Care* **3**(5): 244–8

McLean C (2001) Moving and positioning patients with altered intracranial haemodynamics. *Nurs Crit Care* **6**(5): 239–44

McPherson E, Perlin E, Finke H, Castro O, Pittman J (1990) Patient-controlled analgesia in patients with sickle cell vaso-occlusive crisis. *Am J Med Sci* **299**(1): 10–12

Moorhouse FA, Geissler AC, Doenges ME (1997) *Critical Care Plans — Guidelines for Patient Care*. FA Davies, Philadelphia

Nursing and Midwifery Council (2002a) *Code of Professional Conduct*. NMC, London

Nursing and Midwifery Council (2002b) *Guidelines for Records and Record Keeping*. NMC, London

Oh TE (1997) *Intensive Care Manual*. 4th edn. The Bath Press, Bath

Oztekin D, Weriman A (2001) Weaning from mechanical ventilation. *Crit Care Nurs Eur* **1**(2): 52–58

Pickles A (1999) Nurse versus technician: the dilemma of intensive care nursing. *Nurs Crit Care* **4**(3): 148–50

Pierce LNB (1995) *Guide to Mechanical Ventilation and Intensive Respiratory Care*. WB Sanders, Philadelphia

Riddle MM, Dunston JL, Castanis JL (1996) A rapid recovery programme for cardiac surgery patients. *Am J Crit Care* **5**: 152–9

Robb J (1997) Physiological changes occurring with positive pressure ventilation: part 1. *Intensive Crit Care Nurs* **13**: 293–307

Sawyer N (1997) Back from the twilight zone. *Nurs Times* **93**(7): 28–9

Scheinhorn DJ, Artinian BM, Catlin JL (1994) Weaning from prolonged mechanical ventilation: the experience at a regional weaning centre. *Chest* **105**: 534–539

Sharar S (1995) Weaning and extubation are not the same. *Respir Care* **40**: 239–243

Slutsky AS (1993) Mechanical ventilation. *Chest* **104**: 1833–59

Todres L, Fulbrook P, Albarran J (2000) On the receiving end: a hermeneutic phenomenological analysis of a patient's struggle to cope while going through intensive care. *Nurs Crit Care* **5**: 277–87

Wheeler H (1997) Positioning: one good turn after another? *Nurs Crit Care* **2**(3): 129–31

Glossary	
Continuous positive airway pressure (CPAP)	A positive airway pressure maintained throughout spontaneous breathing (Oh, 1997)
Extubation	The plastic endotracheal tube (ETT) is removed from the patient's trachea to allow patient to breath unaided by mechanical ventilator
Grades of intubation	Grade 1–2 is straightforward/unproblematic and grade 3–4 is a difficult intubation procedure. A consultant anaesthetist should be called to perform any reintubation procedures
Intubation	Provides a route for mechanical ventilation, maintains a clear airway, protects the lungs and allows control of bronchial secretions (Hinds, 1996). A plastic ETT is placed into the trachea by a physician in order to perform mechanical ventilation
Mechanical ventilation breathing	Support via a mechanical ventilator
Nasopharyngeal	Nose to pharynx
Oropharyngeal	Mouth to pharynx
Positive end expiratory pressure (PEEP)	An airway pressure above atmosphere (i.e. positive) at the end of the ventilator cycle, during which spontaneous breathing is absent (Oh, 1997)
Pressure support ventilation (PSV)	Where patients' spontaneous breaths are enhanced using PEEP
Synchronized intermittent mandatory ventilation (SIMV)	Allows unassisted spontaneous breathing along with triggered mechanical breaths (Oh, 1997)

Chapter 13

Integration of critical care and palliative care at end of life

Natalie Pattison

The provision of care at the end of life can be fraught with difficulties. There are numerous ethical issues, and no clear guidelines exist on how the process of moving from acute care to end-of-life care should be carried out. The boundaries of how far life can be sustained have been extended with advances in technology and knowledge to the point where dying may even be postponed. However, mortality in critical care is still significant, with figures ranging from as high as one in three to one in five patients in the UK (Goldhill and Sumner, 1998; Audit Commission, 1999; Intensive Care National Audit and Research Centre, 2000; Wunsch et al, 2005). Therefore, there is a need for end-of-life care in critical care.

Critical care has been defined as the care provided for patients who have a greater level of medical and nursing dependency as a result of a potentially reversible critical illness (Audit Commission, 1999; Department of Health (DoH), 2000). In the UK, critical care encompasses level one, two and three care, which ranges from close monitoring postoperatively (level one), to a patient with multi-organ failure (level three) (DoH, 2000). Palliative care refers to the alleviation of symptoms that accompany the end of life, using 'low-tech' options, such as morphine for dyspnoea (rather than increasing or aggressive respiratory support), for treatment of people dying with advanced disease (Clark and Seymour, 1999).

Critical care nurses face the dilemma of initially trying to prolong and save lives and then, when futility is apparent, having to redefine their care and respond to the needs of a dying patient and his or her loved ones. In fact, critical care practitioners are obliged to help patients and families prepare for death when life-sustaining treatment fails (Danis et al, 1999; Faber-Langendoen and Lanken, 2000).

Formalized palliative care in critical care is rare, such as palliative care consultant ward rounds, even in the US where the Society of Critical Care Medicine has suggested how end-of-life care in critical care should be implemented (Danis et al, 1999; Nelson et al, 2001; Truog et al, 2001). Critical care units are rarely used in palliative care studies and yet nearly every hospital has access to palliative care services. Implementing palliative care tenets within critical care need not mean the transfer of patients out of critical care. Although it is sometimes recommended (Audit Commission, 1999), transfer may be inappropriate if patients are likely to die imminently after treatment has been withdrawn (Seymour, 2001; Marr and Weismann, 2004).

By retaining the core vision of caring for the patient as a whole and by ensuring comfort, principles of the palliative care paradigm can be incorporated into critical care.

There is a division between the two disciplines, which may be because of how they view the patient:

- The palliative care philosophy is more holistic and patient-focused (Doyle, 2003)
- The critical care philosophy fights to retain a patient focus, as emphasis is still placed on life-saving technical skills and medical frameworks (Byock, 1999; Seymour, 2003).

The critical care philosophy is challenged when life can no longer be prolonged and patients are dying. Critical care nurses and doctors often intuitively know when a patient is dying, even before treatment has been reviewed for discontinuation, and experience is the main factor in this intuition (Seymour, 2000).

A new vision of compassionate end-of-life care in critical care has been called for, and a need for acute palliative care has been highlighted (Rocker et al, 2000; Nelson and Danis, 2001; Rushton et al, 2002).

Status quo

One of the reasons for a lack of clarity about end-of-life care in critical care may be a lack of certainty. Patients may be seen to improve initially, and there can be no certainty about who will survive and who will not. Prognostic tools, such as the Applied Physiology and Chronic Health Evaluation (APACHE) scoring system (devised by Knaus et al, 1981), may assist those making decisions but still fail to accurately and consistently predict survival or death (Nelson and Danis, 2001; Higgins et al, 2003).

Seymour (2000, 2003) undertook an ethnographic study of doctors' decision-making in critical care at the end of life. She showed that consultants and registrars frequently and intuitively know, based on experience, when a patient in the critical care unit will die. Part of the process of moving towards a 'natural death', and withdrawal of treatment, was to legitimize this intuition in this study (Seymour, 2000). Although doctors rationalize decisions as they make them, intuition influences the decision-making to some extent; therefore, since doctors try to predict who will die and when beforehand, decisions to move to end-of-life care must be appropriately timed and more frequently considered.

In the UK, advance directives, which determine the patient's wishes about treatment before he or she becomes incapable of decision-making (Oates, 2000), are relatively rare. In the absence of a decision from a capacitous patient, any decisions regarding cessation, withdrawal or withholding of treatments (referred to here under the collective term 'forgoing life-sustaining treatments') within critical care should be discussed with the consultant-in-charge, a senior nurse or the patient's primary nurse and the patient and/or his or her surrogates. In practice, this is often not the case (Ferrand et al, 2003).

It can appear that decision-making about moving the goals of care is often paternalistic. Some doctors may undertake a decision without input from either care-giving colleagues or patients' loved ones and presume that this decision is the most appropriate.

The British Medical Association (BMA, 2001) recommends in its guidelines on withdrawing and withholding treatment that others' views should be considered. However, it is clear in the documentation that doctors still retain jurisdiction over decisions, and therefore the decision-making fails to include all those involved (Ferrand et al, 2003).

Webb (2000) argues that paternalism may have a place in health care. Paternalism is the attitude of certain doctors that takes over patients' responsibility or choice. Consequentialism holds that an action is right or wrong according to whether its consequences are good or bad (Beauchamp and Childress, 2001). Critical care doctors believe their decision-making to be right as they perceive the consequences of their actions to be good. Critical care doctors want critical care beds for those who are likely to survive and benefit (Cassell et al, 2003), using a utilitarian approach of the greatest good for the greatest number. These doctors are ultimately responsible for withdrawing treatment and have to decide what the costs of prolonging treatment are for the family and society, and may want critical care beds for the sickest patients who have the greatest chance of improving.

However, poor decision-making is too frequently observed (Ferrand et al, 2003) and decisions to forgo treatment often leave families and staff dissatisfied, excluded or confused (Faber-Langendoen, 1996; Kirchhoff and Beckstrand, 2000; Kyba, 2002; Prendergast and Puntillo, 2002). In order to move away from this paternalistic style of care to ensure the best possible end-of-life care for patients for whom the goals of care have changed, an approach that encompasses all involved in the care of the patient needs to be implemented.

Goals of care

Comfort *vs* cure is the fundamental difference between palliative and critical care (Truog et al, 2001). Some critical care practitioners may perceive the shift from the acute end of the spectrum in critical care to end-of-life care as failure. Critical care models of care are often reductionist. The patient is compartmentalized into body systems (Robins, 1999; Evans, 2003), which, in the case of critical care, are functioning or failing (Robins, 1999; Helman, 2000), and the patient does not tend to be considered as a whole. Survival is an initial key focus. Once cure is no longer feasible, end-of-life care is considered.

The best care, which is in the patient's best interests, should be what drives decision-making. Faber-Langendoen and Lanken (2000) and Campbell (2002) highlight our responsibility to provide excellent care even when goals have shifted.

It could be argued that critical care nurses are ideally placed as advocates or facilitators for good end-of-life care decisions, as well as having the advantage, through one-to-one care, of being able to be patient-focused.

There is some discussion as to whether palliative care should be a core competency for all practitioners, particularly in critical care where there may be high mortality rates (Goldhill and Sumner, 1998; Audit Commission, 1999). Danis et al (1999) suggest that a formalized study of palliative care should be incorporated into critical care education to improve practice. Charlton and Smith (2000) highlighted that junior doctors in the UK perceive their palliative care skills to be inadequate, as a result of a lack of basic education.

Whether there is a need for specialist palliative care providers for end-of-life care in critical care is subject to debate (Rocker et al, 2000; Rushton et al, 2002). Randall and Downie (1996) outline how the focus of palliative care in critical care is very narrow. The health professional is focusing on alleviating particular symptoms alone, such as intubation and ventilation for respiratory distress, whereas in palliative care the focus is broad and more holistic. The total mental and social wellbeing of the patient is also the focus of the palliative care paradigm. However, end-of-life care in critical care should ideally retain the holistic approach that Randall and Downie (1996) delineated for palliative care.

The SUPPORT study in the US highlighted that, even when designated nurse clinicians discussed goals of care with families and then informed the doctor of those preferences, no change was evident in how decisions to forgo life-sustaining interventions were made (SUPPORT Principal Investigators, 1995). Reasons suggested for this include:

- Patients and families have their own ideas about how far they wish treatment to go and their degree of willingness to even accept the discussion of end-of-life treatment alternatives
- It is difficult to know when a justifiable treatment becomes one that is no longer beneficial and doctors have difficulty in defining 'benefit' (Oliverio and Fraulo, 1998).

Futility and decisions to forgo life-sustaining treatment

Critical care sustains life beyond that which would otherwise be possible and, as technology advances, the expectation for patients to live longer increases. However, it is important to consider what happens when technology is no longer effective.

The concept of futility has become increasingly popular as an argument for decisions about care (Löfmark and Nilstun, 2002; Melia, 2004). When an intervention is no longer useful, it is deemed futile. Practitioners have an obligation to decide whether or not a particular treatment is useful. When futility is apparent, decisions to forgo life-sustaining treatments are made.

This may be the case in critical care, where supportive therapy is withdrawn or withheld. Alternatively, it may be in palliative care where intravenous hydration or even feeding is withdrawn. Nurses are in a prime position to ensure that the practical aspects of withdrawal lead to a smooth transition and that comfort measures are implemented. This may include ensuring the patient is free of pain. Decision-making around withdrawal of treatment can be difficult for both nurses and doctors, who have the ultimate responsibility for those decisions. Some of these difficulties will be addressed later with regard to conflict.

Futility encompasses two notions:

- Quantitative
- Qualitative (ten Have and Janssens, 2002).

Quantitative futility holds that on the basis that treatment is likely to be ineffective, as seen through evidence in the literature or substantial experiential knowledge, then it should not be commenced or continued. Qualitative futility holds that treatment may be regarded as effective but may have no benefit to that patient (ten Have and Janssens, 2002). An example of quantitative futility might be cardiopulmonary resuscitation of a brain-dead patient; an example of qualitative futility could be when a patient is kept alive indefinitely despite multi-organ failure and a deterioration and dependence on critical care.

Futility in palliative care may seem to be a paradox, given that palliative care may begin when the goals have shifted from acute to end-of-life care. Nevertheless, interventions may be started in the end-of-life stage that are not in the patient's best interests, such as intravenous hydration. Even in palliative care where the best models for end-of-life care should be apparent, patients may be subjected to unnecessary treatments, medications, diagnostics and caring processes (ten Have and Janssens, 2002). It is obvious, therefore, that clarity is required in provision of best end-of-life care.

Resources and context

The resources discourse is too vast to explore in great detail here without addressing the ethics of access to health care. Nonetheless, the impact that scant resources have on end-of-life care decisions must be acknowledged. Cassell et al (2003) undertook an ethnographic account of the influence of administrative models on end-of-life care in intensive care. They revealed that some surgeons felt pressurized by critical care doctors to make early decisions to forgo life-sustaining treatment in order to release critical care beds for new admissions.

Critical care is a finite resource; therefore, ethical decisions need to be made about providing care to those who need it most and up to what point that care is provided.

Conflict

Ethical concerns can lead to conflict among the teams making the decisions, leading to unsatisfactory outcomes for patients and their families.

A surgeon may feel his covenant of care means that he has to prolong the life of a patient at all costs, but a critical care doctor may have bed pressures that necessitate early decisions to forgo life-sustaining treatment. The conflict between critical care doctors and surgeons in Cassell et al's (2003) study was tangible to the point where resource arguments superseded what might be appropriate for the patient.

One could extrapolate from this that decisions to forgo treatment are subject to individual doctors' control, rather than necessarily being dependent on patients' best interests.

Conflict also extends to differences of opinion between doctors and nurses. Ferrand et al (2003) found discrepancies between critical care nurses' and doctors' perceptions of end-of-life decisions. Nurses felt excluded from much of the decision-making and felt that lack of cohesion was a major obstacle to timely discussions about decisions to forgo life-sustaining treatments. Families may perceive conflict in end-of-life discussions with health professionals, as in Abbott et al's (2001) study, through poor communication and the behaviour of professionals.

Table 13.1 summarizes the effects of this conflict. *Figure 13.1* gives details of a case study that illustrates some of the above problems.

Table 13.1: Effects of conflict on end-of-life decision making

Fragmentation	Disagreement between disciplines, leading to disjointed care for the patient
Feelings of exclusion	Lack of consideration of opinions of the key people involved in the patient's care
Patient care suffering	As a result of above fragmentation
Dissonance (personal)	Caregivers' own values being challenged
Dissonance (professional)	Caregivers having to provide care inconsistent with their own values, and being tempted to deviate from prescribed care to assuage this dissonance
Confusion and distress	Conflicting opinions leading to families and caregivers not knowing where care is proceeding
Delay	Decision-making delay because of conflict
Poor communication	May result from the conflict

Adapted from Abbott et al (2001); Cassell et al (2003); Ferrand et al (2003)

Case study

Mr X was a 43-year-old man with acute myeloid leukaemia (AML), which was in remission. He was admitted to the critical care unit following acute respiratory distress. The patient was ventilated within 4 hours of admission to critical care, and his ventilation was difficult to manage. The patient then quickly became septic, requiring inotropes in increasing doses.

By day 3, Mr X was on pressure control ventilation with FiO_2 1.0 and on massive inotropic support of 0.7 µg/kg/min of epinephrine and 0.7 µg/kg/min of norepinephrine. By day 6, he was found to have a multiresistant pathogen in his sputum and blood cultures and was deteriorating further; haemofiltration was now in progress. By day 9, despite more than 1 week of antibiotics and critical care, Mr X now had respiratory, cardiovascular, gastrointestinal tract and renal failure.

His family was keen to continue present care. The critical care consultant felt that this care was becoming futile and wished to discuss forgoing life-sustaining treatment. Although the critical care consultant led the decision-making process while Mr X was in critical care, the oncology consultant was aware of the grave prognosis and felt that a discussion should be initiated to decide where the care was headed. There was a conflict between the family, who felt they were being pressurized to make decisions and were not being listened to, and the doctors who felt that by continuing they were prolonging the dying process. Nursing staff were having trouble trying to liaise between the critical care doctors and the family, and there was further disagreement between some of the nurses about where care should be headed.

Figure 13.1: A hypothetical case study

Discussion of case study (*Figure 13.1*)

One of the primary issues is this patient's prognosis. Although Mr X had acute myeloid leukaemia (AML) it was in remission, but the overriding presenting problem was his severe sepsis. The mortality associated with this, particularly in cancer patients, is high (Groeger et al, 1998).

The family needed to be reassured that the decision-making about forging life-sustaining treatment was not solely their responsibility, and that ultimately the consultants were responsible for the patient's care. This might alleviate any feelings of burden or guilt they might experience with regard to feeling as though they were choosing whether the patient lived or died (Prendergast and Puntillo, 2002).

The staff, who have experienced conflict within their team as well as with the family, should be given the opportunity to discuss their concerns, away from the family, so as not to compound confusion.

The oncology consultant and critical care consultant should discuss Mr X's case together, achieving agreement, so that the family does not hear conflicting opinions from the doctors who are ultimately responsible for decision-making. All caregivers, medical and nursing, should attend this discussion, which would ideally be facilitated by an ethicist. This may be, for instance, someone who is a lead on the ethics committee of the hospital or a chaplain experienced with such debates, or even a medical ethics expert from outside the hospital.

No single person's particular view should take precedence over another's, and instead a consensus opinion should be achieved. This may be difficult, as currently nurses, unlike doctors, have no legal liability (although it could be argued they have a moral responsibility) for their contribution to this decision making.

Nurses cannot be held legally accountable in a court of law for a decision to forgo life-sustaining treatment, as they are not, at present, in a position to make or lead such a decision; doctors are ultimately responsible (BMA, 1999). In which case, to what extent should nurses' opinions count? As the caregivers who are closest to the patients, their views should, at least, be carefully considered. Once agreement has been achieved among professionals, a family conference should take place.

Family conferences have been proposed as a solution to poor communication in end-of-life care in critical care (Curtis et al, 2001). A family conference usually includes: the patient's family or surrogates, the primary and/or senior nurse and critical care doctors (and possibly members of the patient's own medical or surgical team), but may also include physiotherapists, social workers, clinical nurse specialists and any other key professional. A pastoral care worker may also be useful. This conference takes place away from the patient's bedside and should not be interrupted.

The futility of the situation needs to be emphasized. In spite of maximum inotropes and ventilation, Mr X's multi-organ failure continued and he had deteriorated further. Mr X was unable to contribute to the decision about whether to forgo life-sustaining treatment, but the views of his family (acting as surrogates) on what they felt Mr X would have wanted should have been heard. According to the BMA (1999) guidelines, the views of families should be an integral part of the decision reached.

Best practice models

Encouraging collaboration is one way of ensuring that palliative care is incorporated into critical care. Where there is a lack of collaboration, good end-of-life decision-making is hindered and often delayed (Kirchhoff et al, 2000). One way of improving an alliance between critical care professionals and patients' families might be a policy change requiring a senior or primary nurse's presence in these discussions. He or she could be part of a formal consensus panel for end-of-life decisions.

Such consensus panels are gaining popularity in some areas, particularly in New Zealand (Ferrand et al, 2003), and perhaps, as alluded to earlier, there may be cases in the future where nurses who are actively involved in the decision do shoulder some of the legal responsibility. The formalized presence of palliative care consultants and ethicists in critical care units has been advocated as a way forward (Danis et al, 1999; Ferrand et al, 2003). They can bring an objectivity and sensitivity to an emotive area, which is often subject to many constraints. Collaboration, therefore, should ideally be a high priority when making decisions regarding end-of-life care (Baggs and Mick, 2000).

By considering some of the precepts of palliative care — respecting patient choices, ensuring good interdisciplinary working, using everybody's strengths, establishing support systems, caring comprehensively and acknowledging caregivers' concerns (Rushton et al, 2002) — a move to better practice in critical care is initiated. The importance of nurses not only doing (as in the predominantly medicalized model of critical care), but also being (establishing 'presence' with patients and viewing care as patient-centred) is emphasized as a best-practice model for end-of-life care (Rushton et al, 2002).

The transition of care from acute, predominantly medical care, which is often fragmented or disintegrated, to holistic palliative care, is summarized in *Figure 13.2*.

Although nurses are responsible for patient comfort in critical care, this sometimes becomes

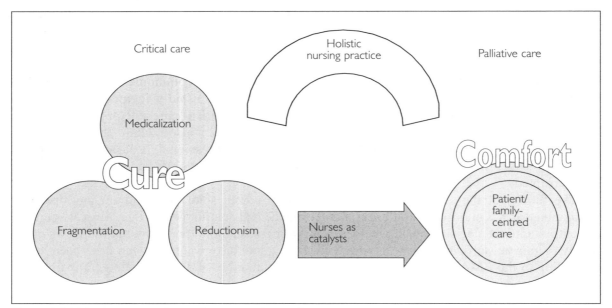

Figure 13.2: The transition of care from critical to palliative care

sidelined by life-sustaining interventions. Nurses must try and move forwards and ensure they act as advocates for patients as they approach end of life, as well as providing holistic care throughout. Comprehensive collaboration between nursing and medical colleagues is required, along with a conscious effort not to 'reduce' a patient to a prognostic probability score, or even worse to a critical care 'failure'. Consistent decision-making is necessary (Nelson and Danis, 2001; Pettila et al, 2002), but each patient's case must also be considered on its own circumstances.

Communication with families and relatives at end of life is identified as one of the most important skills needed at this time (Kirchhoff and Beckstrand, 2000; Levy, 2001). Levy (2001) pinpoints being able to communicate in a clear, straightforward and compassionate manner to the patient's relatives as an essential part of good end-of-life care practice. Kirchhoff and Beckstrand (2000) found that communication between staff members was considered important for best decision-making. Really, both should be routine for nurses caring for dying patients in all settings.

Conclusion

This chapter has considered the literature and where the pitfalls lie in practice, namely, poor nurse-to-doctor collaboration, poor doctor-to-doctor collaboration, poor nurse-to-nurse collaboration and poor health professional-to-relative or surrogate collaboration. This needs to be addressed by further research into measures that can improve these interactions. Critical care nurses must ensure they retain the fundamental nursing characteristics of patient advocate for the dying patient and are not drawn into the reductionist model of care that fragments a patient away from being viewed holistically. Nurses may be responsible for resources as much as doctors in many ways, but this must not detract from providing the right care for a patient.

By responding to changes in a patient's condition and redefining care as appropriate for that condition, nurses can transcend the boundaries of critical care *vs* palliative care. The dichotomy should not lie between the two paradigms if these fundamentals are considered. There should not be a division between critical care and palliative care in end-of-life care provision in the critical care unit. By considering tenets of both paradigms, end-of-life in critical care can be enhanced. While providing critical care to a very sick patient who may well die, nurses should also think about palliative care and retaining the focus of care on what is best for the patient, before any decisions to forgo life-sustaining treatments are made. The critical care nurse should push for timely and appropriate decisions in the patient's best interests and be able to provide excellent end-of-life care.

References

Abbott KH, Sago JG, Breen CM, Abernathy AP, Tulsky JA (2001) Families looking back: one year after discussion of withdrawal or withholding of life-sustaining support. *Crit Care Med* **29**: 197–200

Audit Commission (1999) *Critical to Success: The Place of Efficient and Effective Critical Care Services within the Acute Hospital*. Audit Commission, London

Baggs JG, Mick DJ (2000) Collaboration: a tool addressing ethical issues for elderly patients near the end of life in intensive care units. *J Gerontol Nurs* **26**(9): 41–7

Beauchamp TL, Childress JF (2001) *Principles of Biomedical Ethics*. 5th edn. Oxford University Press, Oxford

British Medical Association (2001) *Withholding and Withdrawing Life-Prolonging Medical Treatment: Guidance for Decision Making*. 2nd edn. BMA, London

Byock IR (1999) Conceptual models and the outcomes of caring. *J Pain Symptom Manage* 17(2): 83–92

Campbell ML (2002) End-of-life care in the ICU: current practice and future hopes. *Crit Care Nurs Clin North Am* **14**: 197–200

Cassell J, Buchman TG, Streat S, Stewart RM (2003) Surgeons, intensivists, and the covenant of care: administrative models and values affecting care at the end of life — updated. *Crit Care Med* **31**: 1551–9

Charlton R, Smith G (2000) Perceived skills in palliative medicine of newly qualified doctors in the UK. *J Palliat Care* **16**(4): 27–32

Clark D, Seymour J (1999) *Reflections on Palliative Care: Sociological and Policy Perspectives*. Open University Press, Buckingham

Curtis JR, Patrick DL, Shannon SE, Treece PD, Engelberg RA, Rubenfeld GD (2001) The family conference as a focus to improve communication about end-of-life care in the intensive care unit: opportunities for improvement. *Crit Care Med* **29**(2 Suppl): N26–33

Danis M, Federman D, Fins J et al (1999) Incorporating palliative care into critical care education: principles, challenges, and opportunities. *Crit Care Med* **27**: 2005–13

Department of Health (2000) *Comprehensive Critical Care: the Review of Adult Critical Care Services*. NHS Executive, London

Doyle D (2003) Proposal for a new name as well as having the new WHO definition of palliative care. *Palliat Med* **17**(1): 9–10

Evans RG (2003) Patient-centred medicine: reason, emotion, and human spirit? Some philosophical reflections on being with patients. *J Med Ethics* **29**(1): 8–15

Faber-Langendoen K (1996) A multi-institutional study of care given to patients dying in hospitals. Ethical practices and implications. *Arch Intern Med* **156**: 2130–6

Faber-Langendoen K, Lanken P (2000) Dying patients in the intensive care unit: forgoing treatment maintaining care. *Ann Intern Med* **133**: 886–93

Ferrand E, Lemaire F, Regnier B et al (2003) Discrepancies between perceptions by physicians and nursing staff of intensive care unit end-of-life decisions. *Am J Respir Crit Care Med* **167**: 1310–15

Fetters MD, Churchill L, Danis M (2001) Conflict resolution at the end of life. *Crit Care Med* **29**(5): 921–5

Goldhill DR, Sumner A (1998) Outcome of intensive care patients in a group of British intensive care units. *Crit Care Med* **26**: 1337–45

Groeger JS, Lemeshow S, Price K et al (1998) Multicenter outcome study of cancer patients admitted to the intensive care unit: a probability of mortality model. *J Clin Oncol* **16**(2): 761–70

Helman CG (2000) *Culture, Health and Illness*. 4th edn. Butterworth Heinemann, Oxford

Higgins TL, McGee WT, Steingrub JS, Rapoport J, Lemeshow S, Teres D (2003) Early indicators of prolonged intensive care unit stay: impact of illness severity, physician staffing, and pre-intensive care unit length of stay. *Crit Care Med* **31**: 45–51

Intensive Care National Audit and Research Centre (2000) *Data Analysis for the Case Mix Program Database*. Issue 5. Intensive Care National Audit and Research Centre, London

Johnson N, Cook D, Giacomini M, Willms D (2000) Towards a 'good' death: End-of-life narratives constructed in an intensive care unit. *Culture, Medicine and Psychiatry* 24: 275–95

Kirchhoff KT, Beckstrand RL (2000) Critical care nurses' perceptions of obstacles and helpful behaviours in providing end-of-life care to dying patients. *Am J Crit Care* **9**(2): 96–105

Kirchhoff KT, Spuhler V, Walker L, Hutton A, Cole BV, Clemmer T (2000) Intensive care nurses' experiences with end-of-life care. *Am J Crit Care* **9**(1): 36–42

Knaus WA, Zimmerman JE, Wagner DP, Draper EA, Lawrence DE (1981) APACHE — acute physiology and chronic health evaluation: a physiologically based classification system. *Crit Care Med* **9**: 591–7

Kyba FC (2002) Legal and ethical issues in end-of-life care. *Crit Care Nurs Clin North Am* **14**: 141–55

Levy M (2001) End-of-life care in the intensive care unit: can we do better? *Crit Care Med* **29**(2 Suppl): 56–61

Löfmark R, Nilstun T (2002) Conditions and consequences of medical futility: from a literature review to a clinical model. *J Med Ethics* **28**(2): 115–19

Marr L, Weismann DE (2004) Withdrawal of ventilatory support from the dying adult patient. *J Supportive Oncology* **2**(3): 283–8

Melia K (2004) *Health Care Ethics: Lessons from Intensive Care*. Sage, London

Nelson J, Danis M (2001) End-of-life care in the intensive care unit: where are we now? *Crit Care Med* **29**(2 Suppl): 2–9

Nelson JE, Meier DE, Oei EJ et al (2001) Self-reported symptom experience of critically ill cancer patients receiving intensive care. *Crit Care Med* **29:** 277–82

Oates L (2000) The courts' role in decisions about medical treatment. *Br Med J* **321:** 1282–4

Oliverio R, Fraulo B (1998) SUPPORT revisited: the nurse clinician's perspective. *Holist Nurs Pract* **13**(1): 1–7

Pettila V, Ala-Kokko T, Varpula T, Laurila J, Hovilehto S (2002) On what are our end-of-life decisions made? *Acta Anaesthesiol Scand* **46:** 947–54

Prendergast TJ, Puntillo KA (2002) Withdrawal of life support: intensive caring at the end of life. *JAMA* **288:** 2732–40

Randall F, Downie RS (1996) *Palliative Care Ethics: a Good Companion*. Oxford University Press, Oxford

Robins JLW (1999) Synthesizing reductionism and holism: integrative health care practice. *Issues in Interdisciplinary Care* **1**(3): 197–202

Rocker GM, Shemie SD, Lacroix J (2000) End-of-life issues in the ICU: a need for acute palliative care? *J Palliat Care* **16**(Suppl): S5–6

Rushton CH, Williams MA, Sabatier KH (2002) The integration of palliative care and critical care: one vision, one voice. *Crit Care Nurs Clin North Am* **14:** 133–40

Seymour JE (2000) Negotiating natural death in intensive care. *Soc Sci Med* **51:** 1241–52

Seymour JE (2001) *Critical Moments: Death and Dying in Intensive Care*. Open University Press, Buckingham

Sprung CL, Cohen SL, Sjokvist P, Baras M, Bulow H, Hovilehto S, Ledoux D, Lippert A, Maia P, Phelan D, Schobersberger W, Wennberg E, Woodcock T (2003) End-of-life practices in European intensive care units: The Ethicus Study. *J Amer Med Assoc* **260**(6): 790–7

SUPPORT Principal Investigators (1995) A controlled trial to improve care for seriously ill hospitalized patients: the study to understand prognoses and preferences for outcomes and risks of treatment (SUPPORT). *JAMA* **274:** 1591–8

ten Have H, Janssens D (2002) Futility, limits and palliative care. In: ten Have H, Clark D, eds. *The Ethics of Palliative Care: European Perspectives*. Open University Press, Buckinghamshire: 212–32

Truog RD, Cist FM, Brackett SE et al (2001) Recommendations for end-of-life care in the intensive care unit: the Ethics Committee of the Society of Critical Care Medicine. *Crit Care Med* **29:** 2332–48

van der Heide A, Deliens L, Faisst K, Nilstun T, Norup M, Paci E, van der Wal G, van der Maas P (2003) End-of-life decision-making in six European countries: Descriptive study. *Lancet* **362**(9381): 345–50

Webb P (2000) Why is the study of ethics important? In: Webb P, ed. *Ethical Issues in Palliative Care: Reflections and Considerations*. Hochland and Hochland, Manchester: 1–12

Wunsch H, Harrison DA, Harvey S, Rowan K (2005) End-of-life decision: A cohort study of the withdrawal of all active treatment in intensive care units in the United Kingdom. *Intensive Care Med* **31:** 823–31

Section 3

Management of patients with long-term neurological conditions

Chapter 14

A practical guide for managing adults with epilepsy

Christine Hayes

Epilepsy is a common condition. The incidence (new cases per year) in studies in most Western populations is about 80 per 100 000 people (Clinical Standards Advisory Group (CSAG), 1999). The prevalence (number of cases at any one time in the population) is between 5–10 per 1000 people (Shorvon, 2000).

Brown et al (1998) describe an epileptic seizure as a brief, usually unprovoked, stereotyped disturbance of consciousness, behaviour, emotion, motor function or sensation resulting from abnormal cortical neuronal discharge. The tonic–clonic seizure (*Table 14.1*) is most typically associated with epilepsy, and approximately 60% of people with epilepsy will have this type of seizure (Brown et al, 1998). However, estimates suggest that there are over 40 different types of epileptic seizure (Epilepsy Action, 2003a).

Table 14.1: Generalized seizures — what may be experienced or observed

Common	
Tonic–clonic	Muscles contract, forcing air out of the lungs. Body stiffens then jerks uncontrollably for 1–2 minutes. There may be irregular breathing, cyanosis of lips, possible incontinence of urine and tongue biting, followed by drowsiness, confusion, then sleep
Typical absence	Brief arrest of activities, may appear vacant for a few seconds
Myoclonic	Sudden, sometimes violent muscle jerk or jerks
Less common and often associated with learning disabilities	
Atypical absence	May last minutes rather than seconds
Tonic	Sudden limb and trunk stiffening
Atonic	A sudden loss of body tone, causing falling

Adapted from Brodie and Schachter (2001)

Reasons for hospital admission may be as an acute emergency following a first seizure, blackout, in those diagnosed with epilepsy where a convulsive seizure lasts longer than normal, where one convulsive seizure follows another, or status epilepticus. It is not uncommon that an ambulance will be called if a person with epilepsy is having a seizure in a public place. This may result in unnecessary attendance at the accident and emergency (A&E) department. Booked hospital admissions are more commonly arranged for periods of seizure observation and/or electroencephalogram (EEG) monitoring either to review or confirm a diagnosis. Main nursing roles for epilepsy are listed in *Table 14.2*.

Table 14.2: Main nursing roles in relation to epilepsy

- To know how to provide first aid for a person having a seizure and when medical assistance is required

- To provide detailed records of any seizures personally witnessed, witnessed by others and experienced by the person with epilepsy

- To encourage the individual to keep a seizure diary at times when seizures are not optimally controlled and when medication changes are being made

- To provide an educational role, giving information and advice about epilepsy, and how this may impact on the individual's lifestyle. If the nurse is unable to provide this role, referral should be made to an appropriate source, e.g. epilepsy specialist nurse or the voluntary sector

---

The aim of this chapter is to appreciate how hospital and practice nurses come into contact with people who have epilepsy or probable epilepsy. Through this contact, however brief, areas are identified in which the nurse provides essential care and treatment in the acute and emergency setting. It also identifies how the nurse may assist adults to self-manage their epilepsy through education.

Defining epilepsy

The term epilepsy is used to indicate the occurrence of recurrent epileptic seizures, which typically involve excessive firing and synchronization of neurones (Jefferys, 2002). There is an imbalance between excitatory and inhibitory neurones, resulting in excessive excitation or excessive inhibition in specific areas of the cerebral cortex or over the entire cerebral cortex (Hickey, 2003). The outward manifestation of the seizure depends on the part of the brain involved in the epileptic neuronal discharge (*Tables 14.1* and *14.3*). Some seizures are subtle and are only apparent to the person experiencing them.

Table 14.3: Types of partial seizure

Partial seizures start at a focus in the brain. There are two types, simple and complex. In a simple partial seizure consciousness is preserved, whereas in a complex partial seizure consciousness is affected. Either of these seizures may progress to a secondary generalized tonic–clonic seizure

Frontal lobe

Frequent brief attacks

Focal motor seizures

Tonic and postural signs and symptoms with preserved consciousness

Frequent falls

Vocalization, gestural automatisms

Complex partial

Temporal lobe (most common partial)

Preceded by aura, e.g. déjà vu, feeling of fear, olfactory or commonly rising epigastric discomfort

Dreamy state

Oral manual automatisms

Parietal lobe

Somatosensory auras

May have distorted body image

Occipital lobe

May have visual auras, visual hallucinations, e.g. flashing lights, coloured lights

Eye blinking

Nystagmus

Head deviation

Adapted from Hickey (2003)

The role of the hospital nurse

The CSAG (1999) found that 25% of people with epilepsy were seen in the A&E department in the previous 12 months because of their epilepsy. Potential reasons for attending A&E were acute seizures, status epilepticus, non-epileptic seizures, accidents in seizures, iatrogenic causes, such as rash from anti-epileptic drugs (AEDs) and overdose or other psychiatric emergencies. Fifteen per cent were admitted overnight, 80% of whom stayed in hospital for 1–5 days.

Emergency admission following a first seizure

The first essential role of the nurse is to provide a safe environment for the patient, to provide first-aid treatment in the event of a seizure and to know when medical intervention is required.

Best practice would suggest that if the patient is on a trolley/bed and left unattended at any time, cot sides (preferably padded) should be used and the trolley/bed left at its lowest height to reduce the risk of injury (Hickey, 2003). During a self-limiting seizure the first-aid treatment is to prevent patients harming themselves and to protect their airway by placing them in the recovery position as soon as that is possible. No action at this stage will prevent the seizure from taking its normal course (see *Table 14.1*). As the patient is already in hospital, the preceding history of seizure activity is important in the continuing management, and medical intervention is likely at an earlier stage to prevent status epilepticus (see below). *Table 14.4* summarizes the first aid required.

Table 14.4: First aid for dealing with a convulsive seizure

DO

Stay calm

Loosen any tight clothing around neck

Protect from injury

Cushion the head if on the ground

Place in the recovery position when convulsive movements subside

Protect airway, stay with person and act as a witness of the seizure

DO NOT

Try to restrain the person

Put anything in mouth or between teeth

Move the person unless in danger

Give anything to drink until fully recovered

From Epilepsy Action (2003a)

Immediate management of convulsive status epilepticus

Shorvon (2000) describes status epilepticus as prolonged or recurrent tonic–clonic seizures persisting for 30 minutes or more. Panayiotopoulos (2005) refers to the World Health Organisation definition of status epilepticus as being charaterized by epileptic seizures that are sufficiently prolonged or repeated at sufficiently brief intervals so as to produce an unvarying and enduring epileptic condition. Where there is pre-existing epilepsy, AED changes, particularly drug withdrawal, or concurrent illness may be the cause. Where there is no previous history of epilepsy the cause is usually an acute cerebral event. Usual seizure patterns may become more frequent or more intense. Shorvon refers to this as the premonitory stage, which if not rectified can result in status epilepticus. Generalized tonic–clonic status epilepticus is a medical emergency as it is associated with significant morbidity and mortality if not treated promptly (National Institute for Clinical Excellence (NICE), 2003a).

The aim of treatment is to stop seizure activity and prevent irreversible cerebral, systemic, metabolic, autonomic and cardiovascular changes (Shorvon, 2000):

- *Compensation*. In phase one (compensation), cerebral metabolism is increased by seizure activity. Physiological mechanisms meet metabolic demands. Major physiological changes relate to increased cerebral blood flow and metabolism, autonomic activity and cardiovascular changes
- *Decompensation*. In phase two (decompensation), if seizure activity continues then cerebral metabolic demands become unsustainable, which may result in hypoxia, hypoglycaemia, acidosis, falling blood pressure and cardiac output and other changes leading to failure of homeostasis.

Immediate measures are to secure the airway, give oxygen, assess cardiac and respiratory function and secure intravenous (IV) access in the large veins. Lorazepam 4 mg IV or diazepam 10 mg IV, if lorazepam is unavailable, should be given and repeated 10 minutes later if there is no response. Benzodiazepines interact specifically with receptor molecules to modulate the efficiency of the inhibitory neurotransmitter gamma-aminobutyric acid (GABA). Lorazepam is a fast-acting benzodiazepine that is longer acting than diazepam and is, therefore, the preferred drug (Rey et al, 1999).

If there is any delay in gaining IV access, give 10–20 mg rectal diazepam (Scottish Intercollegiate Guidelines Network (SIGN), 2003). A full blood analysis may help establish causation and the degree of any physiological changes that may have occurred. Blood should be taken for full blood count, urea and electrolytes, liver function tests, calcium, glucose, coagulation studies and AED levels. Blood gases need to be measured to assess the extent of acidosis and respiratory function (SIGN, 2003). Local protocols will explain how to proceed if status epilepticus continues.

Ongoing care

Whether a patient has established epilepsy or has been admitted as an emergency after a first seizure, the nurse has an important management and educational role. Observing and interacting with the person during the attack to provide an accurate written account is essential to enable a diagnosis to be made.

According to SIGN (2003):

'A clear history from the patient and an eyewitness to the attack give the most important diagnostic information, and should be the mainstay of diagnosis.'

Table 14.5: Recording an attack

- Was there a warning (aura)?

- What behaviour or motor activity occurred?

- Was consciousness lost or diminished?

- How long did the attack last?

- How long did it take to full recovery?

- Was there incontinence?

- Observations of any injuries sustained

- Condition following attack

The nurse should ensure that during the inpatient stay a description of the person's experience of the attack(s) and a witness account of what was observed are recorded (*Table 14.5*). It is far more important to document this accurately than try to categorize the attack into a particular seizure type.

Preparation for discharge

A person may be hospitalized after a first convulsive seizure with loss of consciousness. Establishing whether there have been previous more subtle seizures is important for planning future management (see *Tables 14.1* and *14.3*). The diagnosis of epilepsy has important physical, psychological and economic implications; it is, therefore, important that it is correct, and should be made by a neurologist or other epilepsy specialist (SIGN, 2003). This will also enable informed choices to be made about management strategies and treatment options (NHS Modernisation Agency, 2002). It is important to check that a referral has been made to a neurologist before discharge.

Where established epilepsy exists, the nurse should check concordance with AEDs and any recent medication changes (Greenwood, 2000). Often no cause for the seizure can be found, but sometimes there are triggers, such as illness, sleep deprivation, excess alcohol or stress (Epilepsy Action, 2003a). Photosensitive epilepsy, i.e. being affected by strobe lighting, occurs in only 5% of people with epilepsy (Epilepsy Action, 2003b).

The hospital stay is usually short. Verbal and written advice and a contact number for the epilepsy specialist nurse or self-help group should be provided before discharge. It is important that appropriate information and support for individuals with epilepsy and their family and/or carers is provided at each stage of the care pathway. This should be appropriate to the individual needs considering age, gender and culture (Stokes et al, 2004b). *Figure 14.1* provides useful information for patients who have had a first seizure (Epilepsy Action, 2003a).

What happened to me?

It is normal to be frightened and worried the first time a blackout or epileptic seizure occurs. It may be necessary to have further tests, or to await further events, before it is certain what caused your attack.

When is it safe to go home?

If you have been admitted to hospital, it is usually considered safe to go home 12–24 hours after the attack, as long as the doctors do not think there is any immediate risk of a recurrence.

Could it happen again?

If the seizure is the first sign of an epileptic disorder, you may have further attacks. This is most likely to occur in the first few months after the first one.

Do I need medication?

Anti-epileptic medication is only used if it is certain that the attack was epileptic and that the benefits of treatment outweigh the risks. It is common practice to start treatment only after two definite seizures.

Looking after yourself after discharge from hospital

The seizure may leave you feeling tired and washed out. Sometimes your limbs will ache, your head will feel fuzzy and your memory may be poor. If you are in employment, it is often a good idea to take a few days off work to recuperate.

Can I prevent further attacks?

Most seizures strike completely out of the blue. However, sometimes there are triggers, which can make you more vulnerable to having a seizure. Some of the more common triggers include: late nights and lack of sleep; drinking large amounts of alcohol; illness with fever, e.g. influenza and sore throats. Flickering lights affect about 5% of people with a diagnosis of epilepsy.

General health and safety advice

If you have epilepsy it is safer to shower than have a bath. If you do have a bath, make sure someone else is in the house and knows you are taking a bath. Leave the door unlocked. Avoid dangerous sports such as rock climbing and hang gliding. If you swim inform the pool attendant. Avoid swimming in the sea.

Driving

UK law states that you cannot drive for 1 year after a seizure or any unexplained loss of consciousness.

Figure 14.1: Information following a first seizure. From Epilepsy Action (2003a)

Routine hospital admission

Planned hospital admissions are arranged for seizure monitoring, usually when seizures are continuing despite AED therapy. This may be as part of an epilepsy surgery programme where an exact focus of origin of the seizures needs to be established (Duncan, 2002). These patients will have had previous EEG recordings and high-resolution magnetic resonance imaging (MRI). To ascertain whether the epileptic seizures have a focus of origin and whether this is associated with an operable lesion, the MRI needs to be of high resolution with thin slices to localize the lesion. Presurgical work-up is directed at identifying the functional and structural basis of the seizure disorder (Hickey, 2003).

Other patients may be admitted if there is doubt about the nature of their attacks, and a diagnosis needs to be established to confirm whether the attacks are because of epilepsy or a non-epileptic attack disorder. In the latter, AEDs will be of no benefit and referral to the department of psychological medicine for counselling and therapy is the usual mode of management. The nurse needs to provide a supportive role to manage the transitional period while uncertainty of the diagnosis exists. Listening skills and the ability to allow patients to discuss their life experiences are valuable qualities for the nurse to demonstrate at this time.

Videotelemetry allows for continuous recording of the EEG and video monitoring. Both are synchronized and can continue for several days or longer to capture attacks. A specialized unit has the advantage of optimum observation facilities with multi-skilling of nurses and EEG technicians. Unlike specialist centres, most hospitals do not have a videotelemetry unit but are able to provide some form of video and EEG monitoring.

Inpatient video EEG monitoring is undertaken to establish the anatomical location of the seizure site and to correlate behaviour patterns with abnormal EEG patterns. If this programme is to assess suitability for surgery then the patient also needs to undertake neuropsychological testing as an outpatient. Psychometric assessment is mandatory in all patients being investigated with a view to temporal lobe surgery. The assessment should include tests of general intellectual ability, language and memory (Shorvon, 2004). If both these presurgical investigations are favourable then a sodium amytal test (Wada test) may be performed preoperatively, particularly if an unexpected or significant risk to memory on routine psychological testing has been demonstrated. This test is not an absolute guarantee of postoperative freedom from memory impairment (Shorvon, 2004).

Guidelines for videotelemetry

The EEG and video-monitoring equipment usually restrict the patient's movements. If a side ward is provided, the patient is often confined to the room. Guidelines for management are useful, especially in areas where videotelemetry is not provided on a regular basis.

Before admission

The patient should be informed of the no-smoking policy as he or she may have to go 5 days without a cigarette. Boredom can be a problem, so activities need considering before admission. A risk assessment should be conducted with the aim of providing a safe environment during the patient's stay. This needs to consider the level of observation required and will depend on any AED reduction before admission, seizure type and frequency, particularly if there is no warning.

On admission, document the seizure descriptions and frequency. Check medication and ensure prescribed drugs are clearly written, as doses may be variable. Medication often remains unchanged, and many patients can self-medicate. Local guidelines may vary, but it is usual for the nurse to ensure a venflon has been inserted, a heparin flush has been prescribed to maintain patency and to check the site of insertion daily. A prescription should be written for IV benzodiazepine, e.g. 10 mg diazepam for emergency use, with the prescription indicating under what conditions it is to be administered. When reducing AEDs to try and provoke seizures, there is always the potential of causing a prolonged tonic–clonic seizure that requires emergency intervention.

During the inpatient stay, the nurse should work collaboratively with EEG technicians and ensure documentation is completed and observation periods are agreed. The patient should be fully conversant with what is expected of him or her and how to summon assistance. Owing to the harness and electrodes required for monitoring purposes, assistance may be required with washing and dressing.

At the beginning of the attack the alert button should be pressed to highlight the attack on the EEG recording. Expose as much of the patient as possible. At night pull the bedcovers back and put the lights on. Do not block the camera's view of the patient but do interact.

Ask the patient the following questions:

- Tell me your name
- What is this (show the patient an object)?
- Can you raise your right arm?
- I want you to remember the colour green.

This makes the videorecording more purposeful, and the level of responsiveness can be assessed more accurately. After the event, stay with the person until full recovery. Remember to ask him or her what you wanted him or her to remember, and make sure this is still on camera. Document everything witnessed and the time.

Other forms of monitoring include ambulatory EEG. This does not have the advantage of videorecording and relies on an accurate witness description. Again an event button is pressed. Other units provide a 24–48-hour hospital stay with EEG and videorecording, but these are not synchronized as with videotelemetry.

Finally, one of the easiest and quickest ways to capture attacks is on video using a handheld camcorder. Many families can accomplish this in their own homes and hospitals may provide a lending service. Where this is not possible, a hospital admission may be necessary. Again, interaction with the patient gives useful additional information. Hospital procedures need to be in place for obtaining video consent.

The role of the practice nurse

The new general medical service contract now includes epilepsy as a quality indicator. Financial incentives are available for holding a register of patients over the age of 16 years receiving drug treatment for epilepsy, and also for a record of seizure frequency and medication review in the past 15 months (NHS Confederation, 2003). The aim of the quality indicators is to encourage the establishment and delivery of a structured management plan for people with epilepsy in primary care (Epilepsy Action, 2003c). The practice nurse is likely to have a pivotal role in the recommended annual review of adults with epilepsy (SIGN, 2003). Providing information and advice will be a key element.

Most premature deaths among those with epilepsy are directly related to the epilepsy itself (Hanna et al, 2002). Information about first aid, risks and safety, lifestyles, precipitating factors, medication and treatment options are some of the areas identified as important issues for those with epilepsy (Epilepsy Action, 2003c). The practice nurse may need additional resources to provide this information, and collaboration with an epilepsy specialist nurse or the voluntary sector may be useful. Improved communication between primary and secondary care, access to an epilepsy specialist nurse, shared care protocols, guidelines and the provision of education and training for staff are seen as improving services for epilepsy (CSAG, 1999). Proposed actions that will help to implement the National Service Framework (Department of Health, 2005) include the development of expert patient programmes and courses for the newly diagnosed in conjunction with the voluntary sector. Also there is a commitment to support epilepsy care using the general medical service quality outcomes framework and future performance indicators.

Medication

Modern outcome studies have demonstrated that 60–70% of people with newly diagnosed epilepsy enter long-term remission usually on one AED. However, 30% continue to have seizures despite pharmacological treatment (Brodie and Kwan, 2002).

It is important to keep up-to-date records of medication and dosage. Patients making alterations to their AEDs are most likely to be under specialist review. They should be encouraged to keep a diary of seizure types and frequency during drug changes to establish their effectiveness. Any side-effects should be recorded and dose changes dated. The principle of drug changes is to 'start low and go slow'. Ideally, only one drug change is made at any one time.

NICE (2003b) has guidelines on drug treatment for different seizure types. Goodwin (2003) emphasizes initiating treatment with an appropriate AED, as changes in medication are unlikely to be considered once seizure freedom and driving have been re-established. This has particular implications for women who may need to consider changing an AED because of risk factors in pregnancy. SIGN (2003) provides guidance relating to drug withdrawal, which needs to be discussed with the patient concerned so that he or she can make an informed choice. Withdrawing medication with a view to discontinuing it does have driving implications (Driver and Vehicle Licensing Agency (DVLA), 2003a).

Diagnosis and control of seizures

- If the diagnosis of epilepsy is in doubt, refer to a neurologist for a review
- If the patient plans to conceive and is on anti-epileptic medication, refer to a neurologist or epilepsy nurse for review of treatment
- If the seizures are not well controlled, refer to a neurologist for review of treatment.

Hormonal contraception

Which methods of contraception do anti-epileptic drugs affect?

Oestrogen-based oral contraceptives are affected by topiramate and enzyme inducing anti-epileptic drugs (carbamazepine, phenytoin, phenobarbitone, primidone and oxcarbazepine). For the combined oral contraceptive the dose of ethinyloestradiol should be 50μg daily. The simplest method is to take two contraceptive pills. If breakthrough bleeding occurs increase to 75–100 μg daily or tri-cycle – taking three packets without a break. A barrier method should be used until it is established there is no intermenstrual bleeding. If this occurs, further advice should be sought. The medroxyprogesterone depot injection given every 12 weeks is an alternative.

Pregnancy

What are the risks of anti-epileptic drugs in pregnancy?

Studies have shown that a significant foetal malformation on taking one anti-epileptic drug is about 3% (slightly above background risk). The UK pregnancy register reports major malformation risk of 6.2% for valproate and 5.45% for lamotrigine above 200 mg daily. This risk increases with polytherapy with reports of a risk of 9–12% with a combination of valproate and lamotrigine. Retrospective studies suggest an increased risk of additional educational needs in children conceived while on valproate.

Can anti-epileptic drugs be reduced or withdrawn in pregnancy?

Yes, if the patient is seizure-free and counselled about the risk of relapse. If the patient has occasional non-convulsive seizures, the decision must be taken on the advice of a neurologist. If seizures are poorly controlled, treatment should continue. Withdrawing drugs requires cessation of driving for the withdrawal period plus 6 months. A driving ban of 1 year applies if seizures recur.

Does pregnancy affect anti-epileptic drug levels?

Pregnancy can reduce drug blood levels. Blood monitoring is advised if seizure control deteriorates. Doses are usually changed only on clinical grounds, however, blood monitoring may be appropriate in some cases.

What supplements are recommended before and during pregnancy?

Folic acid   5 mg daily 3 months before conception until the end of the first trimester

Vitamin K   All infants of mothers taking anti-epileptic drugs should be given1 mg vitamin K at birth. If additional risk factors for haemorrhagic disease of newborn, oral vitamin K (10 mg phytomenadione daily) should also be given in the last month of pregnancy (SIGN, 2003).

Figure 14.2: Preconception management for women with epilepsy (a quick guide for professionals). Adapted from Crawford (2005). Continued on next page

Can a mother on anti-epileptic drugs breastfeed?
Yes, as long as the baby is well and she observes the baby for signs of excessive sedation as drug elimination mechanisms are not fully developed in early infancy. Repeated administration of a drug such as lamotrigine via breast milk may lead to accumulation in the infant.

What precautions do mothers with epilepsy need for their baby?
To share the care so as not to become sleep-deprived. To sit with the baby on the floor when feeding. When using a baby chair to ensure it cannot fall over. Never bath the baby alone. Try not to carry the baby up- or downstairs, but if necessary use a carrycot or car seat to provide protection from a fall. Use stair gates at all times. Use a pram with a brake that comes on when the pram handle is released. Always strap the baby in. Use reins strapped securely to mother and child. If seizures are frequent, a formal health and safety assessment of the home may be advisable through the health visitor/community occupational therapist. The risk to the child depends on the mother's seizure type, severity and frequency. Women most at risk are those with uncontrolled juvenile myoclonic epilepsy because children tend to wake early.

Figure 14.2 continued.

Preconception counselling

Women of childbearing age should be offered preconception counselling and encouraged to plan their families based on informed choice. It is never too early to discuss this issue (National Society for Epilepsy, 2003). They need to be informed if their AEDs interfere with the reliability of their method of contraception (Epilepsy Action, 2003d). Allowing 2 years before conception means that there is time to discuss current research on foetal abnormality risks and also allows time for any medication changes to be made. *Figure 14.2* provides preconception management advice for women with epilepsy (Crawford et al, 1999: SIGN, 2003). Betts and Greenhill (2001) have shown that referring a woman to an epilepsy specialist nurse for preconception counselling can be beneficial.

If a woman is already pregnant then it is important for her to feel supported by the nurse and that medication, seizures and pregnancy are managed through a coordinated approach between healthcare professionals. The nurse should be available and supportive throughout to answer questions and enable the woman to make informed choices regarding decisions she needs to make. Providing an educational role may help for planning future pregnancies (Crawford et al, 1999).

Lifestyle

Dilorio and Henry (1995) researched self-management strategies in people with epilepsy. They found general adherence to medication but less to other recommended practices such as safety and lifestyle behaviours. Buelow (2001) identified perceptions of self-management in people with epilepsy. These management strategies fell into three main categories:

- Treatment
- Seizures
- Lifestyle.

All respondents discussed medication as an important part of self-management. Many strategies were developed to avoid seizures, such as getting a good night's sleep and reducing stress. Lifestyle issues related to relationships, employment and the legal regulations pertaining to driving.

Even where services for epilepsy exist, people still have the same concerns (Epilepsy Advisory Board, 1999). This demonstrates that quality of life, lifestyles and decision-making skills around this area are important for those with epilepsy. Long et al (2000) studied people's knowledge of their epilepsy and revealed that people with epilepsy knew little more about their disorder than age-matched controls. This supports the nurse's role as educator and is endorsed by the Government's expert patient programme, which emphasizes a partnership between healthcare professionals and the patient in decision making (DoH, 2001).

Driving

The DVLA states that any unexplained loss of consciousness or seizure, however small, results in a 1-year ban for group one vehicles (motorcars and motorcycles), unless the person fulfils the requirements for sleep-only seizures (DVLA, 2003b). Employment and lifestyle impact on a person, and having the right advice at the right time is an essential quality of the nursing consultation. As the law is specific about driving, this is taken out of the nurse's/doctor's decision making.

The nurse has a duty of care to the patient and society in general to inform those with epilepsy the requirements of the law. This information should be documented, and further written information provided to remind the patient to contact the DVLA. If patients choose to withdraw their AEDs, the law states that they should not drive for the period of withdrawal and for 6 months afterwards (DVLA, 2003a).

Conclusion

Nurses have a key role to play in the care of those with epilepsy. They should be able to respond appropriately when first-aid management is necessary and know when to call for medical assistance. Providing information and advice on first aid, risks, precipitating factors to seizures, lifestyles, particularly employment, family planning and driving, medication and treatment options is useful and has been identified as being important to those with epilepsy (Epilepsy Action, 2003c). The nurse may not be able to provide all the information, but can contact an epilepsy specialist nurse or make appropriate referrals and suggestions as to where information may be found.

References

Betts T, Greenhill L (2001) The cost of everything and the value of nothing: nursing case histories. *Seizure* **10:** 628–32

Brodie MJ, Kwan P (2002) Staged approach to epilepsy management. *Neurology* **58**(Suppl 5): S2–S8

Brodie MJ, Schachter SC (2001) *Fast Facts: Epilepsy.* Health Press, Oxford

Brown S, Betts T, Crawford P, Hall B, Shorvon S, Wallace S (1998) Epilepsy needs revisited: a revised epilepsy needs document for the UK. *Seizure* **7:** 435–46

Buelow JM (2001) Epilepsy management issues and techniques. *J Neurosci Nurs* **33:** 260–9

Crawford P (2005) Best practice guidelines for the management of women with epilepsy. *Epilepsia* **46**(Suppl 9): 117–24.

Crawford P, Appleton R, Betts T, Duncan J, Githrie E, Morrow J (1999) Best practice guidelines for the management of women with epilepsy. *Seizure* **8:** 201–17

Clinical Standards Advisory Group (1999) *Services for Patients with Epilepsy.* Department of Health, London

Department of Health (2001) *The Expert Patient: A New Approach to Chronic Disease Management for the 21st Century.* Department of Health, London

Department of Health (2003) *Long-term Conditions NSF.* Department of Health, London (www.dh.gov.uk/PolicyAndGuidance/ HealthAndSocialCareTopics/LongTermConditions/fs/en) (last accessed 22 March 2004)

Department of Health (2005) T*he National Service Framework for Long-term Conditions* (p 81, Section 7C–D). Department of Health, London

Dilorio C, Henry M (1995) Self-management in persons with epilepsy. *J Neurosci Nurs* **27:** 338–43

Driver and Vehicle Licensing Agency (2003a) *Guidance for Withdrawal of Anti-epileptic Medication Being Withdrawn on Specific Medical Advice.* DVLA, Swansea (www.dvla.gov.uk/at_a_glance/annex_3.htm) (last accessed 22 March 2004)

Driver and Vehicle Licensing Agency (2003b) *At a Glance.* DVLA, Swansea (www.dvla.gov.uk/at_a_glance/content.htm) (last accessed 22 March 2004)

Duncan JS (2002) Temporal lobe epilepsy. In: Duncan JS, Sisodiya SM, Smalls JE, eds. *Epilepsy 2002 from Science to Patient.* International League Against Epilepsy, Bristol

Epilepsy Action (2003a) *Epilepsy and Everyone.* Epilepsy Action, Leeds

Epilepsy Action (2003b) *Photosensitive Epilepsy.* Epilepsy Action, Leeds

Epilepsy Action (2003c) *Epilepsy Resource Pack.* Epilepsy Action, Leeds

Epilepsy Action (2003d) *With Women in Mind: Getting Ahead.* Epilepsy Action, Leeds

Epilepsy Advisory Board (1999) *Epilepsy Care: Making it Happen: A Tool Kit for Today.* British Epilepsy Association, Leeds

Goodwin M (2003) Managing epilepsy in primary care. *Primary Health Care* **13**(7): 35–8

Greenwood RS (2000) Adverse effects of antiepileptic drugs. *Epilepsia* **41**(Suppl): S42–S52

Hanna NJ, Black M, Sander JWL et al (2002) *National Sentinel Clinical Audit of Epilepsy-related Death: Epilepsy: Death in the Shadows.* The Stationery Office, London

Hickey JV (2003) *The Clinical Practice of Neurological and Neurosurgical Nursing.* Lippincott, Williams and Wilkins, Philadelphia

Jefferys J (2002) Basic mechanisms of epilepsy. In: Duncan JS, Sisodiya SM, Smalls JE, eds. *Epilepsy 2002 from Science to Patient.* International League Against Epilepsy, Bristol

Long L, Reeves AL, Moore JL, Roach J, Pickering CT (2000) An assessment of epilepsy patients' knowledge of their disorder. *Epilepsia* **41**(6): 727–31

National Society for Epilepsy (2003) *Pregnancy and Parenting.* National Society for Epilepsy, Chalfont St Peter, Buckinghamshire (www.epilepsynse.org.uk/pages/info/leaflets.preg.cfm) (last accessed 22 March 2004)

NHS Confederation (2003) *Investing in General Practice. The New General Medical Service Contract.* NHS Confederation, London

NHS Modernisation Agency (2002) *PCT Competency Framework.* NHS Modernisation Agency, London (www.natpact.nhs.uk/downloads/cf/framework.pdf) (last accessed 22 March 2004)

National Institute for Clinical Excellence (2003a) *Epilepsy: the Diagnosis and Management of Epilepsy in Children and Adults.* NICE, London (www.nice.org.uk/cat.asp?c=20119) (last accessed 22 March 2004)

National Institute for Clinical Excellence (2003b) *Final Appraisal Determination. Newer Drugs for Epilepsy in Adults.*

NICE, London ([www.nice.org.uk/ Docref.asp?d=92494](www.nice.org.uk/Docref.asp?d=92494)) (last accessed 22 March 2004)

Panayiotopoulos CP (2005) *The Epilepsies*. Bladon Medical Publishers, Oxford

Rey E, Treluyer JM, Pons G (1999) Pharmacokinetic optimization of benzodiazepine therapy for acute seizures. *Clin Pharmacokinet* **36**(6): 409–24

Shorvon S (2000) *Handbook of Epilepsy Treatment*. Blackwell, Oxford

Shorvon S (2004) Introduction to epilepsy surgery and its presurgical assessment. In S Shorvon, E Perucca, D Fish, E Dodson (eds.) *The Treatment of Epilepsy*. Blackwell, Oxford.

Scottish Intercollegiate Guidelines Network (2003) *Diagnosis and Management of Epilepsy in Adults*. SIGN, Edinburgh

Stokes T, Shaw EJ, Juarez-Garcia A, Camosso-Stefinovic J, Baker R (2004b) *Clinical Guidelines and Evidence Review for the Epilepsies: Diagnosis and Management in Adults and Children in Primary and Secondary Care. 1.3.1 Information Needs of Individuals, Families and Carers*. p. 281. Royal College of General Practitioners, London

Chapter 15

Epilepsy: Clinical management and treatment options

Muili Lawal

According to the World Health Organization (WHO, 2001a), epilepsy is a disorder characterized by recurrent seizures resulting from outbursts of excessive electrical activity in either part or the whole of the brain (*Figure 15.1*).

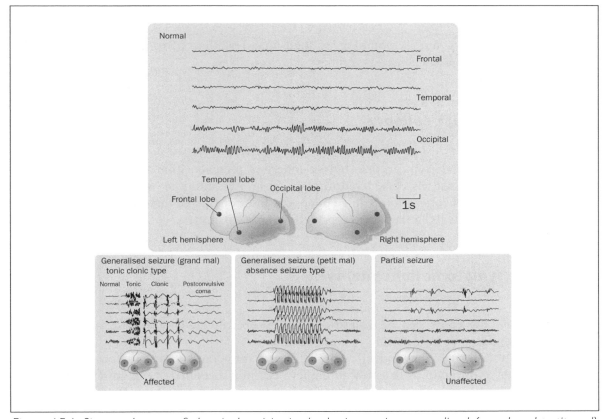

Figure 15.1: Sites and types of electrical activity in the brain causing generalized (grand and petit mal) and partial seizures

Also, Brooker and Nicol (2003) see seizures as abnormal firing of the cerebral neurons. Davies (1999) believes that it is difficult to offer a comprehensive clinical definition of epilepsy owing to various degrees of signs and symptoms exhibited by different patients. According to Davies, epilepsy is an intermittent disturbance of consciousness, behaviour and motor function resulting from cortical neural discharge.

Incidence

Epilepsy is the most common, chronic, disabling, neurological disorder, affecting almost 380 000 people in England with about 800 deaths every year associated with seizures (Department of Health (DoH), 2003). Hampshire (2005) states that epilepsy claims approximately 1000 lives every year in England.

Aetiology

The causes of epilepsy are as complex as their manifestations. Brooker and Nicol (2003) classified epilepsy into two categories, primary and secondary.

Primary (idiopathic) epilepsy

There is no obvious underlying cause, but an inherited predisposition to hypersensitivity and dysrhythmia of the neurons is considered to play a role. According to WHO (2001b), the most commonly acceptable theory of idiopathic epilepsy is low convulsive threshold resulting from an excess of certain chemicals in the brain, especially neurotransmitters.

Secondary (symptomatic) epilepsy

In this category, the cause can be identified. It may be triggered by almost any intracranial pathological condition or by general systemic disorders.

Symptomatic seizures may occur with increased intracranial pressure or brain damage associated with a difficult birth or head injury, cerebral oedema or an intracranial space-occupying lesion, haemorrhage or infection. Brain tumours and metastatic lesions to the brain may also directly irritate brain tissue, setting up an epileptogenic focus (Guyton and Hall, 2000; Brooker and Nicol, 2003).

According to the WHO (2001b), trauma and infection is responsible for a higher incidence of epilepsy in developing countries, and about 3% of children with febrile convulsion tend to develop epilepsy later in life. General systemic conditions in which seizures most commonly occur are listed in *Table 15.1*, and Manford (2003) also recognizes some factors that can trigger seizures (*Table 15.2*).

Table 15.1: General systemic causes of seizures
• Brain diseases, such as tumours, cerebrovascular disease
• Trauma
• Infection, e.g. malaria, meningitis, neurocysticercosis
• Febrile illness
• Hyperthermia
• Hypoglycaemia
• Hyponatraemia and hypocalcaemia
• Eclampsia
From WHO (2001b); Brooker and Nicol (2003)

Table 15.2: Further factors that may trigger seizures
• Emotional stress
• Lack of sleep
• Hormonal changes in menstrual cycle
• Flickering light
• Alcohol withdrawal
From Manford (2003)

Pathophysiology

The brain is a sensitive organ protected by the bony skull. It controls the functions of the body, either by interpreting electrical messages from sensory nerves or by generating electrical impulses for transmission down the motor nerves (Hole, 1993). To fulfil its many functions, the brain's nerve cells (neurons) must work in smooth harmony. The nervous system functions by sending nerve impulses to one another and to muscles and glands (Hole, 1993). The electrical activity of the brain can be measured by an electro-encephalogram (EEG). In individuals with epilepsy, the EEG is abnormal; characteristic wave forms are altered by the appearance of spikes of electrical activity.

The exact cellular mechanism that initiates seizure activity is unclear (Hickey, 2003). However, most epileptic seizures are thought to result from abnormal hyperactive neurons that form an epileptogenic focus (Hickey, 2003). During an epileptic seizure there is abnormal and excessive discharging of impulses originating from brain cells, and some are from epileptogenic focus. This reaches skeletal muscle fibres to stimulate violent contractions, and later subsides owing to a lack of neurotransmitters in the synapse. In time, the seizure stops because of the lack of neurotransmitters in the synapse. According to Hole (1993):

'If nerve impulses reach synaptic knobs at rapid rates, the supplies of neurotransmitters may become exhausted, and impulses cannot be transferred between the neurons involved until more neurotransmitters are synthesized.'

The hyperactivity of an epileptogenic focus can result in partial or generalized seizure activity. Partial seizures may be caused by a localized hyper-excited focus, which eventually ceases, or the hyperactivity may spread to synaptically-related areas but does not involve the entire brain. Enough resistance is offered by adjacent cells so that impulse firing stops. When the rapid, repetitive electrical discharges spread throughout the brain, the resulting seizure is described as a generalized seizure (British Epilepsy Association (BEA), 2003).

Also, Farine (2003) claimed that seizures can result from abnormal neurotransmitter or neuronal membrane properties because both can alter blood ion concentrations, such as those of potassium and calcium, which are known to fluctuate during the onset of hypersynchronous discharge. Neuronal membrane property alteration may be a result of hypoxia, alkalosis, hypoglycaemia and abnormal neurotransmitter properties, which may cause the release of large amounts of neurotransmitters at the synapse and consequently promote seizure.

During a seizure, the cerebral oxygen consumption increases by as much as 60% (Hickey, 2003). In status epilepticus, oxygen and glucose consumption by skeletal muscle contraction, coupled with periods of apnoea, rapidly depletes oxygen delivery and nutritive stores, leading to hypoxaemia, hypercapnia and hypoglycaemia. The increase in cellular lactate associated with anaerobic metabolism further complicates the pathophysiologic state. The end result is an energy debt that rapidly leads to cellular exhaustion (Hole, 1993; Guyton and Hall, 2000; Hickey, 2003).

Diagnosis

In assessment it is important to determine whether the signs and symptoms are, in fact, epileptic seizures or a disorder that mimics epilepsy. A thorough history obtained from the patient, family and/or partner will best describe the seizure type, cause, duration, previous treatment and current status. In addition to eliciting a careful history, the complete physical examination may reveal neurological defects associated with recent or remote neurological lesions (e.g. previous trauma, cranial surgery, cerebrovascular accident, infection or long-standing seizure disorder) (BEA, 2003; Hickey, 2003).

Farine (2003) identified the following useful diagnostic techniques:

- Electroencephalogram (EEG) is a measure of cerebral function and is therefore useful in locating the focus of the abnormal electrical cerebral activity
- Computed axial tomography (CAT or CT scanning) is an enhanced X-ray technique for studying cerebral structure. CT scanning may give a visual demonstration of a structural abnormality causing seizures, such as the presence of mass lesions, such as tumours
- Skull X-ray may help identify the presence of a lesion
- Laboratory tests are conducted to rule out organic lesions, for example to identify metabolic disturbances such as hypoglycaemia and electrolyte imbalance that may underlie seizure activity
- Brooker and Nicol (2003) identified magnetic resonance imaging (MRI) as a useful diagnostic tool. MRI is a technique that identifies structural changes in the brain. The final picture looks similar to a CT scan, but with more structural detail.

Occasionally other types of diagnostic imaging, such as positron emission tomography (PET) and single photon emission computed tomography (SPECT) are required when surgery is proposed (Brooker and Nicol, 2003).

Classification of seizures

There are many different kinds of epilepsy and over 40 different seizure types, which may affect patients in different ways. According to Hickey (2003), there are different classifications of seizures based on causes, symptoms, origin, prognosis or electrical changes involved in the brain. Farine (2003) classified seizures into two main groups with further subgroups (*Figure 15.2*).

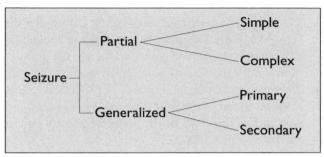

Figure 15.2: Classification of seizures. Farine (2003)

Partial seizures

This is usually unilateral, involving a localized or focal area of the brain, for example Jacksonian seizure. These seizures occur without loss of consciousness and are characterized by a focal onset, for example a twitching of the fingers, and progressively increases to other parts of the body. According to Guyton and Hall (2000):

> '*Focal epilepsy results from some localized organic lesion or functional abnormality, such as a scar that pulls on the neuronal tissue, a tumour that compresses an area of the brain, a destroyed area of brain tissue or congenitally deranged local circuitry.*'

The lesion can promote rapid discharges in the local neurons and, when the discharge rate rises above approximately 1000 per second, synchronous waves begin to spread over the adjacent cortical regions (Guyton and Hall, 2000). Partial seizures are divided into simple and complex seizures:

- *Simple partial seizure*. The presentation of this type of seizure depends on the part of the brain that is affected. The affected person remains conscious and the symptoms include movement of the limbs, experiencing unpleasant smells or perspiring (BEA, 2003)
- *Complex partial*. This involves impairment of consciousness and may take the form of 'automatisms', such as chewing and swallowing, repeatedly scratching the head or searching for an object. Some people may even undress or wander off, recovering full awareness minutes or even hours later, without remembering anything (BEA, 2003).

Generalized seizures

This typical epileptic attack, better known by the name *grand mal*, is characterized by extreme neuronal discharges in all areas of the brain: in the cortex, in the deeper parts of the cerebrum and even in the brain stem and thalamus. According to Farine (2003), generalized seizures affect the entire body and several body functions at once. Generalized seizures can be divided into secondary and primary seizures:

- *Secondary generalized seizures*. Occasionally, the activity that starts as a simple partial or complex partial seizure can progress to the whole brain resulting in a tonic–clonic seizure. Therefore, the person may experience the simple partial seizure as an 'aura' or warning, but sometimes the spread of epileptic activity can be rapid and unnoticed (BEA, 2003)
- *Primary generalized seizures*. This reflects involvement of the entire brain and may be characterized at the onset by a sudden loss of consciousness and immediate bilateral symmetric motor activity. Two of the more frequently occurring types are absence and tonic–clonic seizures (BEA, 2003).

Types of epilepsy

Status epilepticus

Normally, most seizures last for less than 5 minutes. Therefore, in clinical practice, status epilepticus is defined as a seizure occurring continuously or recurrently for a minimum of half an hour without recovery (Manford, 2003). Children are more prone to status epilepticus than adults (Manford, 2003), and a US research study showed that 10% of children diagnosed with epilepsy develop status epilepticus within 8 years of diagnosis (Berg et al, 2004). The researchers also defined status epilepticus as a seizure lasting more than 30 minutes.

In all sufferers, status epilepticus is seen as a life-threatening situation that requires urgent attention, ideally requesting an ambulance if a seizure lasts more than 5 minutes. In hospital, it is quickly controlled by intravenous injection of benzodiazipine; the same can be given rectally by a competent practitioner following permission from the legal guardian of the child (Manford, 2003; Berg et al, 2004).

Catamenial epilepsy

This is an exacerbation of seizures in relation to the menstrual cycle (Manford, 2003). Also, Manford (2003) identified the effect of female sex hormones on epilepsy and states that menarche, menstrual cycle and menopause may alter seizure pattern in women.

Photosensitive epilepsy

This is a form of epilepsy in which seizures are provoked by flickering light, such as television, and reflections from sunlight (Manford, 2003). However, the visual stimuli needs to occupy a large proportion of the visual field to cause a seizure, and therefore sitting a few metres away from the television or wearing sunglasses out of doors on a sunny day will help to prevent this type of light-induced seizure in susceptible people (Manford, 2003).

Epilepsy and alcohol/drugs

Anyone taking drugs that act on the brain, for example anti-epileptic medications, are likely to be more susceptible to the effects of alcohol and illicit drugs (BEA, 2003). Manford (2003) reported that there is an increased risk of seizures in people consuming over 50 g of alcohol daily. Similarly, risk of a seizure increases with high doses of amphetamines. The use of heroin and opiates, and bacteraemic infection also increase the risk of seizure (Manford, 2003).

The social implications of epilepsy

The effects of epilepsy on individuals varies considerably but it generally threatens the sense of wellbeing of the patient. These effects include social isolation, work constraints, altered life-style, psychological problems, such as anger, anxiety and frustration, and coping with prolonged treatment and side-effects of drugs. Lanfear (2002) classified the social impact of epilepsy into four domains (see *Table 15.3*).

Lanfear (2002) argued that schools should have a clear policy to protect students and should provide moral and legal justification to exclude them from any school activities. This is because some students fail to achieve in school due to the attitudes and beliefs of their colleagues and teachers about epilepsy. However, it may be necessary to exclude children with epilepsy from certain sports, and students with photosensitive epilepsy may be cautioned about participating in computer games as these may trigger a seizure. Some employers request that affected people declare epilepsy in the pre-employment questionnaire and people with epilepsy are legally banned from some employment such as the military service.

Table 15.3: Social impact of epilepsy
• Social exclusion from school
• Employment constraints
• Social life and social activity limitations
• Driving restrictions

From Lanfear (2002)

Depending on the frequency and severity of the seizures, some modification may be required in the affected person's life-style, such as using a low level bed to sleep, ensuring life-saving personnel are available during swimming, using a helmet while cycling, and informing proposed partners and life insurance companies of the condition (Lanfear, 2002).

In terms of driving restriction, the DVLA (2006) states that an epileptic patient without a fit for a year qualifies for a driving licence but driving must cease immediately if a driver suffers from any epileptic attack. However, this ban can be reversed if the person can later establish that within the last three years, he or she has been free from attacks while awake.

Treatment options

It is important to treat epilepsy because of its physiological and psychological implications on the affected individual, their working days lost to illness, the economic cost of treating complicated cases, and mortality owing to status epilepticus or sudden unexpected death.

Pharmacological treatment

The standard medical treatment of epilepsy is with anti-epileptic drugs, which are known collectively as anticonvulsants. According to the *British National Formulary* (BNF) (British Medical Association and Royal Pharmaceutical Society of Great Britain, 2004), drugs used to control epilepsy include: carbamazepine, phenytoin, ethosuximide, vigabatrin, lamotrigine, valproic acid, pheno-barbital, levetiracetam and topiramate. A list of the commonly used anti-epileptic drugs is presented in the Appendix. In status epilepticus, lorazepam, diazepam or phenytoin sodium can be given intravenously and paraldehyde rectally. However, facilities for resuscitation should be available to managing this emergency situation.

The objective of treatment is to bring the electrical activity in the brain under control while maintaining quality of life (Galbraith et al, 1999). According to the same group, anticonvulsants act by suppressing the overexcitability of cortical neurons by directly stabilizing the nerve membrane, enhancing the activity of inhibitory transmitter gamma aminobutyric acid (GABA), or a combination of both. GABA is the most common inhibiting transmitter in the brain and functions as an inhibitory agent (*Figure 15.3*). Similarly, Farine (2003) found that anticonvulsants enhance GABA by increasing calcium movement to post-synaptic receptors.

There is a wide choice of effective anti-epileptic drugs available, which usually come in tablet or capsule form, or as a syrup for children. The choice of treatment depends on the type and severity of symptoms. Other relevant considerations are preference of the person being treated, success or failure of previous treatment and drug–drug interaction. All drugs have potential side-effects, and this is especially true of the anti-epileptic drugs (British Medical Association and Royal Pharmaceutical Society of Great Britain, 2004). The most common side-effect of this group of drugs is drowsiness, and it is important to weigh the benefits of the drug against the unwanted effects of large doses.

Farine (2003) classified the side effects into dose-related adverse reactions and non-dose-related drug interactions. The former are drowsiness, irritability, vertigo and diplopia, while the latter is localized or widespread skin rash. In the past, the use of several drugs was embraced, but polytherapy is only used nowadays when monotherapy has proved ineffective.

The *BNF* (British Medical Association and Royal Pharmaceutical Society of Great Britain, 2004) and Farine (2003) state that combination therapy increases the risk of drug-induced complications

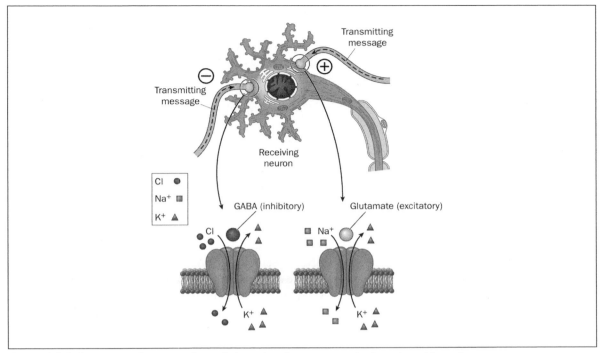

Figure 15.3: Diagram of nerve cells and the role of gamma aminobutyric acid vs glutamate

and drug–drug interactions, and therefore recommend monitoring the plasma concentrations of the drugs, something that is being done routinely in the UK and Europe (Davies, 1999).

Also, anti-epileptic drugs should be withdrawn slowly, and this varies with different drugs (for example, the withdrawl process for barbituates may last for months). The Epilepsy Association of Australia warned against sudden withdrawal of these drugs, as this may lead to life-threatening status epilepticus. Equally, the *BNF* (British Medical Association and Royal Pharmaceutical Society of Great Britain, 2004) recommends against sudden withdrawals, especially of barbiturates and benzodiazepines, as this may precipitate severe rebound seizures.

Complementary therapies

Although, the pharmacological approach is the most effective way of treating seizure (WHO, 2004), complementary therapies have proved to be effective in controlling some forms of epilepsy in certain individuals (Epilepsy Association of Australia, 2004).

Manford (2003) acknowledges patients' increasing interest in using complementary therapies, but warned that they should never be used to supplement conventional treatments without first consulting their physician. Pharmacologically neutral therapies, such as reflexology, massage, homeopathy, biofeedback and spiritual healing, are not likely to be harmful, but pharmacologically active therapies, such as herbs or aromatherapy, require more caution (Manford, 2003). Manford

Table 15.4: Natural remedies contraindicated in epilepsy

- Eucalyptus
- Fennel
- Hyssop
- Pennyroyal
- Rosemary
- Sage
- Tansy
- Turpentine
- Wormwood

From Manford (2003)

further acknowledged that some natural remedies are strong convulsants and are therefore contraindicated for epilepsy owing to their content of highly reactive monoterpene ketones, such as camphor, pinocamphone, thujone, cineole, pulegone, sabinylacetate and fenchone (*Table 15.4*).

Trevelyan and Booth (1994), however, claimed that aromatherapy massage oils, derived from a range of anticonvulsant to anxiolytic essential oils, can reduce seizure frequency.

Manford (2003) also reported the successful use of ketogenic diet (high fat diet) therapy in children and some adults, but said that the potential side-effects for children are thirst, hunger, weight loss and toxicity in polypharmacy. Likewise, in adults it may potentiate cardiovascular complications.

Trevelyan and Booth (1994) claim that the Alexander technique has been used successfully to reduce the number of attacks in patients suffering from epilepsy. This is a form of psychophysical education used to teach patients how to alter their thinking and action and how to support their bodies through appropriate movement.

Generally, Manford (2003) and the Epilepsy Association of Australia (2004) recommend discussing the use of any complementary therapy with a general practitioner or epilepsy specialist. It should be noted that some of these complementary therapies may be contraindicated with the patient's current medication. Any of these complementary therapies should only be provided by a qualified therapist.

Surgical management

This is excision of an epileptogenic focus following lack of response to medical treatment and extensive diagnostic assessment. According to Hickey (2003), it is the treatment of choice for the patient with a unilateral epileptic focus that is impacting on their quality of life. Nevertheless, the aim of surgical intervention is to locate and excise the epileptogenic area without causing more neurological deficit. Surgical therapy is usually followed by the use of anticonvulsants for 1–2 years (Hickey, 2003).

Manford (2003) also claimed that the gamma knife (a form of radiosurgery that involves the use of gamma radiation to kill abnormal brain cells) offers a positive effect, as seizures tend to reduce in number after radiotherapy with fewer complications than surgery. Similarly, Manford (2003) also reported that vagus nerve stimulation is helpful for about 25% of patients with refractory epilepsy.

Nursing management

Nurses have a significant role to play in caring for people affected by epilepsy. The goals of seizure management are to help the patient (BEA, 2003):

- Control the seizures
- Accept the disorder that gives rise to the seizures
- Comply with the medication regimen and recommended modifications in lifestyle
- Cope with the situation and maintain quality of life.

The primary aim of nursing care during a seizure is to prevent injury and to protect the client's airway. The nurse should:

- Position the client on his or her side to promote drainage of secretions and to prevent the tongue from obstructing the airway
- Remove all potentially dangerous articles around the patient
- Never restrain the client during a seizure
- Administer prescribed anticonvulsant drugs
- Keep records of seizures and inform the physician immediately
- If seizures occur in the hospital, suctioning and administration of oxygen may be instituted
- Provide the patient with privacy
- Ensure that appropriate explanations and support are given to the patient.

The nurse should also help the client and family to understand epilepsy by teaching them about the disease, such as precipitating factors, importance of drug compliance, how to live a full life and where to seek help, for example, epilepsy organizations offer a range of services to their members (*Table 15.5*).

Table 15.5: Epilepsy organizations

• *British Epilepsy Association*	Tel: 0808 800 5050	www.epilepsy.org.uk
• *Joint Epilepsy Council*	Tel: 01943 871852	www.jointepilepsycouncil.org.uk
• *National Society for Epilepsy*	Tel: 01494 601400	www.epilepsynse.org.uk
• *Epilepsy Bereaved*	Tel: 01235 772852	www.sudep.org
• *Mersey Region Epilepsy Association*	Tel: 0151 298 2666	www.epilepsymersey.org.uk
• *Epilepsy Action Scotland*	Tel: 0141 427 4911	www.epilepsyscotland.org.uk
• *Wales Epilepsy Association cyf*	Tel: 01745 584444	
• *Brainwave – Irish Epilepsy Association*	Tel: 0035 31 455 7500	

A detailed history and assessment coupled with advice on pregnancy and contraceptive use, complementary therapy options and prompt referral by the primary care nurse to a specialist epilepsy nurse is essential.

It is also important to tell them or a loved one or carer to keep a seizure diary, i.e. dates, time of day or night and circumstances.

Prognosis

Diagnosis of epilepsy is often difficult to deal with and people require some time to come to terms with the news. According to research compiled by the WHO (2001b), about 70% of patients with epilepsy can be pharmacologically treated successfully, while 30% may not respond to treatment owing to underlying brain disease. Davies (1999) identified some factors that may affect prognosis, such as age of onset of epilepsy, early course of treatment and whether seizures are symptomatic (underlying lesion) or asymptomatic.

Manford (2003) claimed that there is an associated risk of morbidity and mortality in patients with epilepsy from causes not directly linked to epilepsy, such as intracranial tumour and metastic lesions to the brain. Nevertheless, some deaths appear to be directly related to epilepsy itself and this is termed 'sudden unexpected death in epilepsy' (SUDEP). Manford (2003) found that severity of the seizure is a significant risk factor in SUDEP.

As a result of the national clinical audit of epilepsy-related deaths (National Institute for Clinical Excellence, 2004), the UK Department of Health issued an epilepsy action plan in 2003, and plans to publish the *National Service Framework* for long-term illness with a particular focus on neurological conditions, including epilepsy. This 10-year implementation programme started in June 2005 sets 11 requirements designed to help patients with neurological conditions to live independent lives.

Conclusion

This chapter provides readers with information about epilepsy and its management with the intention of promoting optimal care of the patient. The subject is considered important because it represents a major and relatively common neurological problem.

Equally, epilepsy has social and physical impacts on affected people who often have a feeling of inferiority, anger or other emotions who therefore require support and guidance.

There are several types of seizures, but status epilepticus is a life-threatening situation that requires urgent treatment. There is need for improvement, and the Department of Health (2003) action plan and its implementation programme is a way forward. Also, in 1992, NICE launched the audit of epilepsy-related death. The ongoing research findings are expected to aid reduction in the number of avoidable deaths.

Finally, in addition to these positive actions, it is important to continue researching complementary approaches, as anecdotal evidence suggests they may have a role in supporting conventional therapy.

References

Berg AT, Shinnar S, Testa FM et al (2004). Status epilepticus after initial diagnosis of epilepsy in children. *Neurology* **63:** 1027–34

British Epilepsy Association (2003) *Seizures Explained*. British Epilepsy Association, Leeds

British Medical Association and Royal Pharmaceutical Society of Great Britain (2004) *British National Formulary*. Number 48. British Medical Association and Royal Pharmaceutical Society of Great Britain, London

Brooker C, Nicol M (2003) *Nursing Adults: The Practice of Caring*. Elsevier, London

Davies N (1999) Epilepsy and blackouts. In: Williams AC, ed. *Patient Care in Neurology*. Oxford University Press, Oxford: 59–92

Department of Health (2003) *Improving Services for People with Epilepsy*. DoH, London (www.dh.gov.uk/assetRoot/04/06/10/62/04061062.pdf) (last accessed 30 August 2005)

DVLA (2006) *Driving Licences: Epilepsy. Ordinary Driving Entitlement*. Available at www.dvla.gov.uk/drivers,dmed/-files/.htm (last accessed 5 April 2006)

Epilepsy Association of Australia (2004) *Complementary Therapies*. Epilepsy Association of Australia (www.epilepsy.com.au/treatment_comp.asp) (last accessed 30 August 2005)

Farine AP (2003) Seizures and epilepsy. In: Thompson T, Mathias P eds. *Lyttle's Mental Health and Disorder*. 3rd edn. Elsevier, Philadelphia: 297–303

Galbraith A, Bullock S, Manis E, Hunt B, Richard A (1999) *Fundamentals of Pharmacology: A Text for Nurses and Health Professionals*. 2nd edn. Addison Wesley Longman, Harlow

Guyton AC, Hall JE (2000) *Textbook of Medical Physiology*. 10th edn. WB Saunders Co, Philadelphia

Hampshire M (2005) Breakthrough in epilepsy care. *Nurs Stand* **19**(23): 20–1

Hickey JV (2003) *The Clinical Practice of Neurological and Neurosurgical Nursing*. 5th edn. Lippincott, Philadelphia

Hole JW (1993) *Human Anatomy and Physiology*. 6th edn. Wm C Brown Communications, Iowa

Lanfear J (2002) The individual with epilepsy. *Nursing Standard* **16**(46): 43–53

Manford M (2003) *Practical Guide to Epilepsy*. Butterworth Heinemann, Oxford

National Institute for Clinical Excellence (2004) *Clinical Audit of Epilepsy-Related Death (SUDEP)*. NICE, London (www.nice.org.uk/page.aspx?o=32146) (last accessed 30 August 2005)

Trevelyan J, Booth B (1994) *Complementary Medicine for Nurses, Midwives and Health Visitors*. Macmillian, London

World Health Organization (2001a) *The World Health Report: Epilepsy*. WHO, Geneva (www.who.int.whr2001/main/en/chapter 2/002e4.htm) (last accessed 30 August 2005)

World Health Organization (2001b) *Epilepsy: Aetiology, Epidemiology and Prognosis*. WHO, Geneva (www.who.int/mediacentre/factsheets/fs165/en/) (last accessed 30 August 2005)

World Health Organization (2004) *Epilepsy: historical overview*. WHO, Geneva (*www.who.int/mediacentre/factsheets/fs168/en/*) (last accessed 30 August 2005)

Appendix

Anti-epileptic drugs

Carbamazepine (Tegretol)
- *Indications:* Partial and secondary generalized tonic-clonic seizures, some primary generalized seizures.
- *Adult dosage*: 0.8–1.2 g daily in divided doses.
- *Side-effects and comments*: Bone marrow depression, nausea, vomiting, headache, urinary retention, oedema, rash and drowsiness. Blood cell counts and haematocrit should be done at least monthly.

Ethosuximide (Zarontin)
- *Indications:* Absence seizures.
- *Adult dosage*: 500 mg daily, increased by 250 mg at intervals of 4–7 days to usual dose of 1–1.5 g daily.
- *Side-effects and comments*: Gastro-intestinal irritation, drowsiness and headache. Should be taken at meal-time with a large amount of fluid. Primarily for use in petit mal epilepsy.

Phenobarbitone (Luminal)
- *Indications:* All forms of epilepsy except absence seizures, status epilepticus.
- *Adult dosage*: 60–180 mg at night. Status epilepticus: 10 mg/kg i/v. Maximum 100 mg/minute.
- *Side-effects and comments*: Rashes, drowsiness, mental slowing, aggressiveness, depression. Children may become hyperactive. Withdrawal seizures may occur if stopped abruptly after prolonged use.

Phenytoin (Epanutin)
- *Indications:* All forms of epilepsy except absence seizures.
- *Adult dosage*: 3–4 mg/kg daily as a single or in two divided doses increased gradually as necessary. Usual dose 200–500 mg daily.
- *Side-effects and comments*: Phenytoin intoxication (dizziness, loss of co-ordination, mental slowing) may occur, especially soon after starting, following a dose increase or after a change in concurrent treatment. Drowsiness, headaches. Nausea, ataxia, diplopia or nystagmus, slurring of speech, gingival hyperplasia, rash and hirsutism. Drug should be taken with meals. Good oral hygiene, gum massage and regular dental supervision are necessary. Serious blood disorders occur, but are very rare. Monitor plasma concentration.

Sodium valproate (Epilim)
- *Indications:* All forms of epilepsy.
- *Adult dosage*: 20–30 mg/kg daily in divided doses. Maximum 35 mg/kg daily.
- *Side-effects and comments*: Weight grain, drowsiness, tremor, hair thinning/loss. Gastrointestinal disturbance. Hormone problems in women. Serious liver and blood disorders occur, but are rare. Drug should be taken with meals. Frequent blood cell count and bleeding time should be done.

Primidone (Mysoline)
- *Indications:* All forms of epilepsy except absence seizures; essential tremor.
- *Adult dosage*: 1.5 g daily in divided doses (to be increased gradually).
- *Side-effects and comments*: Depression, irritability, dizziness, ataxia and, rarely, impotence. If used with symptomatic seizures, dosage decreased gradually before withdrawal.

Topamax (Topiramate)

- *Indications:* Adjunctive treatment of partial seizures with or without secondary generalization not satisfactorily controlled with other anti-epileptics; seizures associated with Lennox Gastaut syndrome; primary generalized tonic-clonic seizures.
- *Adult dosage*: Initially 1–3 mg/kg daily in two divided doses. Maximum 5–9 mg/kg daily in two divided doses.
- *Side-effects and comments*: Mental slowing, confusion, agitation, amnesia, depression, difficulty finding words; all more likely to occur if the dose is increased quickly (reducing the dose by too much too quickly can trigger seizures). Weight loss, headache, dizziness, tremor.

Vigabatrin (Sabril)

- *Indications:* Initiated and supervised by appropriate specialist, adjunctive treatment of partial seizures with or without secondary generalization not satisfactorily controlled by anti-epileptics; monotherapy for management of infantile spasms (West's syndrome).
- *Adult dosage*: Initially 1 g daily in two divided doses. Maximum 2–3 g daily in two divided doses.
- *Side-effects and comments*: This drug is now recommended only for restricted use because of visual (field) problems, potentially resulting in the patient developing 'tunnel' vision, without being aware of the problem at an early stage. Other side-effects include drowsiness, dizziness, headache, mood change, agitation, confusion, psychosis and weight gain.

Clobazam (Frisium)

- *Indications:* Adjunct in epilepsy; anxiety.
- *Adult dosage*: 20–30 mg daily. Maximum 60 mg daily.
- *Side-effects and comments*: Drowsiness, dizzyness, impaired co-ordination. Withdrawal effects (including increased seizures and/or anxiety) may occur, especially if the drug is stopped abruptly following protracted use.

Clonazepam (Rivotril)

- *Indications:* All forms of epilepsy; status epilepticus.
- *Adult dosage*: 4–8 mg daily in divided doses.
- *Side-effects and comments*: Drowsiness (common, may be severe), mental slowing, dizziness, impaired co-ordination. Withdrawal effects (including increased seizures and/or anxiety) especially if the drug is stopped abruptly following protracted use.

Acetazolamide (Diamox)

- *Indications:* A second-line drug for both tonic-clonic and partial seizures. It is occasionally helpful in atypical absence, atonic and tonic seizures.
- *Adult dosage*: 0.25–1.0 g daily in divided doses.
- *Side-effects and comments*: Headache, lethargy, nausea, pins and needles.

Gabapentin (Neurontin)

- *Indications:* Adjunctive treatment of partial seizures with or without secondary generalization not satisfactorily controlled with other anti-epileptics.
- *Adult dosage*: Initially 300 mg once daily. Maximum 800 mg three times daily.
- *Side-effects and comments*: Drowsiness, dizziness.

Lamotrigine (Lamictal)

- *Indications:* Monotherapy and adjunctive treatment of partial seizures and primary and secondary generalized tonic-clonic seizures; seizures associated with Lennox Gastaut syndrome.
- *Adult dosage*: 100–200 mg daily as a single or two divided doses.

- *Side-effects and comments*: Rash (typically soon after starting, sometimes very severe). Headache, dizziness, insomnia. Serious blood disorders occur, but are very rare.

Tiagabine (Gabitril)

- *Indications:* Adjunctive treatment for partial seizures with or without secondary generalization not satisfactorily controlled with other anti-epileptics.
- *Adult dosage*: With enzyme inducers 5–10 mg daily initially, maintenance 30–45 mg daily. Without enzyme inducers 5–10 mg daily initially. Maintenance 15–30 mg daily.
- *Side-effects and comments*: Dizziness, drowsiness, headache, tremor, confusion, depression, psychosis, diarrhoea.

Valproic acid (Convulex)

- *Indications:* All forms of epilepsy.
- *Adult dosage*: Initially 15 mg/kg. Maximum 30 mg/kg daily.
- *Side-effects and comments*: None

Levetiracetam (Keppra)

- *Indications:* Adjunctive therapy in the treatment of partial onset seizures with or without secondary generalization in patients with epilepsy.
- *Adult dosage*: Initially 1 g daily in two divided doses. Maximum 3 g daily in two divided doses.
- *Side-effects and comments*: Drowsiness, dizziness, headache.

Oxcarbazepine (Trileptal)

- *Indications:* Monotherapy and adjunctive treatment of partial seizures with or without secondary generalized tonic-clonic seizures.
- *Adult dosage*: 0.6–2.4 g daily in divided doses.
- *Side-effects and comments*: Rash (typically soon after starting). Drowsiness, dizziness, headaches, nausea, diarrhoea.

Chapter 16

Management of patients who have relapses in multiple sclerosis

Gaynor Williams

Multiple sclerosis (MS) is a chronic neurological condition, which disrupts the typical functions and daily activities of those affected. It is the most common cause of disability among young adults in the UK (Compston, 1998). Relapsing/remitting MS is a subtype of the disease, as identified by Lubin and Reingold (1996). Patients with this type of MS can expect to have episodes of remission, when the disease is not active, countered by disabling episodes of relapse or an exacerbation of the disease and its variety of symptoms.

This chapter explores strategies that are used to manage such episodes and establishes the best evidence-based practice for caring for patients during a relapse. It will begin by briefly discussing MS and establish its definition, effects and the current understanding regarding its cause. Second, it will determine what a relapse is and will explore the knowledge that exists surrounding the triggers of relapse in MS. Favoured methods of treating relapse in MS will then be discussed. Finally, conclusions will be made regarding the current most favoured methodology for treating MS relapses.

Multiple sclerosis

MS is an idiopathic, inflammatory neurological condition, which causes areas of demyelination within the central nervous system (Hickey, 2003) (*Figure 16.1*).

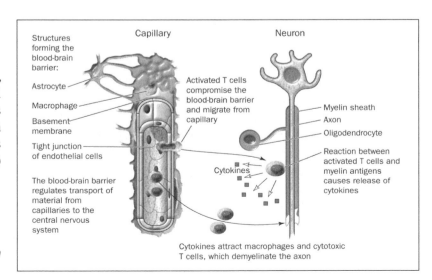

Figure 16.1: Demyelination in MS by autoreactive T cells

Owing to the unpredictable nature of this myelin damage, the symptoms and possible impairments experienced by a patient with the condition may vary dramatically. These can include fatigue, pain, mobility problems, spasticity, visual disturbances, bladder, bowel and sexual dysfunction, tremor, cognitive difficulties and depression (Burgess, 2002).

It has a current prevalence of 1 per 800 population in the UK (Compston and Coles, 2002). The cause of the disease remains unknown, but it is postulated to be an autoimmune condition triggered by a combination of several factors such as the environment, predisposing genes and infectious agents (Martin and McFarland, 1997). It is twice as predominant in women as in men, and worldwide MS becomes more common the further away from the equator travelled (Morrison, 1999). It is current practice to divide the disease into four subtypes differentiated by the rate of relapse in symptoms and the rate of progression (Weinshenker et al, 1989). These subtypes are listed in *Table 16.1*.

Eighty per cent of patients diagnosed with MS will have relapsing/remitting disease at diagnosis (National Institute for Clinical Excellence (NICE), 2003). Their disease is characterized by periods of remission and wellbeing, interspersed by relapses.

Table 16.1: The four multiple sclerosis (MS) subtypes

- Benign MS
- Relapsing/remitting MS
- Secondary/progressive MS
- Primary/progressive MS

From Weinshenker et al (1989)

Relapses in MS

A relapse is defined by Polman et al (2001) as:

> '...the subacute appearance of a neurologic abnormality that must be present for at least 24 hours in the absence of fever or infection.'

Relapses initially occur on average once every 12 months, and generally abate during the course of the disease (Ebers, 1998). Each relapse is unique, with neurological abnormalities of varying severity and duration. Spontaneous recovery is usual, but varies considerably between individuals. Relapses may elicit new symptoms or produce a flare up of older, underlying, symptoms (Hickey, 2003) (*Table 16.2*).

Table 16.2: Symptoms of relapses

- Sensory symptoms, such as burning, pins and needles or reduced sensation in any area of the body
- Motor symptoms that affect the individual's ability to use various muscles
- Visual symptoms such as diplopia (double vision), pain or spots in the field of vision
- Cerebellar symptoms such as vertigo, nausea or ataxia
- Or a combination of any of these

From Hickey (2003)

Individuals may recover completely in episodes of remission or may develop incremental disability following each relapse. In a survey of people with MS undertaken by the Multiple Sclerosis Trust (unpublished), relapses on average lasted approximately 55.3 days. Such relapses can have a huge impact on the physical, social, financial and psychological wellbeing of those affected (Miller, 1997; Baker, 1998; Kroencke et al, 2001).

Triggers of relapse

The triggers of relapse in MS have been well investigated (Sibley, 1997). Although trauma has been implicated in causing relapses, there is no current evidence to support these claims (Goodin et al, 1999). A prospective study by Buljevac et ál (2003), however, was able to demonstrate an association between stressful life events and relapse. It was also able to show that a bacterial or viral infection trebled the risk of relapse in the subsequent 4 weeks from initial infection onset. This study, in relation to infection, reaffirms the findings of another study exploring this area (Metz et al, 1998). Where possible avoiding infections, by being vaccinated against influenza for example, is recommended (NICE, 2003). Questions have been raised regarding the possibility of immunizations triggering a relapse in MS, but to date there has been no evidence to support this (Leary et al, 2004). However, heat intolerance is thought to exacerbate underlying MS symptoms (Hickey, 2003) and prompt a relapse in some susceptible adults (Burgess, 2002).

It was believed up until the 1950s (Kalb and LaRocca, 1997) that pregnancy and childbirth had a negative impact upon MS and disease progression. This belief has now been dispelled, as long-term studies of women who have been pregnant and those who have not have demonstrated no significant difference in both groups' disease course (Thompson et al, 1986; Birk, 1995). A study has however established that following childbirth and during the early postpartum period the risk of relapse is much higher (Confareux et al, 1998), but this is offset by the low risk of relapse during pregnancy itself. The same study also found that breastfeeding and the use of epidural analgesia during labour did not appear to increase the risk of relapse.

Relapse management

The management of relapse can be divided into two categories (NICE, 2003) (*Table 16.3*).

Table 16.3: Management of relapse categories

- First, reducing the length and severity of a relapse by using corticosteroids

- Second, supporting the individual affected by using members of the interdisciplinary team

From NICE (2003)

Corticosteroids

The mainstay of acute relapse management to date is the administration of corticosteroids. This practice has been well established over the past few decades (Filippini et al, 2004). The anti-inflammatory effects of corticosteroids have made them invaluable in reducing the duration and impact of a relapse, although the degree of long-term recovery and ultimate disease course remains unchanged (Compston, 1998). Corticosteroids do not slow down or alter the rate of new lesion development in MS, and therefore do not alter the amount of relapses that could occur. In addition, continued use of corticosteroids may result in side-effects such as weight gain, hypertension, osteoporosis, euphoria and insomnia (Polman et al, 2001). Hence, their long-term use is not supported (Francis, 1999).

Adrenocorticotropic hormone

Adrenocorticotropic hormone (ACTH) was the first derivative of cortisone to be used in the treatment of acute relapse in MS (Miller et al, 1961; Rose et al, 1970). This drug was given via a daily intramuscular injection, but although effective its unfavourable side-effects of weight gain and oedema have rendered it relatively obsolete in current practice (Tremlett et al, 1998; Polman et al, 2001). It is not, therefore, considered to be a recommended method of relapse management.

Prednisolone

There is a dearth of published data using oral prednisolone. Despite this lack of empirical evidence, a study of prescribing patterns for MS in Wales showed that over 80% of the corticosteroids prescribed in general practice were oral prednisolone (Tremlett et al, 2001). It is surmised that the reason for this is that GPs may feel pressurized to administer chronic courses of corticosteroids when little else can be offered. It was not possible in this study to evaluate at what stage of the MS disease process the patients' prescribed oral prednisolone were at, but as pointed out by Hawkins and Wolinksy (2000), corticosteroids should only be prescribed in the most severe of relapses.

Methylprednisolone

Methylprednisolone can be given via an oral or intravenous (IV) route, while prednisolone can only be administered orally (Royal Pharmaceutical Society of Great Britain and British Medical Association, 2004). Studies have been completed that compare the effects of methylprednisolone, ACTH and placebo (Barnes et al, 1985; Milligan et al, 1987; Thompson et al, 1989), and overall these studies have supported the use of methylprednisolone. In addition, a meta-analysis of methylprednisolone and corticosteroids respectively (Miller et al, 2000; Filippini et al, 2004) found that methylprednisolone is an effective agent in MS relapse management. The findings of these studies have prompted others to examine the most effective dose, route of administration and length of methylprednisolone treatment.

Alam et al (1993), in a double-blind, placebo-controlled trial of oral and IV methylprednisolone, were able to show no significant difference between patients in relapse given IV methylprednisolone and those given oral methylprednisolone. In this study, both groups of patients were given 500 mg of methylprednisolone over a 5-day course. The first group (*n*=20) were given IV active treatment with an oral placebo, and the second group (*n*=15) were given IV placebo with oral active treatment. Both groups were similar in age, gender, duration of disease and severity of disability on entry to the study.

The groups were assessed by a blinded assessor on days 0, 5 and 28 using the functional and disability score devised by Kurtzke (1983). Both groups improved by days 5 and 28, with no significant difference between the two groups on their Kurtzke scores. The scale is an incremental scale ranging from 0.0–10.0, where 0.0 denotes an individual with no impairments and 10.0 denotes death from MS. Scores above 4 rely heavily upon mobility as its main measure of disability, where scores less than 4 require a more detailed neurological examination to elicit any impairment. Its reliance upon mobility as its main measure of disability, to the detriment of other signs such as visual damage or upper limb weakness, has resulted in criticism from some authors (Thompson and Hobart, 1998).

The findings of the above study are echoed by a similar multicentre study reported by Barnes et al (1997). Eighty patients were randomized into two groups; one group received oral methylprednisolone, and the other group received IV methylprednisolone. In broad terms, the study was unable to find any difference between the two groups at weeks 1, 4, 12 or 24 when assessed using Kurtzke's (1983) Expanded Disability Status Scale.

The small sample sizes in both these studies may have reduced the power of the studies to disclose any differences between the two groups and their respective treatment regimens. Therefore, the findings of both these studies are that high-dose oral methylprednisolone may be just as effective as IV in the treatment of MS relapses. Prescribing oral medication is less costly, less of an infection risk to the patient as cannulation is not required and does not require the patient to attend hospital. No head-to-head studies of dosage regimens have been published to date.

It would appear, therefore, that oral methylprednisolone can be used in MS relapses (Polman et al, 2001). However, this recommendation may lead to a potential abuse of the drug in MS relapse, as already noted with the use of prednisolone in Wales. It may, however, be difficult to influence current practice, and there may be some credence in prescribing and recommending IV corticosteroids for relapses as a way of monitoring the use of corticosteroids in MS (Barkhof and Polman, 1997). Efforts should be made to educate physicians, who prescribe such medication, and patients, who may unwittingly place undue pressure on their physicians to prescribe them corticosteroids, that such medication should only be used in the most disabling of circumstances.

The term 'disabling relapse' is a subjective phrase as symptoms one individual may find disabling may not be troublesome to another. While motor relapse symptoms are relatively easy to assess and their impact can be appreciated, other relapse symptoms that fall outside this domain are more difficult to assess and comprehend. In such cases, a full assessment of an individual may elicit aspects of their life that is severely affected by their hidden symptoms. For example, a scientist's ability to use a microscope would be severely hindered by an episode of optic neuritis. Likewise, a mother would find it difficult to care for her baby if she were experiencing pins and needles and numbness in her hands as a result of a sensory relapse. Hence, an individualized assessment of symptoms and problems is an essential part of the decision process when the use of corticosteroids is being considered.

Other treatments

The use of plasma exchange has been assessed in the treatment of acute MS relapses (Weiner et al, 1989; Weinshenker et al, 1999), while immunoglobulins have shown some effect in relapse reduction (Achiron et al, 1998). Although both treatments did appear to have some positive impact upon relapse in MS, the high cost of both drugs when compared with the benefits demonstrated, relinquished them as inferior to traditional corticosteroid therapy.

Prevention of relapse

As an adjunct to the use of medication to reduce the impact of relapse in MS, drugs also exist that aim to modify the disease process by reducing or eliminating relapses.

There are currently four licensed disease-modifying drugs, three interferon betas (Avonex, Betaferon, Rebif) and one glatiramer acetate product (Copaxone). These drugs, when used in suitable adults, reduce relapses on average by one-third and relapses, if they do occur, appear to be less severe (Association of British Neurologists, 2001). The availability of these drugs across the UK was a fragmented affair (Keenan and Porter, 2003) and there has been much debate about the cost-effectiveness of these drugs (NICE, 2002). In response to these issues, the Department of Health (DoH), in collaboration with the pharmaceutical companies concerned, drew up a risk sharing scheme which will monitor the efficacy of these drugs over a 10-year period. Within the remit of this scheme, all eligible patients will be offered disease-modifying treatments (DoH, 2002).

Other, more aggressive medications, are being used to treat MS or are under development. To date the most effective of these have been monoclonal antibodies, in particular alemtuzumab (Campath 1H) and natalizumab (Tysabri). These drugs, while they remain at the clinical trial stage, appear to reduce significantly the relapse rate in MS, but are not without significant side-effects. Current thinking would suggest that their use is best reserved for patients following a more aggressive disease trajectory although identifying those patients is difficult due to the unpredictability of the condition (Zajicek, 2005).

Rehabilitation

The benefits of physiotherapy in chronic MS have been established (Lord et al, 1998; Wiles et al, 2001). Rehabilitation of individuals is a key aim of physiotherapy in MS, and in acute disabling relapses the need for swift intervention is self-evident. What has been more difficult to establish is the benefit that patients obtain when cared for by a team of specialists, such as physiotherapists, occupational therapists, clinical nurse specialists and neurologists.

A recent study completed in Liverpool (Craig et al, 2003) examined the impact of planned interdisciplinary rehabilitation compared with standard care when used in conjunction with corticosteroids in MS relapse. The sample was identified by neurologists via the general neurology and specialist MS outpatient clinics. Patients with a confirmed diagnosis of MS and deemed to have a disabling relapse requiring IV methylprednisolone as inpatient or day cases were included. Forty patients were identified over a 17-month period and were randomized into two groups. There was no statistical difference between the demographic data of the two cohorts. Baseline data collated also included Expanded Disability Status Scale (EDSS) (Kurtzke, 1983) scores.

Group one (*n*=20) received IV methylprednisolone 1000 mg for 3 days and current standard ward care. Standard care was described as IV infusion of methylprednisolone in conjunction with referral to other disciplines, such as physiotherapy or occupational therapy, within the general neurology ward resources. Outpatient follow-up therapy was organized if appropriate and available. Group two (*n*=20) had a planned interdisciplinary assessment along with their 3 days of IV methylprednisolone. Therapy interventions were focused on meeting the individual's specific needs at the time, and ranged from health promotion information, continence advice or passive exercises for the more severely disabled.

Seven valid and reliable outcome measures were used to assess the effects of the intervention on both groups. The primary measures used were the Guy's Neurological Disability Scale (Sharrack et al, 1999) and the Amended Motor Club Assessment (De Souza and Ashburn, 1996). Both these questionnaires focused on symptoms related to MS. The former was self-reported by the patient and the subsequent scale completed by the research physiotherapist. Secondary measures in the form of the Barthel Index, the Human Activity Profile and the SF-36 quality-of-life questionnaires were used to assess quality of life and activity associated with MS. All these measures were self-reporting. Questionnaires were completed at baseline, 1 month and 3 months.

Data of normal distribution were tested parametrically using the univariate analysis of variance. Other data and results from the secondary measures were tested non-parametrically using the Mann-Whitney test. Analysis was conducted on baseline and 3-month data. Results were statistically significant at $P<0.05$. Both groups showed improvement at 1 month, but the control group had not sustained that improvement by 3 months. The treatment group, however, did sustain a trend of improvement by 3 months. The treatment group, on average, were also referred to more members of the interdisciplinary team and had therapy for a longer duration. The main finding of the study therefore was that focused, planned, interdisciplinary intervention, when combined with IV methylprednisolone, did appear to be beneficial to patients with MS as opposed to standardized care and IV methylprednisolone alone.

There were limitations to the study, which are articulated in the paper. There was the inability, because of staff constraints, to blind the physiotherapy assessor. In this study the assessor was also the treating therapist. The small sample reduces the power of the study and a longer period of follow up may have allowed for more changes to be noted in the quality-of-life scores of both cohorts.

The finding of this small study does demonstrate that, in Liverpool, interdisciplinary management of a patient during relapse is superior to standard management. Indeed, NICE (2003) recognizes the benefit patients obtain from a specialist neurological rehabilitation service and urge that patients in relapse should be referred to such a team as soon as deemed necessary. Other authors have supported the development of a responsive, specialist MS relapse clinic, the aim of which is to assess and manage patients and their new symptoms within the shortest time possible (Leary et al, 2005; Warner et al, 2005). Ideally, patients should be actively involved during their clinic appointments and given the opportunity to discuss their symptoms and the impact of these symptoms. Köpke et al (2004) advocate a shared decision-making approach to relapse management, where patients and health care professionals discuss the possible options and evidence for treatment and reach a mutually agreeable plan of management.

As part of such a team, the MS specialist nurse's role is invaluable. As an expert resource, the nurse is able to anticipate issues that could arise as a result of a patient's relapse. These may include a difficulty in managing activities of living or an inability to fulfil his or her normal role within society, for example as a main carer for an elderly relative. Part of the nursing role in such a situation will include appropriate onward referral to colleagues within the health and social care settings.

Caring for patients during relapse, however, will also involve assisting patients to come to terms with their new symptoms and the impact these symptoms may have on their emotional and psychological wellbeing. The uncertain nature of recovery from a relapse can be a difficult time for patients (Baker, 1998; Vaughan et al, 2003), and a nurse sensitive to these issues can provide the communication and counselling skills needed during this time.

To this end an interdisciplinary relapse clinic would allow patients to access a group of expert individuals who would be able to assess all their needs and provide prompt and individualized care when they need it (Craig, 2002). Corticosteroids have an appropriate place in relapse management and physiotherapy can be useful when motor symptoms dominate the relapse. Most of the research to date has examined how disabling motor relapses can be managed. An interdisciplinary assessment will also allow for patients with predominately sensory and optic relapses, which do not respond to traditional interventions, to also have their needs assessed. Further research is needed to evaluate how healthcare professionals can help these individuals with a less obviously disabling relapse, but nevertheless with an impact that can be just as detrimental.

Conclusion

Relapse management to date is exposed to the personal preferences of the physician involved (Tremlett et al, 1998, 2001). There is a need to standardize the care of patients during relapse so that the best care may be established for this group of patients (Embrey et al, 2003). From this brief literature review it would appear that the most appropriate way of managing acute disabling relapses would be to ensure the patient is assessed by experts in MS management, i.e. an MS interdisciplinary team, and to administer methylprednisolone if appropriate. More work is needed to examine the needs of patients who fall outside this treatment remit but whose relapse remains a difficult personal event.

References

Achiron A, Gabbay U, Gilad R et al (1998) Intravenous immunoglobulin treatment in multiple sclerosis. Effect on relapses. *Neurology* **50**(2): 398–402

Alam SM, Kyriakides T, Lawden M, Newman PK (1993) Methylprednisolone in multiple sclerosis: a comparison of oral with intravenous therapy at equivalent high doses. *J Neurol Neurosurg Psychiatr* **56**: 1219–20

Association of British Neurologists (2001) *Guidelines for the Use of Beta Interferons and Glatiramer Acetate in Multiple Sclerosis*. Association of British Neurologists, London (www.theabn.org/downloads/msdoc.pdf) (accessed 6 September 2004)

Baker LM (1998) Sense making in multiple sclerosis: the information needs of people during an acute exacerbation. *Qual Health Res* **8**(1): 106–20

Barkhof F, Polman C (1997) Oral or intravenous methylprednisolone for acute relapses of MS? *Lancet* **349**: 893

Barnes D, Hughes RAC, Morris RW, Wade-Jones O, Brown P, Britton T, Francis DA, Perkin GD, Rudge P, Swash M, Katifi H, Farmer S, Frankel J (1997) Randomized trial of oral and intravenous methylprednisolone in acute relapses of multiple sclerosis. *Lancet* **349**: 902–6

Barnes MP, Bateman DE, Cleland PG et al (1985) Intravenous methylprednisolone for multiple sclerosis in relapse. *J Neurol Neurosurg Psychiatr* **48**: 157–9

Birk K (1995) Reproductive issues in multiple sclerosis. *Clinical Issues* **2**(3): 2–5

Buljevac D, Hop WCJ, Reedeker W et al (2003) Self-reported stressful life events and exacerbations in multiple sclerosis: prospective study. *Br Med J* **327**: 646–9

Burgess M (2002) *Multiple Sclerosis: Theory & Practice for Nurses*. Whurr Publishers, London

Compston A (1998) Treatment and management of multiple sclerosis. In: Compston A, Ebers G, Lassmann H, McDonald I, Matthews B, Wekerle H, eds. *McAlpine's Multiple Sclerosis*. 3rd edn. Churchill Livingstone, London: 437–98

Compston A, Coles A (2002) Multiple sclerosis. *Lancet* **359**: 1221–31

Confareux C, Hutchinson M, Hours MM, Cortinovis-Tourniaire P, Moreau T (1998) Rate of pregnancy-related relapse in multiple sclerosis. *N Engl J Med* **339**(5): 285–91

Craig J (2002) Development of a relapse clinic for people with multiple sclerosis. *Br J Ther Rehabil* **9**(9): 333

Craig J, Young CA, Ennis M, Baker G, Boggild M (2003) A randomized controlled trial comparing rehabilitation against standard therapy in multiple sclerosis patients receiving intravenous steroid treatment. *J Neurol Neurosurg Psychiatr* **74**: 1225–30

De Souza LH, Ashburn A (1996) Assessment of motor function in people with MS. *Physiother Res Int* **1**: 98–111

Department of Health (2002) *Cost-Effective Provision of Disease Modifying Therapies for People with Multiple Sclerosis*. Health Service Circular (2002/04). The Stationery Office, London

Ebers G (1998) Natural history of multiple sclerosis. In: Compston A, Ebers G, Lassmann H, McDonald I, Matthews B, Wekerle H, eds. *McAlpine's Multiple Sclerosis*. 3rd edn. Churchill Livingstone, London: 191–221

Embrey N, Lowndes C, Warner R (2003) Benchmarking best practice in relapse management of multiple sclerosis. *Nurs Stand* **17**(22): 38–42

Filippini G, Brusaferri F, Sibley WA, Citterio A, Ciucci G, Midgard R, Candelise L (2004) Corticosteroids or ACTH for acute exacerbation in multiple sclerosis (Cochrane Review). In: *Cochrane Library*. Issue 1. John Wiley and Sons, Chichester

Francis DA (1999) Multiple sclerosis. In: Williams AC, ed. *Patient Care in Neurology*. Oxford University Press, Oxford: 111–26

Goodin DS, Ebers GC, Johnson KP, Rodriguez M, Sibley WA, Wolinsky JS (1999) The relationship of MS to physical trauma and psychological stress. *Neurology* **52**: 1737–45

Hawkins C, Wolinsky J (2000) *Principles of Treatment in Multiple Sclerosis*. Butterworth Heinemann, Oxford

Hickey J (2003) *The Clinical Practice of Neurological and Neurosurgical Nursing*. 5th edn. Lippincott Williams and Wilkins, Philadelphia

Kalb RC, LaRocca NG (1997) Sexuality and family planning. In: Halper J, Holland N, eds. *Comprehensive Nursing Care in Multiple Sclerosis*. Desmos Vermande, New York: 109–25

Keenan E, Porter B (2003) Disease-modifying drugs in multiple sclerosis. *Nurs Stand* **17**(30): 39–45

Köpke S, Heesen C, Kasper J, Muhlhaüser I (2004) Steroid treatment for relapses in multiple sclerosis: The evidence urges shared decision-making. *Acta Neurologica Scand* **111**: 1–5

Kroencke DC, Denney DR, Lynch SG (2001) Depression during exacerbations in multiple sclerosis: the importance of uncertainty. *Mult Scler* **7**: 237–42

Kurtzke JF (1983) Rating neurologic impairment in multiple sclerosis: an expanded disability status scale (EDSS). *Neurology* **33**: 1444–52

Leary MS, Porter B, Thompson AJ (2005) Multiple sclerosis: Diagnosis and the management of acute relapses. *Postgrad Med J* **81**: 302–8

Lord SE, Wade DT, Halligan PW (1998) A comparison of two physiotherapy treatment approaches to improve walking in MS: a pilot randomized control study. *Clin Rehabil* **12**: 477–86

Lubin FD, Reingold SC (1996) Defining the clinical course of multiple sclerosis: results of an international survey. *Neurology* **46:** 907–11

Martin R, McFarland HF (1997) Immunology of multiple sclerosis and experimental allergic encephalomyelitis. In: Raine CS, McFarland HF, Tourtellotte WW, eds. *Multiple Sclerosis Clinical and Pathogenetic Basis*. Chapman and Hall Medical, London: 221–42

Metz LM, McGuinness SD, Harris C (1998) Urinary tract infections may trigger relapse in multiple sclerosis. *Axone* **19**(4): 67–70

Miller CM (1997) The lived experience of relapsing multiple sclerosis: a phenomenological study. *J Neurosci Nurs* **29**(5): 294–304

Miller H, Newell DJ, Ridley A (1961) Treatment of acute exacerbations with corticotrophin (ACTH). *Lancet* **2:** 1120–2

Miller DM, Weinstock-Guttman B, Bethoux F et al (2000) A meta-analysis of methylprednisolone in recovery from multiple sclerosis exacerbations. *Mult Scler* **6:** 257–73

Milligan NM, Newcombe R, Compston DAS (1987) A double-blind controlled trial of high dose methylprednisolone in patients with multiple sclerosis. *J Neurol Neurosurg Psychiatr* **50:** 511–6

Morrison W (1999) Multiple sclerosis: an overview for nurses. *Axone* **20**(3): 55–62

National Institute of Clinical Excellence (2002) *Beta Interferon and Glatiramer Acetate for the Treatment of Multiple Sclerosis*. Technology Appraisal Guidance No 32. NICE, London

National Institute of Clinical Excellence (2003) *Multiple Sclerosis: Management of Multiple Sclerosis in Primary and Secondary Care*. NICE, London

Polman CH, Thompson AJ, Murray TJ, McDonald WI (2001) *Multiple Sclerosis: The Guide to Treatment and Management*. 5th edn. Desmos Medical Publishing, New York

Rose AS, Kuzma JW, Kurtzke JF, Namerow NS, Sibley WA, Tourtellotte WW (1970) Cooperative study in the evaluation of therapy in multiple sclerosis. ACTH *vs* placebo. Final report. *Neurology* **20**(5 Part 2): 1–59

Royal Pharmaceutical Society of Great Britain and British Medical Association (2004) *British National Formulary*. Royal Pharmaceutical Society of Great Britain and British Medical Association, London

Sharrack B, Hughes RA, Soudain S et al (1999) The psychometric properties of clinical rating scales used in multiple sclerosis. *Brain* **122:** 141–59

Sibley WA (1997) Risk factors in multiple sclerosis. In: Raine CS, McFarland HF, Tourtellotte WW, eds. *Multiple Sclerosis Clinical and Pathogenetic Basis*. Chapman and Hall Medical, London: 141–8

Thompson AJ, Hobart JC (1998) Multiple sclerosis: assessment of disability and disability scales. *J Neurol* **245:** 189–96

Thompson DS, Nelson LM, Burns A, Burks JS, Franklin GM (1986) The effects of pregnancy in multiple sclerosis: a retrospective study. *Neurology* **36:** 1097–9

Thompson AJ, Kennard C, Swash M et al (1989) Intravenous methylprednisolone and ACTH in the treatment of acute relapses in MS. *Neurology* **39:** 969–71

Tremlett HL, Luscombe DK, Wiles CM (1998) Use of corticosteroids in multiple sclerosis by consultant neurologists in the United Kingdom. *J Neurol Neurosurg Psychiatr* **65:** 362–5

Tremlett HL, Luscombe DK, Wiles CM (2001) Prescribing for multiple sclerosis patients in general practice: a case-control study. *J Clin Pharm Ther* **26:** 437–44

Vaughan R, Morrison L, Miller E (2003) The illness representations of multiple sclerosis and their relations to outcome. *Br J Health Psychol* **8:** 287–301

Warner R, Thomas D, Martin R (2005) Improving service delivery for relapse management in multiple sclerosis. *Br J Nurs* **14**(14): 746–53

Weiner HL, Dau PC, Khatri BO et al (1989) Double-blind study of true *vs* sham plasma exchange in patients treated with immunosuppression for acute attacks of multiple sclerosis. *Neurology* **39**(9): 1143–9

Weinshenker BG, Bass B, Rice GPA, Noseworthy J, Carriere W, Baskerville J, Ebers GC (1989) The natural history of multiple sclerosis: a geographically based study. 1: Clinical course and disability. *Brain* **112:** 133–46

Weinshenker BG, O'Brien PC, Petterson TM, Noseworthy JH, Lucchinetti CF, Dodick DW, Pineda AA, Stevens LN, Rodriguez M (1999) A randomised trial of plasma exchange in acute central nervous system inflammatory demyelinating disease. *Ann Neurol* **46**(6): 878–86

Wiles CM, Newcombe RG, Fuller RG, Shaw S, Furnival-Doran J, Pickersgill TP, Morgan A (2001) Controlled randomization crossover trial of the effects of physiotherapy on mobility in chronic multiple sclerosis. *J Neurol Neurosurg Psychiatr* **70**(2): 174–9

Zajicek J (2005) Diagnosis and disease modifying treatments in multiple sclerosis. *Postgrad Med J* **81:** 556–61

Chapter 17

The management of pain in multiple sclerosis: A care-study approach

Elizabeth Gray

The purpose of this chapter is to discuss pain management for people with multiple sclerosis (MS). It gives an overview of current literature and considers a case study. It includes a discussion of the lessons that can be learnt from the case study and concludes with suggestions for ensuring good pain management for people with MS.

The reported prevalence of pain in MS differs considerably between studies. Svendsen et al (2003) found studies with figures for prevalence of pain in people with MS ranging between 30–90%. As with many other symptoms of MS, pain can fluctuate throughout the course of the disease.

Patients generally fall into two groups:

- Those who have musculoskeletal pain that may or may not be related to MS
- Those who have neuropathic pain from their MS (Howarth, 2001).

Musculoskeletal pain can be exacerbated by reduced mobility, weakness, spasticity and lack of coordination (Heckman-Stone and Stone, 2001). Neuropathic pain can be characterized by burning and occasional shooting pains accompanied by sensory changes. It occurs as a result of damage to neural tissue, either peripherally or via the central nervous system (Wilson, 2002).

Nursing role

Nurses have an important role in the management of pain as they are often able to spend time with the patient to gain a thorough assessment, which is the first step towards successful treatment (Wilson, 2002). Pain assessment not only allows practitioners to identify the site, intensity and extent of the pain, but also provides an opportunity to identify factors that exacerbate or relieve pain, as well as any related psychological problems (Wilson, 2002). It also provides an opportunity to assess the effectiveness of pain-management techniques, both pharmacological and non-pharmacological, which have been used in the past or with the current episode of pain.

The Health Technology Review (Beard et al, 2003) was not able to identify any formal review of current clinical practice regarding the treatment of pain in MS. It found evidence that few patients are referred to pain specialists (Beard et al, 2003); however, this does not necessarily mean their pain is not being managed. Many chronic pain teams have a waiting list, and it may be that the neurologist and/or GP manage pain symptoms for people with MS. Also, the fluctuating nature of pain in MS may mean it is difficult to arrange a timely appointment with a chronic pain team. The Health Technology Review (Beard et al, 2003) suggests there are many variables in how pain related to MS is managed, and point out that most of the drugs used to treat pain in MS are being used out of license, i.e. many of the drugs used are not licensed for pain relief in MS in the UK.

The presence of pain may influence quality of life and daily activities (Svendsen et al, 2003). Pain of any description can have a dramatic effect on all aspects of a person's quality of life (Wilson, 2002). People can develop problems with general mobility and experience difficulty sleeping and loss of appetite (Wilson, 2002). Encouraging self-care is particularly important for adaptive coping and helps patients feel more in control in the face of the uncertainty of their disease and symptoms (Heckman-Stone and Stone, 2001). The assessment of pain and other symptoms is needed for diagnosis and to guide therapy (Dworkin et al, 2003). Some symptoms may exacerbate the pain experience, whereas others may be present as a direct result of untreated pain. Patients often have trouble describing the unusual nature of their symptoms and fear that they will not be believed (Dworkin et al, 2003).

In a postal survey, Svendsen et al (2003) found a higher prevalence of pain among people with MS than in matched reference subjects without MS. The reported pain was more likely to be rated as moderate or severe in the group with MS, and was often reported at more than one location. Patients with MS were more likely to have had physiotherapy treatment. For MS patients who had not had physiotherapy, their analgesic intake was higher than for reference subjects; whereas those who had had physiotherapy had a similar analgesic intake to reference subjects. This suggests that physiotherapy is often an important part of pain-management regimens. The benefits of physiotherapy for musculoskeletal pain are probably most evident; however, neuropathic pain can often be exacerbated by poor posture or maladaptive movements that have become habit, which were initially used by the patient to control symptoms.

More MS patients than reference subjects reported that pain interfered with daily life 'all the time'. Patients with MS reported a lower prevalence of muscle/joint disease than reference subjects; otherwise the groups were similar concerning other diseases.

Svendsen et al (2003) suggest musculoskeletal disease may be underdiagnosed in patients with MS because symptoms are wrongly connected to MS. They concluded that the frequency of reported pain in a Danish sample of MS patients was similar to that reported by a sample from the general population. However, pain intensity, treatment requirement, number of pain sites and the influence of pain on daily life were higher in patients with MS than in reference subjects.

Neuropathic pain usually responds well to antidepressant medication, such as amitriptyline, and anticonvulsant therapy, such as gabapentin and carbamazepine (Wilson, 2002). Antidepressants have an analgesic effect on neuropathic pain by altering monoamine neurotransmitter activity at the synapse (Wilson, 2002). Anticonvulsants stabilize excitable cell membranes and are useful in treating shooting neuropathic pain (Wilson, 2002). These drugs have side-effects that can usually be controlled by introducing the drug at small doses and increasing the dose every few days until adequate pain control is achieved. Amitriptyline, gabapentin and

Table 17.1: Drugs used for neuropathic pain

Drug	Common side-effects	Recommended starting dose	Regimen for increasing dose
Amitriptyline	Sedation, dry mouth, increased heart rate, blurred vision. Occasionally urinary retention	10–25 mg at night	In 10 mg or 25 mg increments, depending on starting dose. Increase every 3–4 days
Carbamazepine	Sedation, blurred vision, ataxia, vertigo	100 mg at night	In 100 mg increments every 3–4 days. Can be taken in divided doses, twice daily
Gabapentin	Somnolence, dizziness. Occasionally gastrointestinal symptoms, mild peripheral oedema	300 mg at night	In 300 mg increments every 3–4 days. Can be taken in divided doses three times daily. Stated maximum dose 2400 mg; however, has been used in doses up to 3600 mg to control neuropathic pain

From Wilson (2002), Dworkin et al (2003)

carbamazepine are often used as firstline management for neuropathic pain, and therefore a brief overview of their common side-effects and dosing regimens is given in *Table 17.1*.

The side-effects of these drugs need monitoring and can usually be resolved with dosage adjustment (Dworkin et al, 2003). The final dosage should be determined either by achieving complete pain relief or by the development of unacceptable adverse effects that do not resolve promptly. Gabapentin may cause or exacerbate gait and balance problems as well as cognitive impairment in elderly patients (Dworkin et al, 2003). However, generally excellent tolerability, safety and lack of drug interactions distinguish gabapentin from most other oral medication used for the treatment of chronic neuropathic pain (Dworkin et al, 2003).

Case study

Tracy is a 48-year-old woman with relapsing remitting MS diagnosed in 1990. She described pain in her legs as discomfort with shooting pain at times. She experienced muscle spasms in her legs and was on 10 mg baclofen. Over a period of a few months the pain in her legs became more problematic and she described it as a constant aching pain that was not relieved by paracetamol or ibuprofen. She also reported increasing weakness in her legs.

She was referred to the physiotherapist and reviewed by the rehabilitation consultant. It was decided that the pain was not linked to spasticity, but more likely to be neurogenic in nature. The baclofen was stopped and she was commenced on gabapentin 300 mg daily. It was agreed that she would be reviewed by the MS nurse to assess how well she was tolerating the gabapentin. It was also agreed that the gabapentin could be increased by 300 mg weekly as necessary, up to a maximum dose of 600 mg three times daily. She was seen by the MS nurse 2 weeks after commencing gabapentin. She did not report any side-effects and felt the pain had been controlled in the first week, but then had become worse. She was advised to increase her gabapentin to 300 mg twice daily, and reminded that she could increase further if necessary.

Her next review by the MS nurse was a month later. Tracy was still getting on well with the gabapentin and did not report any side-effects, although she reported the pain was still not fully controlled. She had remained on 600 mg daily. She was advised to increase the dose to 900 mg and then further in a week's time if the pain remained uncontrolled. Over the next month she increased the dose to 1800 mg and felt the pain was under control. After another month she felt the pain was well controlled and started reducing the gabapentin, settling at a level of 300 mg at night. Her pain has remained well controlled since.

Discussion

Tracy's pain was initially thought to be musculoskeletal in nature exacerbated by muscle spasms, hence the firstline treatment of baclofen and referral to the physiotherapist. It was during one of her physiotherapy sessions that a review by the rehabilitation consultant was requested. This was because there seemed to be little spasticity in her legs and the baclofen was making little difference to her pain. This highlights the necessity of involving the multidisciplinary team to gain good pain management. When gabapentin was initiated, it was decided that the MS nurse would be best placed to monitor side-effects and dose titration, as she could maintain regular contact with Tracy.

The potential side-effects of gabapentin and the process of increasing the dose were explained to Tracy. In retrospect, it would have been beneficial if Tracy had had contact with the MS nurse a week after commencing gabapentin, rather than 2 weeks later, as she had not felt able to increase the dose herself despite experiencing an increase in pain intensity during the second week of treatment. The process of increasing the dose was again explained to Tracy at this point and she was encouraged to contact the MS nurse if she needed any further advice before her next planned appointment a month later.

Again, at the next appointment, the MS nurse found that Tracy had not increased the dose of gabapentin despite reporting that her pain was still not well controlled. A weekly telephone call from the nurse may have allowed Tracy to gain good pain control over a shorter period. The fact that Tracy was able to reduce the dose of gabapentin could be taken to demonstrate the fluctuating nature of pain in MS. It could also be suggested that as Tracy felt more in control of the pain, her perception of its intensity and impact on her daily life changed, meaning that she felt able to cope with a lower dose of medication.

This would suggest that it is beneficial for patients with MS to have early assessment when they experience exacerbations of pain in order to achieve good pain management quickly and thus reduce the impact of pain on their quality of life.

In the current system of health care in the UK, this means that a specialist pain team may not be the most appropriate referral point because of the current waiting lists. The quickest point of access for a person with MS is usually via his or her MS nurse or GP.

Non-pharmacological approaches should be used to complement drug therapies and to ensure a comprehensive approach to pain management (Wilson, 2002). There is a strong link between anxiety and pain intensity; therefore, it is essential that strategies to reduce anxiety and stress are implemented (Wilson, 2002). Often, the fact that someone listens and believes the patient's report of pain, and offers strategies to help manage the pain, will have an impact on the level of anxiety and stress. The MS nurse is often ideally placed to offer this support.

Other non-drug-related methods of pain relief might include relaxation, breathing exercises, visualization and distraction, heat and cold therapy, complementary therapies and transcutaneous electrical nerve stimulation (TENS). A discussion of these techniques is beyond the scope of this chapter, but they use the principles of the gate control theory (Melzack and Wall, 1996), which are effective in the treatment of neuropathic pain (Wilson, 2002).

It must be made clear to patients that the drugs used have some potential to reduce pain, but that they are not typical analgesics and should be taken on a regular basis to have a predictable effect (Wilson, 2002). However, it is also important that patients have an understanding of the nature of pain in MS and gain the confidence to take control of their own pain management. This may mean the introduction of flexible prescriptions that allow patients to increase their medication to an agreed maximum dose when they experience exacerbation of pain. Common concerns focus on the amount of medication taken and the number of tablets.

In Wilson's (2002) experience, patients will often report not taking medicines because they were not in pain at the time. People require education regarding their medication so they understand how to reduce the dose if possible. This may help allay fears regarding the number of tablets taken as the patient can gain an understanding of how to reduce doses gradually in order to maintain good pain control. Through experimentation, patients will often find the baseline level of a given medication that is needed to keep their pain under control between exacerbations. The MS nurse is ideally placed to offer the education and support required. This will potentially be time consuming initially, but with continued support patients are able to take control of their symptoms, which can ultimately increase wellbeing and have a positive impact on their experience of living with MS.

The Health Technology Review (Beard et al, 2003) reported a glaring dissociation between the published evidence regarding the effectiveness of treatments for pain and what appears to be current clinical practice. It is suggested that this does not mean that treatments currently being used are not evidence-based, still less that they are ineffective; however, the evidence on which they are based is largely clinical experience, the teaching of others and anecdote. This could mean effective treatments are not being used consistently throughout the NHS (Beard et al, 2003).

The Review summarizes the literature available to March 2002 and gives a good overview of the evidence supporting each drug currently used to treat pain in MS. It concludes that there is a lack of research evidence on the effectiveness of drugs to treat pain in MS; however, it cautions this should not be taken to imply that there are not effective treatments available.

Conclusion

This case study and the discussion surrounding it has demonstrated the need for good pain assessment and the implementation of pain-management techniques involving the multidisciplinary team. However, it is suggested that one of the most important factors in maintaining good pain control is to allow the person with pain to take responsibility for its management. In order for this to be successful, the patient needs to have a supportive relationship with a healthcare professional whom they can turn to for advice as necessary. The MS nurse is often best placed to take on this role.

The development of protocols for managing pain linked to MS may prove useful; however, pain is often an individualized experience requiring individualized management. The development of a system where a patient experiencing pain can be assessed by the MS nurse, who can then liaise with appropriate members of the multidisciplinary team in order to implement appropriate pain management promptly, may help improve the experience for MS patients who experience pain.

References

Beard S, Hunn A, Wight J (2003) Treatments for spasticity and pain in multiple sclerosis: a systematic review. *Health Technol Assess* **7**(40): 1–111

Dworkin RH, Backonja M, Rowbotham MC et al (2003) Advances in neuropathic pain. *Arch Neurol* **60**: 1524–34

Heckman-Stone C, Stone C (2001) Pain management techniques used by patients with multiple sclerosis. *J Pain* **2**(4): 205–8

Howarth A (2001) Changing lives. *Nurs Stand* **16**(7): 15–16

Melzack R, Wall PD (1996) *The Challenge of Pain.* 2nd edn. Penguin Books, London

Svendsen KB, Jensen TS, Overyad K, Hansen HJ, Koch-Henriksen N, Bach FW (2003) Pain in patients with multiple sclerosis. *Arch Neurol* **60**: 1089–94

Wilson M (2002) Overcoming the challenges of neuropathic pain. *Nurs Stand* **16**(33): 47–53

Chapter 18

A nurse-led, patient-centred mitoxantrone service in neurology

Emily Harrison, Bernadette Porter

Multiple sclerosis (MS) is an incurable, autoimmune-mediated, inflammatory disease of the central nervous system that usually presents with a history of acute onset of neurological symptoms (relapses) or progressive neurological impairment (Compston and Coles, 2002). The cause is unknown, although it is believed that a non-specific viral infection may trigger an autoimmune reaction in a genetically susceptible individual (Compston, 1997). The disease process effects myelinated nerve fibres, such as the optic nerve and the white matter tracts of the brain and spinal cord. This may lead to a variety of symptoms, for example visual disturbances, weakness and sensory symptoms (Toosy and Thompson, 2000).

It is estimated that between 52 000–62 000 people have MS in the UK (National Institute for Clinical Excellence (NICE), 2003), and around 2.5 million people are affected worldwide (Compston and Coles, 2002). MS typically presents between 20–40 years of age. Females are more susceptible than males by a factor that approaches 2:1 (McDonald, 1998). Race and geography also affect susceptibility to the disease (Sadovnick and Ebers, 1993).

MS nurses are able to empower those affected by MS by providing information, support and advice about the condition from time of diagnosis and throughout the disease spectrum. The MS nurse is pivotal in providing a greater understanding of the condition, and by adapting a holistic, collaborative and coordinated approach can help individuals, where possible, reach their goals of self-management (UK Multiple Sclerosis Specialist Nurse Association et al, 2001).

Disease-modifying drugs in MS

There are four disease-modifying drugs (DMDs) available to patients with MS. The double-blind, placebo-controlled trials of these drugs have demonstrated a reduction in the severity and frequency of relapse rate by approximately 30% in patients with relapsing/remitting MS (RRMS) or in patients with secondary progressive MS (SPMS) with superimposed relapses (Association of British Neurologists, 2001). The drugs that are available include interferon beta (Avonex, Betaferon, Rebif) and glatiramer acetate (Copaxone). Currently, DMDs are the only form of licensed treatments in the UK that influence the disease course. Unfortunately for some MS patients, these treatments are not effective, and rapid deterioration in their condition continues. Many centres are now using a potent cytotoxic preparation called mitoxantrone for patients who have failed DMDs or have a more aggressive form of the disease.

The role of immunosuppressants in MS

MS immunosuppressant therapies focus on the modulation or suppression of the immune system, which underscores the major role the inflammatory response plays in the pathology of the disease (Porter et al, 2004). Immunosuppressants used in MS include azathioprine, ciclosporin, methotrexate and mitoxantrone (Toosy and Thompson, 2000). These drugs may be used in isolation or in combination; however, mitoxantrone is fast becoming the first-line cytotoxic drug of choice in many centres (personal communication).

Mitoxantrone (Novantrone) is an anti-neoplastic agent, which exerts potent immunomodulating effects on the immune system, including suppression of B-cell immunity and reduction of T-cell number (Morrissey et al, 2005). The recommended dose is $12 \, mg/m^2$ administered by intravenous infusion trimonthly (Hartung et al, 2002) or 20 mg administered monthly for 6 months (Edan et al, 1997). Mitoxantrone has the potential to cause cardiotoxicity, and therefore the total cumulative dose should not exceed $140 \, mg/m^2$ of mitoxantrone (Ghalie et al, 2002). It is licensed for the use in MS in the USA, but as yet has not been licensed in the UK.

Clinical trial results

To date there have been three important pivotal trials carried out to measure the effectiveness and safety of mitoxantrone in patients with worsening MS. In 1997, Millefiorini et al carried out a phase ll, placebo-controlled trial that involved 51 patients with relapsing/remitting MS. Patients were randomized to receive either mitoxantrone $8 \, mg/m^2$ or placebo for 1 year. Results showed a significant reduction in the annual number of exacerbations and a significant increase in the proportion of exacerbation-free patients in the mitoxantrone group compared with the placebo group.

In the same year, a collaboration of French neurologists (Edan et al, 1997) undertook another phase ll study with 42 patients with RRMS and SPMS. The patients were randomized to either receive mitoxantrone 20 mg and methylprednisolone 1 g, or methyprednisolone 1 g alone. Results showed an improvement in Expanded Disability Status Score (EDSS) (Kurtzke, 1983) by one point from baseline and also a reduction in relapse rates. The EDSS is a quantitative clinical scale of neurological impairment ranging from 1–10. Increasing increments on the scale represent increasing disability (Toosy and Thompson, 2000).

More recently, Hartung et al (2002) conducted a larger, phase lll, controlled, randomized, double-blind study of 194 patients with RRMS and SPMS. Patients were randomly assigned to receive placebo mitoxantrone 5 mg/m^2 or mitoxantrone 12 mg/m^2. A total number of 188 patients were able to be assessed at 24 months. At 24 months, the mitroxantrone group compared with the placebo group experienced benefits on the EDSS and a number of outcome measures. This study suggests that mitoxantrone was well tolerated and reduced progression of disability and clinical exacerbations.

Side-effect profile

As a potent cyctoxic drug, mitoxantrone, like any chemotherapy agent, has the potential to cause harmful and potentially fatal side-effects. The most common side-effects reported throughout the three pivotal trials included bone marrow depression, nausea and vomiting, alopecia, amenorrhoea and urinary and upper respiratory tract infection (Edan et al, 1997; Millefiorini et al, 1997; Hartung et al, 2002). Mitoxantrone has also been associated with cardiotoxicity (Ghalie et al, 2002), can cause fertility problems for both males and females (CancerBacup, 2000) and has the potential to cause therapy-related acute leukaemia (Morrisset et al, 2005).

Introduction of mitoxantrone in a neurological environment

The immunosuppressive action and side-effect profile of mitoxantrone means that this drug should be used with caution. At a large teaching hospital in London, mitoxantrone was introduced within a haphazard medical model. A nurse-led audit initiative of the first cohort of treated patients identified a number of complications, including neutropenia and severe urinary tract and skin infections, among this patient group. The MS nursing team raised concerns regarding safe practice and highlighted a number of areas that needed to be explored within a clinical governance framework. Examples of the areas of concern include: lack of co-ordination; lack of named, trained staff; lack of advice on potential infertility and risk of developing secondary leukaemia; lack of pregnancy screening; and poor documentation.

It is recognized that, as a clinical expert, the MS specialist nurse must be able to:

- Identify areas for improvements
- Lead service development
- Design care pathways appropriate to people with MS across the trajectory of the disease course (UK Multiple Sclerosis Specialist Nurse Association et al, 2001).

In an effort to ensure best practice, the MS nursing team at the National Hospital for Neurology and Neurosurgery, University College London Hospitals NHS Foundation Trust (UCLH), completed a literature search and spent time discussing the use of mitoxantrone with colleagues in the cancer team. In discussion, the option of the cancer team delivering mitoxantrone in isolation of the MS services and the option of mitoxantrone being delivered by the neurology team following specialist education and training were explored. In any clinical situation the benefits of treatments must be weighed against the risks. When the risks of therapy include irreversible cardiac damage, infertility, development of treatment-related leukaemia and infection, the decision to treat and the process of so doing becomes considerably more complex. In an effort to deliver care in a holistic rather than task-oriented framework, a decision was made that these complicated MS patients would receive this treatment in a neurological setting following staff training and support from cancer services.

Introducing standards

In order to design a safe service, standards of care need to be formulated. At the authors' hospital, the

---

Table 18.1: Standards of care*

- There should be a named neurology team to head the service, who should be MS experts
- There should be a timely and appropriate approach to starting treatment
- Inpatients' chemotherapy should only be given where it is agreed as part of a named neurological ward's activities
- A nurse key-worker should be identified for each patient
- Patients should receive the optimal treatment regimen as approved by the trust's pharmaceutical board
- There should be a named lead pharmacist attached to the mitoxantrone MS service
- There should be written guidelines/protocols for mitoxantrone use. These should include protocols for the prevention and treatment of complications and side-effects arising from chemotherapy, and should include acceptable blood test parameters
- There should be written guidelines/protocols that should be made available to primary care practitioners for the management of complications arising from mitoxantrone
- There should be documented evidence of informed consent in all patients
- Pre-treatment investigations must be documented as normal in the medical notes of all patients
- There should be documented evidence of good baseline cardiac function for all patients
- Chemotherapy should be administered by appropriately trained neurological staff
- Chemotherapy administration documentation must be clear and comprehensive
- Every set of patient notes should contain the mitoxantrone integrated care pathway with all variances recorded

*Adapted from the Department of Health (2000)

MS nursing team adopted the standards from the *Manual of Cancer Services Standards* (Department of Health, 2000), to reflect safe practice within a neurological setting (*Table 18.1*).

Although these standards have helped create a framework for safe drug administration, they have also highlighted the need for a more patient-centred, coordinated approach to care delivery in order to improve the quality of the service offered. A multidisciplinary, integrated care pathway (ICP) was agreed to be the most appropriate way of improving the quality of the service.

Integrated care pathways

Middleton et al (2001) state that:

'An integrated care pathway (ICP) is a multidisciplinary outline of anticipated care, placed in an appropriate timeframe, to help a patient with a specific condition or set of symptoms move progressively through a clinical experience to positive outcomes.'

Kitchiner and Bundred (1996) suggest that ICPs use multidisciplinary guidelines to develop and implement clinical plans, which represent current local best practice for specific conditions. ICPs also incorporate national guidelines, evidence-based practice and benchmarking. Pathways are devised into time intervals during which specific goals are expected, together with guidance on the optimal timing of appropriate investigations, advice on side-effect management and treatment options.

The ICP forms part of the clinical record, and in some cases it replaces other forms of documentation, such as nursing care plans (UCLH, 2003). While patients' progress follows the pathway, the appropriate health professional signs for the care he or she has delivered. If the patient's care or progress varies from the pathway then it is recorded as a variance, together with the reason and the action that has been taken.

Members of the team can choose to deviate from the pathway, but this must be clinically justified, for example deterioration in the patient's condition or intolerable side-effects (Kitchiner and Bundred, 1996). This encourages staff to adhere to the guidelines specified on the pathway, thus reducing variations in the care provided. ICPs allow innovative and creative ways of improving quality of care, allowing quality assurance to flourish. Onslow et al (2003) recognize that NHS trusts are increasingly requiring ICPs to be developed for reasons of finance, bed management and to meet the requirements of clinical governance.

The main strength of the mitoxantrone multidisciplinary ICP is that it is patient focused as the delivery of care focuses on the patient's journey, thus improving coordination and consistency. By having explicit evidence-based standards, unnecessary variations to care are reduced. It also allows the clinical team to identify strengths and weaknesses within the area of practice, and ensures that clinical guidelines and evidence are incorporated into everyday practice (Middleton et al, 2001). The mitoxantrone ICP also provides a framework to allow prospective audit against local and national MS guidelines (NICE, 2003).

NICE guidelines state that mitoxantrone should only be used in the following circumstances:

- After full discussion and consideration of all the risks
- With formal evaluation, preferably in a randomized or other prospective study
- By an expert in the use of these medicines in MS.

The lead clinician assesses patients against predetermined eligibility criteria, as approved by the trust pharmaceutical board. A complete neurological examination, including a review of functional systems and an EDSS, is completed. On completion, patients are provided with an information booklet, which provides evidence-based information outlining the risks and benefits of the treatment and side-effect profile to help make an informed decision about proceeding with treatment. Patients who wish to proceed are referred to the nurse-led pre-infusion assessment clinic, which is the starting point of the mitoxantrone ICP.

The clinical nurse specialist (CNS) plays an important role at this stage, by gaining a baseline measure of the impact of MS on each individual using a new patient-based outcome measure known as the Multiple Sclerosis Impact Scale (MSIS-29) (Hobart et al, 2001). The MSIS-29 is an instrument that measures the physical (20 items) and psychological (9 items) impact of MS. In addition, the patient's general health including history of infections, cardiac disease, tissue viability and understanding of the treatment trial results and potential side-effects are all discussed. The CNS also orders baseline investigations including blood screening, electrocardiogram and X-rays, while discussing options for sperm or egg donation as appropriate. In addition, referrals to other multidisciplinary team members as necessary are made, and the GP is informed of the treatment plan and shared care guidelines are discussed.

This screening clinic allows the nurse to make vital nursing assessments of patients' physical, psychosocial, emotional and social functioning. The CNS provides education to the patients, checks their level of understanding and gains insight into their expectations from therapy as well as providing answers to their many questions. Following this clinic, a follow-up telephone call is made by the CNS to inform patients of their test results and to check that they wish to proceed. If patients do not wish to proceed they return to the care of their neurologist to discuss other treatment options and management.

In order to ensure that the MS nurse specialists up-skilled, rather than de-skilled, staff on the designated unit, a training programme was designed in collaboration with the cancer team. The nursing staff on the designated unit undertook training specific to the administration of mitoxantrone in MS. The unit nurses were highly motivated and competent, and volunteered to become key workers taking responsibility for the overall delivery of treatment and coordination of care during each individual's treatment cycle.

Patients who wish to proceed with treatment are therefore given the contact details of a key nurse from the designated infusion unit who arranges a suitable date and time for admission. The drug is administered over six to eight cycles in accordance with the clinical care guidelines of the ICP, which include protocols for communication with the GP and referral back to the CNS-MS and neurology team.

Patients are provided with a mitoxantrone patient handheld record, which records information that other health professionals can access should the patient present or if complications arise. Once the final treatment has been completed, the patients return to the CNS-MS for an overall review of their health, a summary of their treatment and remeasurement of their individual impact of MS scale. Patients are then referred back to the neurologist for long-term neurological management.

Summary

The delivery of mitoxantrone in a neurological setting requires a sound infrastructure based on evidence-based practice within a clinical governance framework. Nurse specialists are well placed to learn from other specialist colleagues to ensure that practice is safe and patient centred. The introduction of a nurse-led multidisciplinary mitoxantrone ICP at the National Hospital for Neurology and Neurosurgery, UCLH NHS Foundation Trust, is an example of nursing collaboration and leadership where vision, courage, reality and ethics were balanced to create a service that directly improves the patient experience and quality of care delivered.

The authors wish to offer their thanks to their colleagues, Kay Eaton (Nurse Consultant/Lead Cancer Nurse), Evelyn Frank (Pharmacist), Ellen Butler (Ward Sister), Professor Alan Thompson (Neurologist), Dr Gavin Giovannoni (Neurologist) and Liz Keenan CNS-MS, for their support in assisting with this project.

References

Association of British Neurologists (2001) *Guidelines for the Use of Beta Interferons and Glatiramer Acetate in Multiple Sclerosis*. Association of British Neurologists, London

CancerBacup (2000) *Factsheet 2001 Mitoxantrone* (Novantrone). CancerBacup, London

Compston A (1997) Genetic epidemiology of multiple sclerosis. *J Neurol Neurosurg Psych* **62**: 553–61

Compston A, Coles A (2002) Multiple sclerosis: seminar. *Lancet* **359**: 1221-31

Dalton J (1999) The case for mitoxantrone in multiple sclerosis. *Inpharma* **1193**: 9–10

Department of Health (2000) *Manual of Cancer Services Standards*. DoH, London

Edan G, Miller D, Clanet M et al (1997) Therapeutic effect of mitoxantrone combined with methylprednisolone in multiple sclerosis: a randomized multicentre study of active disease using MRI and clinical criteria. *J Neurol Neurosurg Psych* **62**: 112–18

Ghalie RG, Edan G, Laurent M et al (2002) Cardiac adverse effects associated with mitoxantrone (Novantrone) therapy in patients with MS. *Neurology* **59**(6): 909–13

Hartung HP, Gonsette R, Konig N et al (2002) Mitoxantrone in progressive multiple sclerosis: a placebo-controlled, double blind, randomized, mulitcentre trial. *Lancet* **360**: 2018–25

Hobart J, Lamping D, Fikpatrick R, Riazi A, Thompson A (2001) The Multiple Sclerosis Impact Scale (MSIS-29): a new patient-based outcome measure. *Brain* **124**(5): 962–73

Kitchiner D, Bundred P (1996) Integrated care pathways. Archives of disease in childhood. *Arch Dis Child* **75**(2): 166–168

Kurtzke JF (1983) Rating neurologic impairment in multiple sclerosis: an expanded disability status scale (EDSS). *Neurology* **33**: 1444–52

McDonald I (1998) Diagnostic methods and investigation in multiple sclerosis. In: Compston A, ed. *Mcalpine's Multiple Sclerosis*. Churchill, London

Middleton S, Barnett J, Reeves D (2001) What is an integrated care pathway? *Evidence-based Med* **3**(3) (http://www.evidence-based-medicine.co.uk/ebmfiles/WhatisanICP.pdf) (accessed 6 September 2004)

Millefiorini E, Gasperini C, Pozzilli C et al (1997) Randomized placebo-controlled trial of mitoxantrone in relapsing-remitting multiple sclerosis: 24-month clinical and MRI outcome. *J Neurol* **224**: 153–59

Morrissey SP, Le Page E, Edan G (2005) Mitoxantrone in the treatment of multiple sclerosis. *Int MS J* **12**(3): 75–87

National Institute for Clinical Excellence (2003) *Multiple Sclerosis: Management in Primary and Secondary Care*. The National Collaborating Centre for Chronic Conditions, London

Onslow L, Roberts H, Steiner A, Powell J, Pickering R (2003) An integrated care pathway for fractured neck of femur patients. *Prof Nurse* **18**(5): 265–8

Porter B, International Multiple Sclerosis Nursing Coalition (2004) *Topics in Multiple Sclerosis (1): An Immunological Perspective*. Multiple Sclerosis Colloquium, University of Minnesota, Minnesota, USA

Sadovnick AD, Ebers GC (1993) Epidemiology of multiple sclerosis: a critical overview. *Can J Neurol Sci* **20**: 17–29

Toosy A, Thompson A (2000) Multiple sclerosis: the disease and its treatment. *The Pharmaceutical J* **264**: 695–700

UCLH (2003) *Integrated Care Pathways: Guidebook for UCLH Staff*. UCLH, London

UK Multiple Sclerosis Specialist Nurse Association, RCN, MS Research Trust (2001) *The Key Elements for Developing MS Specialist Nurse Services in the UK*. MS Research Trust, Letchworth

Chapter 19

Current management of neurogenic bladder in patients with multiple sclerosis

Sue Woodward

Multiple sclerosis (MS) is a common neurological condition affecting between 50–100 people per 100 000 (Hinson and Boone, 1996). Symptoms are caused by demyelination in the white matter of the central nervous system, and can affect the tracts that control bladder function (Ciancio et al, 2001).

One of the main areas of interest in the management of MS in recent years has been around the development of disease-modifying therapies, which reduce disease activity and delay disease progression (Calabresi, 2002). These therapies, however, are not curative and many patients continue to suffer from disabling symptoms, such as bladder symptoms, which still need to be treated to provide symptomatic relief (Clanet and Brassat, 2000; Calabresi, 2002).

Urological problems are common in patients with MS; it is estimated that up to 80% of people with MS will suffer symptoms of urinary dysfunction during the course of their disease (Bennett et al, 2004), which significantly impact on their quality of life and social lives (Clanet and Brassat, 2000). The incidence of bladder dysfunction in patients with MS has been reported to be 33–52%, and it is related to disability status (Araki et al, 2003).

Management of continence symptoms usually falls within the domain of nursing, and it is, therefore, important that nurses are aware of current treatment options that are available for patients. By helping patients to manage their bladder symptoms and regain some control over their pattern of voiding, nurses can positively impact on their quality of life, which has been shown to collapse early in the disease before patients become severely disabled (Canadian Burden of Illness Study Group, 1998).

A range of treatments are available, from simple behavioural methods such as bladder retraining through to invasive surgical procedures, depending on the nature of the bladder problem. This chapter briefly reviews the neurobiology of micturition and the pathophysiology of neurogenic bladder problems that occur in patients with MS. Behavioural, pharmacological and surgical interventions are then discussed and current research developments are identified.

This review of the current management of neurogenic bladder dysfunction in patients with MS was conducted using CINAHL and Medline databases from 1996 to March 2004. The search was limited to papers published in English, and key words used included: 'multiple sclerosis'; 'urinary'; 'neurogenic bladder'; and 'incontinence'.

Review of related anatomy and pathophysiology

Normal micturition requires an intact central and peripheral nervous system to coordinate both the filling and voiding phases (Woodward, 1996) (*Figures 19.1* and *19.2*).

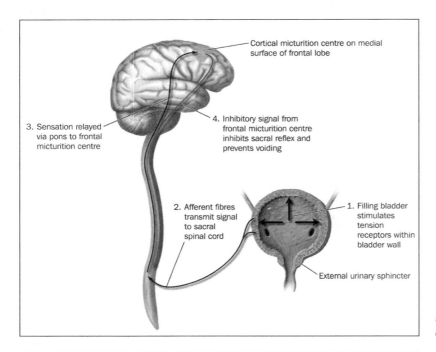

Figure 19.1: *Voluntary inhibition of sacral voiding reflex*

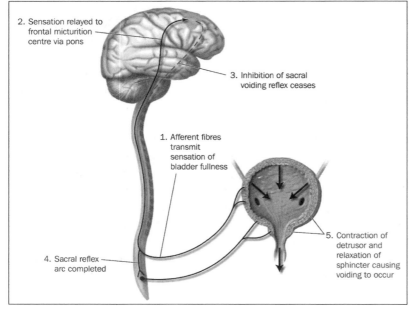

Figure 19.2: *Voluntary control of voiding: micturition (when an appropriate place to void has been selected and reached)*

Micturition is controlled through reflexes and autonomic fibres, but is modulated by voluntary control from the cerebral hemispheres. Micturition pathways pass through peripheral sympathetic and parasympathetic fibres to and from the bladder and spinal cord through sacral segments S2–S4 (*Figure 19.3*). From here they pass upwards to the brain through the spinothalamic tract, pontine micturition centre and thalamus to the frontal micturition centre in the frontal lobes.

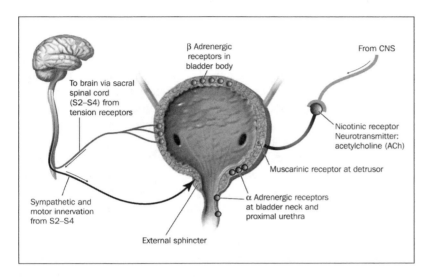

Figure 19.3: Neurological control of bladder function. CNS=central nervous system

During filling, stretch receptors in the detrusor muscle wall of the bladder send an impulse to the sacral spinal cord, and ß-adrenergic receptors in the bladder body are stimulated to increase accommodation of urine by relaxation of the smooth muscle of the detrusor. Also, α-adrenergic receptors are stimulated at the bladder neck and proximal urethra, promoting smooth muscle contraction in this area; while the sympathetic stimulation to the external sphincter is maintained, promoting this ring of skeletal muscle to contract. Bladder contraction is mediated through the stimulation of muscarinic receptors on the detrusor muscle (Abrams et al, 1998) from the central nervous system (see *Figure 19.3*). During voiding, parasympathetic stimulation via sacral segments S2–S4 causes the bladder to contract, while sympathetic tone is reduced to the external urethral sphincter, allowing the bladder neck to open (Getliffe and Dolman, 1997).

Pathophysiology

The cerebral cortex, brainstem and sacral-spinal cord are the main components of the central nervous system responsible for bladder function (Araki et al, 2003). Lesions at different points along this micturition pathway produce different effects on voiding function; for example a cerebral lesion will often result in detrusor hyperreflexia and overactive bladder symptoms of urgency, frequency and urge incontinence (Araki et al, 2003). Detrusor hyperreflexia is characterized by involuntary detrusor contractions during bladder filling that cannot be consciously suppressed and produce an increase in intravesical pressure greater than 15 cm water (Bates et al, 1977).

A lesion in the pons or sacral spinal cord can result in detrusor hyporeflexia, with resulting bladder-emptying problems (Araki et al, 2003). Lesions above the sacral spinal cord (suprasacral lesions) may result in detrusor hyperreflexia with detrusor–sphincter dyssynergia (Araki et al, 2003). This occurs when the contraction of the detrusor muscle and relaxation of the external sphincter are uncoordinated, resulting in incomplete bladder emptying because of interruption of the pathways between the pons and the sacral cord (DasGupta and Fowler, 2002).

There have been some reports of ethnic differences in patterns of bladder problems experienced by MS sufferers, with filling and overactive bladder symptoms of detrusor hyperreflexia being more predominant in Western countries (Koldewijn et al, 1995; Hinson and Boone, 1996), while emptying symptoms are more prevalent in Japan (Araki et al, 2003). It has also been shown that urological problems can change over time with the changing pattern of the disease process itself (Ciancio et al, 2001; DasGupta and Fowler, 2002). Regardless of the disease stage, the risk of emptying symptoms are higher during an exacerbation of the MS (Koldewijn et al, 1995) and once detrusor–sphincter dyssynergia has developed it usually persists (Ciancio et al, 2001).

The lesion site in the central nervous system may be a major determinant of bladder and urethral sphincter dysfunction in patients with MS, but most patients with MS have multiple lesions at multiple sites so it is not always possible to determine which lesion has resulted in the bladder dysfunction. This is probably less important to determine than the nature of the bladder problem being experienced and its impact on the patient's quality of life, so that appropriate treatment can be given.

The onus of initiating assessment of bladder symptoms often falls to nursing staff, and a thorough assessment of bladder function and urinary symptoms should be undertaken. This should include taking a thorough history from the patient as well as aspects of physical examination and basic investigations (*Table 19.1*) (Woodward, 1995; Weiss, 1998; Scientific Committee of the First International Consultation on Incontinence, 2000).

Table 19.1: Factors to be considered during continence assessment, and highly recommended diagnostic tests

Factors to consider when taking the patient's history

- Characteristics of the incontinence/bladder problem, including the nature and duration of symptoms
- How the problem is currently managed
- Past medical, surgical and obstetric history, including drug history
- Bowel habit
- Nutritional and fluid intake
- Functional and cognitive abilities
- The patient's and carer's perceptions and expectations
- Effect on quality of life
- Social and environmental factors

Physical examination and diagnostic investigations that should be performed

- Physical examination of abdomen, perineum, vagina and rectum; simple neurological examination
- Quantification of symptoms using a bladder diary
- Urinalysis
- Midstream specimen of urine if urinary tract infection is suspected
- Measurement of post-void residual volume

Specifically, follow-up of patients with MS should include measurement of the extent of residual urine volumes, preferably by transabdominal ultrasound or by catheterization (DasGupta and Fowler, 2003). This is important because of the changing nature of the disease and urinary dysfunction over time.

It has been argued that the most commonly experienced overactive bladder symptoms (frequency, urgency and urge incontinence) can be assumed to result from detrusor hyperreflexia, and therefore treatment can be initiated based on symptoms and without undertaking detailed urodynamic investigations in all cases (Clanet and Brassat, 2000; DasGupta and Fowler, 2002, 2003). However, Ciancio and colleagues (2001) demonstrated changes in urodynamic pattern over time without a change in urinary symptoms, and they argued that urodynamic evaluation was, therefore, necessary to treat voiding symptoms properly in patients with MS.

Behavioural management

Bladder retraining

Bladder retraining is effective in treating overactive bladder symptoms of urinary frequency, urgency and urge incontinence (Anders, 1999). The reassurance and encouragement that nurses can provide to patients with MS undergoing a programme of bladder retraining cannot be underestimated. The principles of bladder retraining are based on suppressing urinary urge and extending the intervals between voiding (Anders, 1999). Patients should be carefully selected as most success is achieved in patients who are motivated, ideally self-ambulant and cognitively aware (Anders, 1999). This therapy may, therefore, be less appropriate for some patients with MS who have more severe symptoms.

Lower abdominal pressure

Obstructive symptoms and incomplete voiding are evident in 33–50% of MS patients with bladder symptoms, resulting in elevated post-void residual urine volumes greater than 100 ml in many cases (Prasad et al, 2003). This could be caused by either detrusor hypocontractility or detrusor–sphincter dyssynergia and, in turn, can lead to worsening symptoms (DasGupta et al, 1997). For many years, suprapubic bladder compression using the hands (Crede's manoeuvre) has been practised by patients with MS to assist in emptying the neurogenic bladder (Prasad et al, 2003).

The bladder can also be induced to empty more fully if vibration is applied instead of pressure, and a hand-held battery-operated device was developed to achieve this aim (the Queen Square bladder stimulator) (DasGupta et al, 1997). This early work with vibration was criticized as the initial studies were uncontrolled and it was suggested that the results were attributable to the application of pressure using the device, rather than vibration (Hextall et al, 1998). More recently, however, controlled studies have demonstrated that the application of percutaneous vibration produced a significant fall in residual volume, whereas pressure alone did not (Prasad et al, 2003).

Patients have also reported improvement in quality-of-life scores after using this vibration device and have experienced improvement in their symptoms (DasGupta et al, 1997), once again emphasizing the need for nurses to manage urinary symptoms effectively. No serious side-effects have been reported by patients using the device, although some will not use it in public toilets because of the noise it makes (DasGupta et al, 1997).

Clean, intermittent self-catheterization

Self-catheterization is recommended for patients with incomplete bladder emptying and a post-void residual volume greater than 100 ml (Clanet and Brassat, 2000). It is essential to empty the bladder, as any treatment for overactivity is unlikely to succeed with the presence of high residual volumes (DasGupta and Fowler, 2002). Since its introduction by Lapides and colleagues (1972), the management of bladder-emptying problems has been revolutionized; however, it is not a technique that is either practicable or acceptable to many patients with MS, and many will still use the Queen Square bladder stimulator as described previously (DasGupta et al, 1997).

The process of clean, intermittent self-catheterization (CISC) and the advantages and disadvantages of this technique have been discussed in detail elsewhere (Woodward and Rew, 2003). Optimal management would include a combination of CISC and anticholinergic medication; however, increased urgency and intractable urinary incontinence may eventually require management with an indwelling catheter (DasGupta and Fowler, 2002). If this is required, it would be preferable to use a suprapubic rather than a urethral catheter (DasGupta and Fowler, 2002).

Some advantages of suprapubic catheterization include:

- No risk of urethral trauma
- Greater comfort, especially in chairbound patients
- Greater freedom for expression of sexuality (Getliffe and Dolman, 1997).

Pharmacological interventions

Anticholinergic medications

Therapeutic strategy is aimed at providing symptomatic relief of detrusor overactivity, while ensuring complete bladder emptying (DasGupta and Fowler, 2002).

Anticholinergic drugs have been the most effective and commonly used medications available to date to control overactive bladder symptoms, such as urgency, urinary frequency and urge incontinence (Bennett et al, 2004). These drugs include oxybutynin and tolterodine and act by blocking the muscarinic receptors on the detrusor muscle that respond to the neurotransmitter acetylcholine (DasGupta and Fowler, 2002), thereby reducing the unstable bladder contractions that frequently affect patients with MS.

Oxybutynin hydrochloride (oxybutynin)

Oxybutynin is a potent antimuscarinic agent and has pronounced muscle relaxant activity, with some antispasmodic, analgesic and local anaesthetic effects (Birns et al, 2000; Bennett et al, 2004). Treatment with oxybutynin not only improves subjective symptoms reported by patients, but also has been shown to improve objective measures of bladder function as demonstrated on urodynamic assessment (Birns et al, 2000). It has been available in an immediate-release preparation for many years, but is not always well tolerated because of unpleasant side-effects; it also interacts at muscarinic receptors elsewhere in the body, causing symptoms such as dry mouth and constipation (DasGupta and Fowler, 2002; Bennett et al, 2004).

The immediate-release preparation has to be taken regularly throughout the day because of extensive first-pass effects, i.e. it is rapidly absorbed through the gastrointestinal tract and metabolized by the liver (Birns et al, 2000). The mean half-life of oxybutynin is 1.6 hours and it is rapidly eliminated leading to peaks and troughs in dose effects and contributing to the marked side-effects, which may result in poor compliance or discontinuation of the therapy (Abrams et al, 1998). The starting dose for oxybutynin is 2.5 mg twice a day, which may be increased up to a maximum of 20 mg per day in divided doses (DasGupta and Fowler, 2002).

More recently, a controlled-release formulation has been developed that maintains a consistent release of the drug over a 24-hour period, avoiding the peaks seen with immediate-release oxybutynin (Bennett et al, 2004) and maintaining therapeutic blood levels over much of any 24-hour period (Birns et al, 2000). This has been shown to reduce the incidence of dry mouth, and the controlled-release preparation is better tolerated as well as being more convenient for the patient (Birns et al, 2000). It has been shown to have equal efficacy as the immediate-release preparation (Birns et al, 2000), but additional improvement in symptoms has also been shown for patients taking the controlled-release preparation over immediate-release oxybutynin (Gleason et al, 1999).

The single, daily dose of oxybutynin XL can range between 5–30 mg (DasGupta and Fowler, 2003). This development may mean that more patients with MS can be successfully treated with oxybutynin, especially those who require a higher dose and for whom the associated side-effects were intolerable.

Intravesical oxybutynin has also been tried, with good effect. While this is well tolerated, it is rarely used in practice as it requires repeated catheterization to instil the normal dose of 5 mg three times a day into the bladder (DasGupta and Fowler, 2002). Clinical trials are also under way to compare the efficacy of intravesical atropine with other anticholinergics. Early work has demonstrated that this increases bladder capacity and reduces detrusor overactivity in patients with MS (Deaney et al, 1998).

Tolterodine

Tolterodine is a relatively new antimuscarinic agent that was specifically developed for the treatment of the overactive bladder. It is more 'bladder selective' than oxybutynin (DasGupta and Fowler, 2002). Abrams et al (1998) reported the results of a phase III trial to compare the efficacy and safety of tolterodine with oxybutynin. This study showed that both tolterodine and oxybutynin were effective in reducing symptoms and that tolterodine was consistently better tolerated than oxybutynin.

Tolterodine 2 mg twice daily was shown to be as effective as oxybutynin but more tolerable, especially with regard to dry mouth side-effects. This allowed more patients to remain on effective therapy for their urinary symptoms of overactive bladder that negatively impact on quality of life (Abrams et al, 1998). Tolterodine is often recommended for the management of such symptoms in patients with MS.

Tricyclic antidepressants

Some tricyclic antidepressants, such as imipramine, amitriptyline and nortriptyline, also have antimuscarinic properties and can sometimes be a useful addition for patients who fail to respond to oxybutynin alone (DasGupta and Fowler, 2002).

Desmopressin

Desmopressin is an analogue of antidiuretic hormone and can be used to reduce daytime frequency and nocturia in patients who do not respond to anticholinergics alone (DasGupta and Fowler, 2002). It acts on the collecting tubules in the kidneys, promoting reabsorption of water and reduction of urine production. There are risks of hyponatraemia associated with this, thus serum sodium levels should be monitored (DasGupta and Fowler, 2002). Desmopressin may be taken at night to help with problems of nocturia and, if so, fluid intake in the evening should also be reduced (DasGupta and Fowler, 2003).

Capsaicin and other vanilloids

Capsaicin is an ingredient of red-hot chilli peppers and is one of a group of structures called vanilloids. It has been shown to increase bladder capacity and reduce hyperreflexia, as it is toxic to the neurones responsible for triggering detrusor activity, with effects lasting for 3–4 months (DasGupta and Fowler, 2002). It was never produced as a pharmaceutical preparation because of concerns over its pungency and systemic effects (DasGupta and Fowler, 2003) and it has been superceded by another of the vanilloids, resiniferatoxin. Initial studies are promising (Silva et al, 2000) and further trials are ongoing, but these treatments remain controversial (Leippold et al, 2003). There have also been some problems with administration because of its adsorption to plastic (DasGupta and Fowler, 2003).

Botulinum toxin

There are seven known distinct botulinum neurotoxins; however, only types A and B are available for clinical use (Dykstra et al, 2003). Botulinum-A toxin is a neuromuscular blocking agent that inhibits the release of acetylcholine and has been used to treat a range of neuromuscular disorders, such as dystonias, focal muscle spasm and spasticity (DasGupta and Fowler, 2002). It has more recently been used to treat neurogenic bladder problems in patients with MS and spinal-cord injury (Phelan et al, 2001; Leippold et al, 2003). The chemical denervation that results is reversible, with the effects lasting 3–6 months. Once the axons regrow the effects wear off, so repeated injections are necessary (Phelan et al, 2001).

Botulinum-A toxin has been used to treat patients with MS who have either detrusor–sphincter dyssynergia or emptying problems as a result of an acontractile bladder, and who wish to void using the Valsalva manoeuvre by injecting the toxin directly into the external urethral sphincter (Phelan et al, 2001). This enables patients to void successfully without the need for catheterization or a more irreversible solution, such as sphincterotomy. Botulinum-A toxin has also been used to treat overactive bladder symptoms by injection directly into the detrusor smooth muscle (Schurch et al, 2000; Leippold et al, 2003).

Botulinum-B toxin has been used recently for the treatment of detrusor hyperreflexia in a patient with MS (Dykstra et al, 2003). This B toxin has only been available for clinical use for 5 years and, as yet, little research has been undertaken into its use. The toxin in this case was injected into the bladder wall at 10 different points and a positive response was noted within 24 hours. The patient experienced no side-effects and the results of treatment lasted for 4 months (Dykstra et al, 2003).

Botulinum toxin is a promising therapy for patients with MS and emptying problems for whom CISC is not an option. It may also prove beneficial for patients who would otherwise be considering surgical procedures, such as enterocystoplasty or ileal conduit for long-term management of overactive detrusor symptoms. It must be considered, however, that this is an innovative therapy, and results from controlled or long-term follow-up studies have yet to be published, although some are under way (Leippold et al, 2003).

Cannabis-based preparations

There have been many anecdotal reports of patients with MS receiving symptomatic relief after taking cannabis (Consroe et al, 1997), and clinical trials are now under way to test the efficacy of cannabis plant extracts. It has only become possible to undertake clinical research into the effects of cannabis with the recent development of standardized whole-plant cannabis medicinal extracts, and research design is still limited because of various legal considerations (Wade et al, 2003).

The mechanism of action is not clearly understood; however, preliminary studies have shown promising benefits in patients with MS (DasGupta and Fowler, 2003). In one recent study, most patients had the drug administered through a sublingual route and they reported benefits with symptoms of bladder and bowel control, among others (Wade et al, 2003). However, Wade et al also reported that the dose needed to be titrated carefully and introduced gradually to avoid intoxication, which patients disliked.

Further research in this area appears warranted.

Surgical interventions

It has already been highlighted that the most common bladder problems experienced by MS patients are owing to hyperreflexia caused by spinal pathology. In patients whose problems are not successfully treated with anticholinergics and more conservative management, such as CISC or catheterization, surgery is often the next option and includes procedures such as augmentation ileocystoplasty and various urinary diversions such as ileal conduit (Ruud Bosch and Groen, 1996), external sphincterotomy or ileovesicostomy (Gudziak et al, 1999). Surgical procedures are always a last resort and in the main are irreversible (Chartier-Kastler et al, 2000). More innovative and less drastic therapies, such as sacral nerve stimulation, are also gaining in popularity (Ruud Bosch and Groen, 1996; Chartier-Kastler et al, 2000).

The guiding principle of intervention is to maintain low bladder storage pressures, which protect the upper urinary tract from reflux-associated problems such as hydronephrosis, upper urinary tract infection and stone formation, all of which could effect renal function (Gudziak et al, 1999). Transurethral external sphincterotomy is an option and ensures the bladder empties with low pressure, but results in total loss of continence. As such, it is useful for male patients, but not for females as no suitable urine collection device is available (Gudziak et al, 1999).

External sphincterotomy and use of urinary sheaths has also been associated with urinary tract infection, poor urine drainage and skin problems (Perkash, 1993). Ileal conduit is a surgical procedure in which an isolated segment of ileum serves as a replacement for the bladder. The ureters are then implanted into this tubular section of bowel and the normal flow of urine is diverted to drain via a stoma that is created in the abdominal wall. Ileal conduit is not always a good long-term solution and has been associated with high rates of pyelonephritis, renal scarring and stone formation (Gudziak et al, 1999). A couple of the more promising surgical options will now be considered in more detail.

Sacral nerve stimulation

Sacral nerve stimulation involves the implantation of a permanent electrode attached to the third sacral nerve root (S3) and generator placed subcutaneously in the abdomen, following extensive percutaneous testing (Ruud Bosch and Groen, 1996). This pilot study demonstrated that treatment of refractory urge incontinence was possible by S3 sacral spinal nerve stimulation in selected MS patients as it was possible to stimulate spinal inhibitory systems that were capable of interrupting a detrusor contraction (Ruud Bosch and Groen, 1996). Long-term studies were conducted over 5 years, and again both clinical and urodynamic improvement were reported after stimulator activation (Chartier-Kastler et al, 2000).

Early work in this area has shown positive benefits for patients with MS, with low complication rates and durable urodynamic and clinical effects (Ruud Bosch and Groen, 1996; Chartier-Kastler et al, 2000). This therapy is non-destructive and does not compromise future treatment options; however, to date its use has only been reported in a small number of patients with MS (mostly female), and it remains to be seen whether this will be a long-term solution, considering the progressive nature of the disease.

More recently, posterior tibial nerve stimulation has also been used to treat chronic urge incontinence and urinary frequency with a statistically significant decrease in incontinence and urinary frequency being reported (Govier et al, 2001; van Balken et al, 2001), but research in this area remains limited. One such study was reported by Amarenco et al (2003), which included 13 patients with MS in the sample. Stimulation was achieved using a self-adhesive surface electrode on the skin overlying the posterior tibial nerve. The authors found that during stimulation there was significant improvement in bladder capacity, although there were also many failures, and this is a therapy where further research is warranted.

Ileovesicostomy

Ileovesicostomy has successfully been performed for patients with MS and neurogenic bladder-emptying problems (Gudziak et al, 1999). This procedure, unlike formation of an ileal conduit, avoids removal of the bladder and, therefore, has significantly less bleeding, sexual dysfunction and ureteral stricture formation (Atan et al, 1999). This procedure is also reversible in cases of neurological recovery, although this is a lesser consideration in patients with MS, for whom this is unlikely.

During this procedure 10–12 cm ileum is removed and the two ends of the bowel are anastamosed (Atan et al, 1999). The segment of ileum should be long enough to join the top of the bladder to the abdominal wall. The bladder is then freed from its attachments to the pelvic wall and a U-shaped flap is opened into the dome of the bladder. Part of the ileal segment is opened and anastamosed to the flap from the bladder. The other end of the ileal segment is kept as a tube and brought out to form a stoma on the abdominal wall.

Some postoperative complications have been reported, such as stomal stenosis, wound infection and paralytic ileus (Gudziak et al, 1999). However, it has been reported that this is a safe and effective method of bladder drainage in patients with neurogenic bladder dysfunction and emptying symptoms (Atan et al, 1999; Gudziak et al, 1999).

Conclusion

This chapter has reviewed current treatment options for the management of neurogenic bladder symptoms in patients suffering from MS. It is important that nurses working with MS patients remain up to date with current innovations and developments in this area as patients are becoming increasingly expert about their disease and questioning about treatment options. This will enable nurses and patients to work in partnership to manage symptoms effectively based on informed decision-making and, therefore, to optimize the patient's quality of life.

While this review has focused on the management of neurogenic bladder symptoms, nurses also need to consider that bladder problems may not necessarily be the result of the MS disease process. Incontinence can result from other pathological processes that may occur coincidentally alongside MS, and thorough assessment is required in order to rule out other types of incontinence such as genuine stress incontinence.

References

Abrams P, Freeman R, Anderstrom C, Mattiasson A (1998) Tolterodine, a new antimuscarinic agent: as effective but better tolerated than oxybutynin in patients with an overactive bladder. *Br J Urol* **81:** 801–10

Amarenco G, Sheik Ismael S, Even-Schneider A et al (2003) Urodynamic effect of acute transcutaneous posterior tibial nerve stimulation in overactive bladder. *J Urol* **169:** 2210–15

Anders K (1999) Bladder retraining. *Prof Nurse* **14:** 334–6

Araki I, Matsui M, Ozawa K, Takeda M, Kuno S (2003) Relationship of bladder dysfunction to lesion site in multiple sclerosis. *J Urol* **169:** 1384–7

Atan A, Konety BR, Nangia A, Chancellor MB (1999) Advantages and risks of ileovesicostomy for the management of the neuropathic bladder. *Urology* **54:** 636–40

Bates P, Bradley WE, Glen E, Griffiths D (1977) Standardization of terminology of lower urinary tract function. *Urology* **9:** 237–41

Bennett N, O'Leary M, Patel AS, Xavier M, Erikson JR, Chancellor MB (2004) Can higher doses of oxybutynin improve efficacy in neurogenic bladder? *J Urol* **171:** 749–51

Birns J, Lukkari E, Malone-Lee JG (2000) A randomized controlled trial comparing the efficacy of controlled-release oxybutynin tablets (10 mg once daily) with conventional oxybutynin tablets (5 mg twice daily) in patients whose symptoms were stabilized on 5 mg daily of oxybutynin. *Br J Urol Int* **85:** 793–8

Calabresi PA (2002) Considerations in the treatment of relapsing–remitting multiple sclerosis. *Neurology* **58**(Suppl 4): S10–S22

Canadian Burden of Illness Study Group (1998) Burden of illness in multiple sclerosis: part II. Quality of life. *Can J Neurol Sci* **25:** 31–8

Chartier-Kastler EJ, Ruud Bosch JLH, Perrigot M, Chancellor MB, Richard F, Denys P (2000) Long-term results of sacral nerve stimulation (S3) for the treatment of neurogenic refractory urge incontinence related to detrusor hyperreflexia. *J Urol* **164:** 1476–80

Ciancio Sj, Mutchnik SE, Rivera VM, Boone TB (2001) Urodynamic pattern changes in multiple sclerosis. *Urology* **57:** 239–45

Clanet MG, Brassat D (2000) The management of multiple sclerosis patients. *Curr Opin Neurol* **13:** 263–70

Consroe P, Musty R, Rein J, Tillery W, Pertwee R (1997) The perceived effects of smoked cannabis on patients with multiple sclerosis. *Eur Neurol* **38:** 44–8

DasGupta R, Fowler CJ (2002) Sexual and urological dysfunction in multiple sclerosis: better understanding and improved therapies. *Curr Opin Neurol* **15:** 271–8

DasGupta R, Fowler CJ (2003) Bladder, bowel and sexual dysfunction in multiple sclerosis. *Drugs* **63**(2): 153–66

DasGupta P, Haslam C, Goodwin R, Fowler CJ (1997) The 'Queen Square bladder stimulator': a device for assisting emptying of the neurogenic bladder. *Br J Urol* **80:** 234–7

Deaney C, Glickman S, Gluck T, Malone-Lee J (1998) Intravesical atropine suppression of detrusor hyperreflexia in multiple sclerosis. *J Neurol Neurosurg Psych* **65:** 957–8

Dykstra DD, Pryor J, Goldish G (2003) Use of botulinum toxin type B for the treatment of detrusor hyperreflexia in a patient with multiple sclerosis: a case report. *Arch Phys Med Rehabil* **84:** 1399–400

Getliffe K, Dolman M (1997) *Promoting Continence: a Clinical Research Resource*. Baillière Tindall, London

Gleason DM, Susset, J, White C, Munoz DR, Sand PK (1999) Evaluation of a new once-daily formulation of oxybutynin for the treatment of urinary urge incontinence. *Urology* **54:** 420–3

Govier FE, Litwiller S, Nitti V, Kreder KJ, Rosenblatt P (2001) Percutaneous afferent neuromodulation for the refractory overactive bladder: results of a multicentre study. *J Urol* **165:** 1193–8

Gudziak MR, Tiguert R, Puri K, Gheiler EL, Triest JA (1999) Management of neurogenic bladder dysfunction with incontinent ileovesicostomy. *Urology* **54:** 1008–11

Hextall A, Boos K, Cardozo L, Allen K (1998) The 'Queen Square' bladder stimulator. *Br J Urol* **81:** 178–83

Hinson JL, Boone TB (1996) Urodynamics and multiple sclerosis. *Urol Clin North Am* **23:** 475–81

Koldewijn EL, Hommes OR, Lemmens WAJG, Debruyne FMJ, Van Kerrebroeck PEV (1995) Relationship between lower urinary tract abnormalities and disease-related parameters in multiple sclerosis. *J Urol* **154:** 169–73

Lapides J, Diolmo C, Silber SJ, Lowe BS (1972) Clean intermittent self-catheterization in the treatment of urinary tract disease. *J Urol* **107:** 458–61

Leippold T, Reitz A, Schurch B (2003) Botulinum toxin as a new therapy option for voiding disorders: current state of the art. *Eur Urol* **44:** 165–74

Perkash I (1993) Long-term urologic management of the patient with spinal cord injury. *Urol Clin North Am* **20:** 423–34

Phelan MW, Franks M, Somogyi GT et al (2001) Botulinum toxin urethral sphincter injection to restore bladder emptying in men and women with voiding dysfunction. *J Urol* **165:** 1107–10

Prasad RS, Smith SJ, Wright H (2003) Lower abdominal pressure versus external bladder stimulation to aid bladder emptying in multiple sclerosis: a randomized controlled trial. *Clin Rehabil* **17:** 42–7

Ruud Bosch JLH, Groen J (1996) Treatment of refractory urge incontinence with sacral spinal nerve stimulation in multiple sclerosis patients. *Lancet* **348:** 717–19

Schurch B, Schmid DM, Stohrer M (2000) Treatment of neurogenic incontinence with botulinum toxin A. *N Engl J Med* **342:** 665

Scientific Committee of the First International Consultation on Incontinence (2000) Consensus: assessment and treatment of urinary incontinence. *Lancet* **355:** 2153–8

Silva C, Rio ME, Cruz, F (2000) Desensitization of bladder sensory fibres by intravesical resiniferatoxin, a capsaicin analogue: long-term results for the treatment of detrusor hyperreflexia. *Eur Urol* **38:** 444–52

van Balken MR, Vandoninck V, Gisolf KWH et al (2001) Posterior tibial nerve stimulation as neuromodulative treatment of lower urinary tract dysfunction. *J Urol* **166:** 914–18

Wade DT, Robson P, House H, Makela P, Aram J (2003) A preliminary controlled study to determine whether whole-plant cannabis extracts can improve intractable neurogenic symptoms. *Clin Rehabil* **17:** 21–9

Weiss BD (1998) Diagnostic evaluation of urinary incontinence in geriatric patients. *Am Fam Physician* **57**: 2675–90

Woodward S (1995) Assessment of urinary incontinence in neuroscience patients. *Br J Nurs* **4:** 254–8

Woodward S (1996) Impact of neurological problems on urinary continence. *Br J Nurs* **5:** 906–13

Woodward S, Rew M (2003) Patients' quality of life and clean intermittent self-catheterization. *Br J Nurs* **12:** 1066–74

Using action research to develop a responsive service for patients with multiple sclerosis in relapse

Richard Warner, Del Thomas, Roswell Martin

This chapter describes our experience of using action research to develop services for patients with multiple sclerosis (MS). The issue of relapse became important in the UK, in part because of the instigation of the Department of Health (2002) risk sharing scheme. This scheme provided a mechanism for the NHS to prescribe disease-modifying treatments to people with MS. These treatments are effective in reducing the rate of relapses. The Department of Health (2002) adopted the Association of British Neurologists' guidelines for identifying patients who were thought to benefit from this form of treatment. A major feature of this process is to identify people who have had at least two relapses within the preceding two year period. Clinical evaluation again looks to whether the patient is continuing to experience relapse. Like other neurology teams throughout the UK we felt a responsibility to people with MS, who used our service, to ensure that they had access to these treatments. The identification and treatment of relapse needed to become more systematic.

MS is a chronic disease of the central nervous system. Approximately 80% of people with this condition will experience relapses or attacks of symptoms, followed by periods of relative stability or remission (Williams, 2004). The conventionally accepted treatment for such an attack is pharmacological, with corticosteroids given by intravenous infusion over 3–5 days (National Institute for Clinical Excellence (NICE), 2003; Filippini et al, 2004). There is a growing body of evidence that suggests that such treatments should also be combined with access to a team of health professionals with knowledge about MS (Craig et al, 2003).

It is unclear whether certain models of service delivery are more effective than others (NICE, 2003). It remains unclear whether certain presenting features of relapse may respond to intervention more effectively than others. There is no clear evidence to suggest how quickly a person should receive treatment and therapy once symptoms develop (Miller et al, 2000). This raises certain challenges in determining how to evaluate the quality of service provision. The difficulty with an evidence base limited in this way is that it could lead to operational ambiguity in terms of how relapse is defined, and whether some types of relapse are treated and others not. Despite these limitations, the NICE guidance, *Multiple Sclerosis: Management in Primary and Secondary Care* (2003), suggests that people should receive treatment as soon as possible after the onset relapse that causes distressing symptoms or a limitation to normal activities. Clearly there is a responsibility to respond to this guidance and to maximize the effectiveness of the service for the benefit of the local people with MS.

The West Midlands MS Nurse Group has begun to address some of the issues associated with this by developing a benchmark for the provision of intravenous methylprednisolone (IVMP) (Embrey et al, 2003). In an attempt to apply this thinking and develop the relapse management service, we designed an action research study. This chapter describes this research study.

Action research

The various approaches of action research have been described, and it is not the purpose of this chapter to enter into a detailed debate over research design (Hart and Bond, 1995). This particular example of action research could be thought of as moving between the professionalizing and organizational typologies characterized by Hart and Bond (1995). Action research is often attributed with satisfying the ideals of cooperation, emancipation or participatory research practice (Morrow and Brown, 1994; Reason, 1988). Robson (2002) expands on this characterization by suggesting that action research not only adds the notion of change to the traditional research purpose of description, understanding and explanation, but also that change should be characterized by the ideas of improvement and involvement. So action research should improve practice in some observable way, and also improve the understanding of that practice by those involved and improve the context in which that practice occurs (Robson, 2002). Rolfe et al (2001) make the connection between this broader aim of action research and the idea of the reflective practitioner as espoused by Schon (1983). We have tried to incorporate some of these reflective notions of skill and knowledge acquisition into the educational aspects of the project to both nursing staff and people with MS in identifying relapse.

Application of action research methodology

Our specific interpretation and application of these key characteristics of action research is illustrated in *Figure 20.1*.

We have recognized the cyclic nature of action research, which attempts to balance periods of change with evaluation (Rolfe et al, 2001). The initial starting point for the project was to retrospectively audit the patient pathway into treatment. This audit was sufficient to identify certain key time markers in the pathway, such as outpatient appointment with neurologist and time to inpatient or day-case patient hospital attendance.

It was not possible to consistently establish the way in which patients accessed clinic appointments or the length of time they had been experiencing symptoms. Although it was possible to identify some examples of documented presentation and recovery from symptoms, again, this was not consistent. In this sense the audit revealed as much about the service by the lack of documented evidence as it did by presence of such recorded data. The findings from the initial audit are listed in *Table 20.1*.

This data was used to inform various discussions and to produce an action plan. This was presented to the hospital trust board in order to change service delivery (see *Figure 20.1*). This consultation process identified several concerns (*Table 20.2*).

An important consideration was that any service developments should not negatively impact on occupancy of acute neurological beds. The majority of inpatient cases seemed to be discharged quickly, suggesting relatively non-complex clinical management. Given the reality of the internal pressures on acute hospital beds, it was decided that by developing outpatient and day-case services this would safely meet the clinical needs of most of this patient group without compromising access to acute inpatient-based service, where appropriate.

The conclusions of this consultation process had numerous implications. The first obvious concern, recognized by the NICE guidelines, is the fact that there is no sound empirical evidence on which to understand whether prolonged time to treatment failed patients' chances to access a proven treatment that might enhance the speed of their recovery (NICE, 2003). We recognized that the converse of this also applied; there is no evidence to show that rapid treatment is more effective (and not harmful in some way), although this is offered as the preferred opinion (NICE, 2003).

A second concern was that if the service failed to systematically monitor frequency of relapse, we would not be in a position to proactively identify those individuals falling within the Association of British Neurologists guidelines for disease-modifying therapy.

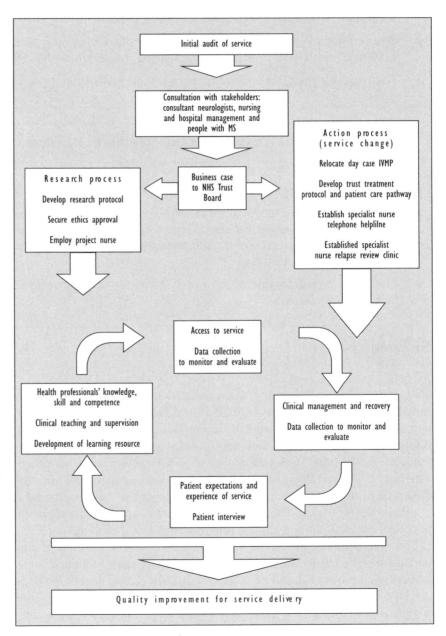

Figure 20.1: Action research project diagram

Table 20.1: Findings of initial audit

- 46 patients requiring treatment were identified over a 12-month period
- 33 patients were treated as day cases and 13 as inpatients
- Route of access to the service was unclear
- Mean time to day-case treatment from neurologist appointment was 24 days (range 4–64 days), with only five patients achieving treatment within 10 days
- Mean time to inpatient treatment from neurologist appointment was 34 days (range 1–88 days), with only four patients achieving treatment within 10 days
- The majority (62%) of inpatients were discharged within 1 week

Table 20.2: Concerns identified by the consultation process

- People with MS might be experiencing difficulty accessing the service in a timely manner
- If these time delays, which are experienced by the majority of patients, impact on the time window of effectiveness for steroids, this could have serious consequences for the therapeutic value of treatment and potentially adversely shift the risk–benefit ratio of high-dose steroid treatment
- The neurology department was not systematically monitoring post-treatment recovery and frequency of relapses

Service change

The current day-case service was provided in a haematology day-case setting. The service was moved, following board approval, to Ermin House, Gloucestershire. This clinical area is part of the neurology department but is off the main Gloucestershire Royal Hospital site. Ermin House provides NHS respite care to people with neurological conditions and has only ever required limited access to medical staff. In this sense the day-case IVMP service is, in all practical purposes, nurse managed. This move allowed neurology to establish a dedicated clinical area for the provision of this service. Research protocols were developed, ethical approval was sought and research grants were obtained.

A project nurse, Del Thomas (DT), was employed for the duration of the research study. Her role was to collect data and act as a clinical role model and mentor to the nursing staff. At the time of the project, DT worked both as a project nurse and as a sister within the clinical area. The lead researcher role was undertaken by Richard Warner (RW). The addition of a project nurse allowed the various clinical practice and research project roles to be more clearly defined and negotiated between the us.

Patients were encouraged to telephone the specialist nursing service if experiencing new symptoms suggestive of relapse. The nurse (RW) would take a history of symptoms. We recognize that at present patients' relapse should be confirmed by the presence of objective neurological signs identified by the individual patient's neurologist (Liu and Blumhardt, 1999). RW organized clinic appointments and scheduled treatment sessions. The neurologist would diagnose relapse and advise on the appropriate environment for treatment, i.e. day-case or inpatient. The patients were reviewed, following treatment, in a nurse-led clinic by DT. The project nurse administered methylprednisolone within the clinical area while nursing staff completed training and supervision.

We have audited the day-case service following the completion of the study. This showed that the clinic treated 100 patients within a 12-month period, compared with the treatment of 33 patients before the project. This represents a three-fold increase in treatment capacity while continuing to maintain the efficiencies in time to treatment created by the project.

Data collection

The project received ethical approval before proceeding to data collection (Department of Health, 2003). Evaluation of the project focused on four distinct areas (see *Figure 20.1*). These areas of data collection were informed by the benchmark for relapse management and the initial audit (Embrey et al, 2003). Data collection forms were designed as part of the research protocol. We collected specific demographic data as well as data that reflected time markers of the patient pathway to treatment and recovery. We also collected data to reflect the clinical condition and the patient experience of the day-case service. All nursing staff attended teaching sessions, received mentorship and training for cannulation and administration of IVMP. However, the educational aspects of the project were not formally evaluated.

Clinical recovery

To evaluate clinical recovery we used the UK Disability Scale and the MS Impact Scale (MSIS-29) (Sharrack and Hughes, 1999; Hobart et el, 2004). Both of these scales have been used in other studies involving relapsing MS (Craig et al, 2003). The experience of fatigue was recorded using the Fatigue Severity Scale (FSS) (Krupp et al, 1989). Also used was a single question telephone interview protocol. Participants were telephoned weekly from receiving IVMP until 6-week review, and asked 'Do you think you are still recovering'? Participants responded 'Yes', 'Not sure' or 'No'.

Patient experience and quality issues

A structured interview protocol was developed, based on Commission for Health Improvement questionnaires designed to test the satisfaction of relapsing patients with outpatient services. The interview covered various themes associated with service delivery. These included coordinated care, access and waiting, information and communication, relationships with healthcare professionals and the clinical environment.

Sampling and analysis

Although we have collected numerical data and used descriptive statistical techniques to present some data, they consider this a primarily qualitative form of research study. Given this, the general principles of qualitative data analysis of data reduction, data display, followed by conclusion drawing and verification have been used (Miles and Huberman, 1994). We considered the patient journey into, through and out of the service, as the boundaries around the 'case' of the relapse service (Miles and Huberman, 1994; Yin, 1994). Data collection points were identified to demonstrate this process. Flow diagrams were used as a method of data display for each case. Cases were purposively selected and recruited to the study as exemplars of service users (Miles and Huberman, 1994). Three main groups of service user were identified:

- Acute relapse
- Newly diagnosed
- Progressive.

These are established techniques of data management for case studies and it is recognized that such techniques are a useful model on which to base action research projects (Robson, 2002).

Issues associated with the application of the methodology

Although the project has clearly travelled through phases of audit, intervention, reflection and evaluation, it was initially anticipated that there would be three monthly episodes of action and evaluation punctuated by reflection (Hart and Bond, 1995). This did occur through limited meetings with key stakeholders and through teaching sessions, but in a more informal and flexible way than originally anticipated. This approach seemed to work well with the various personalities involved.

The lead researcher (RW) was aware of this so-called 'political aspect' of this type of action research study, and this led to a need to constantly negotiate a balance between the aspirations of quality improvement, central to the project, and the need to maintain the interest and involvement of individuals associated with the project (Coghlan and Brannick, 2001). In part, on a practical day-to-day basis, this was addressed by differentiating the various roles demanded by the project between the lead researcher and the project nurse. We felt that this also allowed people (including patients) participating in the project a clearer and perhaps more ethical understanding of the nature of their interaction with these individuals (Williamson and Prosser, 2002). Therefore, although the project maintained a broad collaborative emphasis because of the complexity and volume of the data, priority constantly had to be given, during evaluation, to time for treatment. This non-empirical and reflexive process is as essential to the validity of the study even if the data collection ambition was difficult to manage (Morrow and Brown, 1994).

Overall it is felt that the project gained from using a range of data collection points and techniques and that this, as well as cyclic reflexive management, is an essential feature of action research (Hart and Bond, 1995). In particular, it was felt that it was important to allow patients to voice their impressions of the service.

The majority of patient interviews were conducted by the project nurse and analyzed by the lead researcher. This structured approach seemed to adequately provide consistency across certain fields of questioning, but limited a more in-depth exploration of the emotional experience of waiting for hospital services while experiencing symptoms or uncertainty. The hope was to encourage the idea that the project nurse was removed from both the clinical and service operation of relapse management. This might allow patient participants to feel more relaxed in openly discussing the service that they were using. The success of this aspiration, and whether it is genuinely necessary or achievable, clearly echos the larger researcher–practitioner debate (Hart and Bond, 1995).

Findings

Access to service

We found that, in general, patients responded well to the nursing staff, which may be because the nurses were able to shorten the patients' time to treatment. Some key findings are that:

- Patients reported their symptoms to a nurse sooner (within 10 days of onset), compared with a mean reporting time of 51 days to their GP
- The nurse was able to organize a neurologist appointment in a mean of 6 days (GP 13.8 days) and for treatment to commence, from appointment, in a mean of 4.78 days (GP 5.16 days). Through the nurse route of access, at least 85% of patients were able to be treated within 10 days of reporting symptoms
- Day-case admission for IVMP had some impact on paid employment, both for the patients and for their friends/family who provided transport
- Specialist nurses were able to effectively organize and instigate, if appropriate, day-case admission for relapsing patients.

Distance travelled to the service varied enormously. The hospital is located within the largest conurbation of a diverse geographical area that includes a large expanse of rural areas with market towns. Unsurprisingly, attendance at the unit reflected the demographic spread of people throughout this area. Approximately 50% of people relied on others to provide transport. Some patients expressed concern regarding car parking availability and the distance from the car park to hospital units. Interestingly, there did not seem to be any clear pattern emerging between these grievances and distance travelled. Patients within the progressive group and those with motor relapses seemed to comment more. This was interpreted as reflecting the association between the presence of impaired walking ability and the physical demand of accessing transport and clinical areas.

The NICE guidelines, *Multiple Sclerosis: Management in Primary and Secondary Care* (2003), raise the question concerning the provision of inpatient, day-case care and home delivery of relapse services. NICE (2003) discusses evidence (or the lack of evidence) of these as distinct service models. NICE also recognize the difficulty that district general hospitals may have in delivering day-case services. In our experience at a district general hospital, the most difficult aspect of day-case delivery has been the coordination of the multidisciplinary team (MDT) (particularly physiotherapy) with the administration of steroids. If it is accepted that MDT involvement should commence with treatment, to move most of the service to a home-based delivery service would have considerable resource and operational implications in our rural geographical area.

Within the acute relapse group only half required physiotherapy intervention. It is possible that a specific subgroup of relapsing patient could be identified whose optimal recovery is exclusively based on steroid treatment rather than on steroid treatment and physiotherapy. If this is true then a limited home-based treatment model could be developed and implemented for those individuals, based on either oral or intravenous methylprednisolone. Rather than contriving inpatient, day-case and home delivery as distinct service models, it may be more appropriate for district general hospital neurology services to become more sophisticated in targeting mode of service delivery to patient subgroups.

Clinical recovery and management

We found that most patients perceive their recovery continuing for up to 4 weeks following administration of IVMP. This finding allows for a more detailed explanation of their recovery to be given to patients commencing steroid treatment. It also supports the notion that patients should be reviewed at 6 weeks following administration of IVMP, to review the progress of their recovery and the need for symptomatic treatments. The majority of patients experienced recovery from their relapse as measured by the MSIS-29 and UK Disability Scale.

In this series of patients, 48% required physiotherapy intervention, and then commenced with treatment of IVMP. Of these patients, 8% required specialist continence advice. These additional interventions by the multidisciplinary team were effectively organized by liaison between the specialist nurses and the day-case clinical staff.

Patient expectation and experience of service

Analysis of transcripts of patient interviews suggests that patients value:

- Contact with a specialist nurse during relapse
- A close working relationship between specialist nurses and the consultant neurologist
- Explanation of the nature of relapse
- The specialist nurses' ability to effectively organize appointments with consultant neurologists and treatment sessions
- Easy physical access to the clinical area where IVMP is provided
- Clinical staff who were knowledgeable and had the ability and time to discuss issues
- Treatment within 1 week of reporting symptoms.

Psychological stress

In response to the question 'What was your experience of waiting for clinic appointments when you felt your condition was changing?', most participants seemed initially puzzled by the question. With further

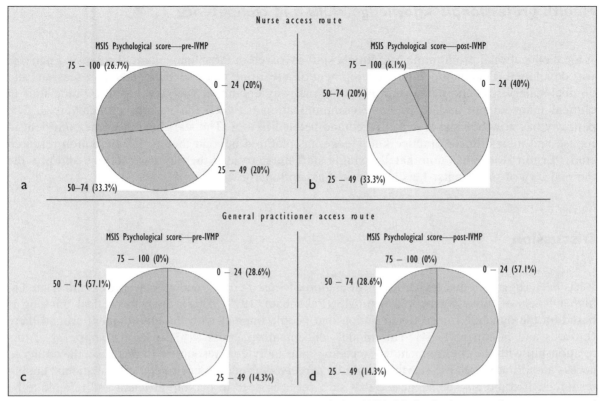

Figure 20.2 (a–d): Data for the psychological element of the MSIS-29 for both general practitioner and specialist nurse routes of access into the service for patients with acute relapse

prompting, relapsing and progressive patients associated the question with the time between contacts with the various services within the hospital. We were surprised by this finding. In this series of patients, only one who was newly diagnosed revealed any suggestion of coping characterized by heightened emotion during interview. In other words, all acute relapse patients did not associate waiting for appointments or treatments with distress. Although they may have distress, in relation to the presence of relapse symptoms, this system of access to treatment, from nurse or GP to neurologist, did not seem to exacerbate this.

Figures 20.2a–d present data for the psychological element of the MSIS-29 for both GP and specialist nurse routes of access into the service for patients with acute relapse. This data is of interest because, despite the route of access, most patients seem to benefit from a 30% reduction in the psychological impact of their MS following treatment for relapse. The patient profile for these two routes seems to be subtlety different.

The specialist nursing route seemed to attract a greater range of MSIS-29 psychological impact, with at least 25% of these patients in the range 75–100 (scale 0–100; higher scores indicate worse health). This high range was not present in the GP access group. Following treatment, this high range only accounted for 6.7% of the nurse access route, suggesting recovery. This pattern is further demonstrated by the consultant neurologist route to treatment. Although discouraged, some patients waited for routine follow-up appointments to report symptoms. Again, this high range of psychological impact was not present within this group.

Health professionals' knowledge, skills and competence

A local educational programme for clinical staff involved in the management of relapsing patients was developed. This included the development of a learning resource pack, teaching sessions and clinical supervision and mentoring. A patient pathway document was developed to guide staff in clinical management and to improve communication between the various clinical areas. The pathway has now become an established and bedded in tool. The staff have become confident in its use and their clinical practice knowledge has matured beyond the end of the action research study. Ermin House has nominated a single staff nurse to lead the day case service and provide the majority of treatments. This has worked exceptionally well.

Discussion

It has been suggested that higher levels of emotion-focused coping and greater distress are related to higher levels of threat for people with MS (Pakenham, 1999, 2001). Such theoretical thinking is based on the dynamic transactional notion that people interact with the environment around them (Lazarus and Folkman, 1984). This model conceptualizes stress as the person's appraisal of this relationship with the environment as exceeding their individual resources. In this case, the ability to access authoritative relapse services could be perceived as adding positively to the patients' coping resources. It could also be suggested that such services need to be both efficient and reliable to be conceptualized by the patient as part of their repertoire of realistic problem-focused coping strategies.

Relapses are understood to be stressful, and the NICE guidelines recommend treatment of relapses characterized by distressing symptoms (Baker, 1998; Kroencke and Denney, 1999; NICE, 2003). It should be noted that, theoretically at least, there is the suggestion that the construction of illness identity by the patient may well contribute or influence the way in which the person adjusts to living with MS (Foote et al, 1990; Wineman, 1990; Miller, 1993; Schwartz et al, 1999). Given this, it is suggested that there are aspects of service delivery that could contribute to aspects of the coping mechanism of people in relapse, and that there is a persuasive ethical argument that relapse services should be flexible enough to accommodate the range of coping responses that people with MS will experience. The question is, when designing services in this way, will there be a clinical difference in recovery and, more importantly, would this influence any longer term psychosocial adjustment of this patient group?

It seems reasonable to suggest that access to treatment, irrespective of route, is dependent on the practitioner's clinical ability to accurately identify a relapse. This is of particular importance to nursing, as 55% of our series of patients chose this route of access into treatment.

During the project there was an attempt to introduce a Patient Group Directive (PGD) to allow the nurse (RW) to initiate treatment. This was rejected by the hospital trust on an interpretation of PGD as being designed for singular one-off events. Although it seems reasonable to expect specialist nurses to be able to effectively identify patients in relapse, there is no evidence, that we are aware of, to support this claim. This expectation is clearly different from a nurse going on to initiate treatment. Both of these situations raise questions about the clinical preparation and supervision of specialist nurses to be able to competently identify relapse, grade relapse severity and initiate treatment within the context of adverse affects associated with steroids. If it is practical and desirable to enable nurses to advance their practice in this manner, this may result in improved access to treatment for patients in relapse.

Conclusion

We found that a nurse working at an advanced level can develop specialist practice, which significantly contributes to the effective clinical management of patients with relapsing MS. Additionally, patients with a relapse of MS expect and value an effective and efficient response to the reporting of the onset of symptoms, such as the nurses were able to provide. This study has demonstrated that most relapsing patients can be successfully identified, treated with IVMP and have appropriate MDT intervention through a day-case system, with patients reporting continuing recovery from relapse for up to 4 weeks following steroid treatment.

It is suggested that, to attain these results, relapsing patients may require access to specialist nurses through a telephone helpline. These specialist nurses need a close working relationship with a consultant neurologist, who needs to offer clinic time to relapsing patients in a responsive manner. It was also found that there needs to be a dedicated clinical area to provide day-case service, where staff are supported by the specialist nurse and have received education and clinical supervision and access to the physiotherapy service to facilitate recovery.

This study raises questions regarding the ability of nurses, working within this area of specialist practice, to be able to safely and accurately identify people who are in relapse. This requires the nurse to exercise an advanced level of clinical judgment. They need to be able to effectively communicate with their patients to build a reliable clinical history of the relapse experience. However, the question of how nurses exercise and learn this clinical skill requires further study. We would also suggest that the psychological impact of service design should also be investigated more thoroughly to determine whether this impacts on acute recovery or longer term adjustment to illness.

This chapter was runner up in the Multiple Sclerosis category at the 2005 British Journal of Nursing *Clinical Practice Awards.*

References

Baker LM (1998) Sense making in multiple sclerosis: the information needs of people during an acute exacerbation. *Qual Health Res* **8**(1): 106–20

Coghlan D, Brannick T (2001) *Doing Action Research in Your Own Organisation*. Sage, London.

Craig J, Young CA, Ennis M, Baker G, Boggild M (2003) A randomized controlled trial comparing rehabilitation against standard therapy in multiple sclerosis patients receiving intravenous steroid treatment. *J Neurol Neurosurg Psych* **74**: 1225–30

Department of Health (2002) *HSC 2002/004. Cost-effective Provision of Disease Modifying Therapies for People with Multiple Sclerosis*. Department of Health, London.

Department of Health (2003) *Research Governance Framework from Health and Social Care*. Department of Health, London

Embrey N, Lowndes C, Warner R (2003) Benchmarking for best practice in relapse management of multiple sclerosis. *Nurs Stand* **17**(22): 38–42

Filippini G, Brusaferri F, Sibley WA et al (2004) Corticosteroids or ACTH for the acute exacerbation in multiple sclerosis (Cochrane Review). In *Cochrane Library*. Issue 1. John Wiley and Sons, Chichester

Foote AW, Piazza D, Holcombe J, Paul P, Daffin P (1990) Hope, self esteem and social support in persons with multiple sclerosis. *J Neurosci Nurs* **22**(3): 155–9

Hart E, Bond M (1995) *Action Research for Health and Social Care*. Open University Press, Buckingham

Hobart JC, Riazi A, Lamping DL, Fitzpatrick R, Thompson AJ (2004) Improving the evaluation of therapeutic interventions in multiple sclerosis: development of a patient-based measure of outcome. *Health Technol Assess* **8**(9): 1–48

Kroencke DC, Denney DR (1999) Stress and coping in multiple sclerosis: exacerbation, remission and chronic subgroups. *Mul Scler* **5**: 89–93

Krupp LB, LaRocca NG, Muir-Nash J, Steinberg AD (1989) The fatigue severity scale: application to patients with multiple sclerosis and systemic lupus erythematosus. *Arch Neruol* **46**(10): 1121–3

Lazarus RS, Folkman S (1984) *Stress, Appraisal and Coping*. Springer, New York

Liu C, Blumhardt LD (1999) Assessing relapses in treatment trials of relapsing and remitting multiple sclerosis; can we do better? *Mult Scler* **5**: 22–8

Miles MB, Huberman AM (1994) *Qualitative Data Analysis: An Expanded Sourcebook*. 2nd edn. SAGE Publications, California

Miller CM (1993) Trajectory and empowerment theory applied to care of patients with multiple sclerosis. *J Neurosci Nurs* **25**(6): 343–8

Miller DM, Weinstock-Guttman B, Bethoux F et al (2000) A meta-analysis of methylprednisolone in recovery from multiple sclerosis exacerbations. *Mult Scler* **6**: 267–73

Morrow R, Brown DD (1994) *Critical Theory and Methodology*. SAGE Publications, California

National Institute for Clinical Excellence (2003) *Multiple Sclerosis: Management in Primary and Secondary Care*. The National Collaborating Centre for Chronic Conditions, London

Pakenham KI (1999) Adjustment to multiple sclerosis: application of a stress and coping model. *Health Psychol* **18**(4): 383–92

Pakenham KI (2001) Application of a stress and coping model to caregiving in multiple sclerosis. *Psychol Health Med* **6**(1): 13–27

Reason P (ed) (1988) *Human Inquiry: A Sourcebook of New Paradigm Research*. SAGE Publications, London

Robson C (2002) *Real World Research: A Resource for Social Scientists and Practitioner-Researchers*. 2nd edn. Blackwell Publishers, Oxford

Rolfe G, Freshwater D, Jasper M (2001) *Critical Reflection for Nursing and the Helping Professions: A Users Guide*. Palgrave, Hampshire

Schon D (1983) *The Reflective Practitioner*. Temple Smith, London

Schwartz CE, Foley FW, Rao SM, Bernardin LJ, Lee H, Genderson MW (1999) Stress and course of disease in multiple sclerosis. *Behav Med* **25**(3): 110–16

Sharrack B, Hughes RAC (1999) The guy's Neurological Disability Scale – a new disability scale for MS. *Mult Scler* **5**: 223–33

Williams G (2004) Management of patients who have relapses in multiple sclerosis. *Br J Nurs* **13**(17): 1012–6

Williamson GR, Prosser S (2002) Illustrating the ethical dimensions of action research. *Nurse Res* **10**(2): 38–49

Wineman NM (1990) Adaptation to multiple sclerosis: the role of social support, functional disability and perceived uncertainty. *Nurs Res* **39**(5): 294–9

Yin RK (1994) *Case Study Research: Designs and Methods*. Sage Publications, CA

Innovative ways of responding to the information needs of people with multiple sclerosis

Rhona MacLean, Andrew Russell

Multiple sclerosis (MS) is a chronic, progressive disease of the central nervous system that typically presents in early adulthood. While it is an autoimmune disease that occurs in a genetically susceptible person, the 'trigger' that causes MS to develop in the individual is, as yet, unknown (Compston and Coles, 2002).

The early disease process is characterized by periods of inflammation within the central nervous system, causing demyelination of the axons (*Figure 21.1*). As the disease progresses, there can be axonal loss. In the early stages of the disease remyelination can occur. Although the individual may perceive that full recovery has taken place, there may be a delay in nerve conduction when tested (McDonald and Ron, 1999).

At some point, for an unknown reason, the inflammatory process stops and gliosis occurs, with sclerotic

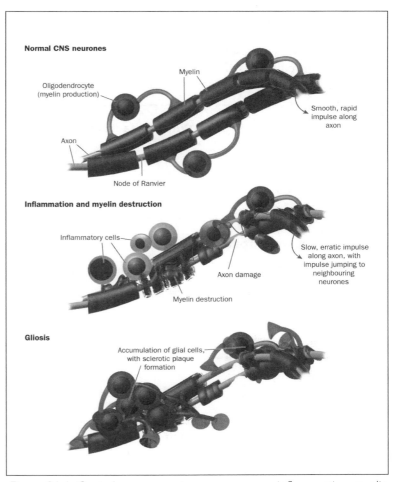

Figure 21.1: Central nervous system neurones — inflammation, myelin destruction and gliosis

plaque formation. Over a period of time, the individual fails to make a complete recovery from the attacks and will be left with residual difficulties. The disease becomes more progressive and the individual accumulates more difficulties (Compston and Coles, 2002).

The rate of progression is variable, with some individuals having little or no disability many years after diagnosis, while others having a progressive disease pattern from the onset (McDonald and Ron, 1999). Approximately 80% of people diagnosed will start with a relapsing-remitting form of MS (Compston and Coles, 2002). A proportion of this group will have a benign disease pattern, with limited difficulties. There will also be a proportion of the relapsing-remitting group who will have an aggressive disease pattern with resulting difficulties within a short space of time (Compston and Coles, 2002).

Approximately 50% of the people who start with a relapsing-remitting disease pattern will enter a secondary progressive phase within 10 years (Thompson, 2003). Some of this group will continue to have relapses, but all will have ongoing progression and accumulation of difficulties over a period of time. Up to 20% of people diagnosed with MS will have progressive disease from the onset (Compston and Coles, 2002).

When an individual is diagnosed with MS, it is not always possible to predict accurately what type of MS the individual has, or the course that the disease will take. Natural history studies point to factors that may be used as prognostic indicators (*Table 21.1*) (Ebers, 1999). However, as MS is such an unpredictable disease, these are not always reliable (Burgess, 2002).

Table 21.1: Summary of prognostic factors in multiple sclerosis

Better	Worse
Female	Male
Onset: monosymptomatic; sensory/optic neuritis	Onset: polysymptomatic; motor disturbance
Complete recovery from attacks	Incomplete recovery from attacks
Long time between attacks	Short time between attacks
Low number of attacks in early years	High number of attacks in early years
Younger age	Older age

Adapted from Ebers (1999)

The prevalence of MS in the UK is between 100–120 per 100 000 of the population. This means that there are between 52 000–62 000 people with MS in England and Wales (National Institute for Clinical Excellence (NICE), 2003), or a total of 85 000 for the whole of the UK (MS Society, 2004; MS Trust, 2004). MS is the largest cause of neurological disability in young adults, and all these people have to live with the variability and uncertainty of MS on a day-to-day basis (UK MS Specialist Nurse Association (UKMSSNA) et al, 2001).

Role of the MS nurse

The role of the MS specialist nurse has been described by the UKMSSNA as to:

> '...*empower those affected by MS by providing information, support and advice about the condition from the time of diagnosis and throughout the disease spectrum. The MS specialist nurse is pivotal in providing a greater understanding of the condition and, by adopting a holistic, collaborative and coordinated approach, can help those individuals, where possible, reach their goals of self-management. The role also involves acting as a consultant and educational resource for staff striving towards greater awareness and knowledge of MS in the health and social arena.*'

Over the past decade, there has been a rapid increase in the number of MS nurses in the UK. The figure is currently in the region of 180, which is still far short of the 300 estimated to be needed (Jones, 2004). There has been a lot of interest in the development and working practices of MS nurses, with a number of published studies evaluating the role of the MS nurse (Kirker et al, 1995; Campion, 1996; De Broe et al, 2001; Johnson et al, 2001).

Educational needs of MS nurses

Both the education needs of MS nurses and the information/education initiatives for people with MS and their significant others, which are provided by the MS nurses, have been highlighted in the above mentioned studies, in varying degrees.

The UKMSSNA document, *The Key Elements for Developing MS Specialist Nurse Services in the UK* (2001), also highlights the need for continuing professional development, education, clinical supervision and peer support for MS nurses to enable them to develop, work effectively and facilitate improvements in clinical practice.

Developments in education and support for MS nursing have improved as a result of all this research. MS nurses who are newly appointed are encouraged to attend a residential development module in MS, accredited to Leeds Metropolitan University.

Throughout the UK, MS nurses meet in regional groups for peer support, supervision and to participate in educational programmes. This has been shown to improve the practice of MS nurses through bench-marking and networking (Ward et al, 2002; Embrey et al, 2003). The UKMSSNA has also done much to advance the role and profile of MS nurses, working with the MS Society, the MS Trust, the RCN, the Association of British Neurologists and members of the pharmaceutical industry in producing publications and other supportive items (*Table 21.2*). The information and education needs of MS nurses are very much at the forefront of this work. Both education and support are needed for practice development, which in turn relies on evidence-based practice (Joyce, 1999).

Table 21.2: Publications/supportive items by the UK MS Specialist Nurse Association (UKMSSNA) and other organizations

UKMSSNA, RCN, MS Research Trust	2001	*The Key Elements for Developing MS Specialist Nurse Services in the UK.* MS Research Trust, Letchworth
UKMSSNA, RCN, MS Trust	2003	*Competencies for MS Specialist Nurses.* MS Trust, Letchworth
UKMSSNA and Serono Symposia International	2003	*The United Kingdom Multiple Sclerosis Clinical Management Manual: Care Across the Disease Trajectory.* UKMSSNA and Serono Symposia International (place of publication unknown)
MS Society, UKMSSNA, NHNN, ABN	2004	*Helping You Explain MS: A Teaching Resource for Healthcare Professionals.* MS Society, London
UKMSSNA and Teva Aventis	2004	Slide library for UKMSSNA members

Information/education needs of people with MS

In 1998, a health needs assessment was conducted on people with MS living in Leeds (Ford et al, 2000). The needs and views of service users were obtained through the use of focus groups and interviews. This research highlighted a need for information that was available when the user wanted it. A resource file on services available in the Leeds area has resulted from this (currently in print). A second need identified in this research was for increased MS nurse support, and this has been actioned with the appointment of two more nurses.

Two further areas of need that were identified were social worker support and the need for a link worker/helpline nurse (with extensive knowledge of MS). The appointment of a specialist MS social worker, who is based in the community but has extensive links with the specialist MS team in the hospital, has helped to bridge that gap in service provision. Regular meetings of a steering group, which includes service users, ensures that this service continues to meet the users' needs. Close liaison and inter-team collaboration and referral have resulted in close links between health and social services being developed and maintained. This is an excellent example of the multidisciplinary and interdisciplinary working discussed in *The National Service Framework (NSF) for Long-term Conditions* (Department of Health (DoH), 2005), as well as the recommendation regarding good communication between health and social services (NICE, 2003).

The neuroscience department in York has supported a social worker post for 8 years. Until recently, the post-holder did not have formal links with the local social services department. This created various problems, including difficulties liaising with the social services departments and issues concerning the support, management and supervision needs of the post-holder. As these issues became more evident, a complete review of the job structure was undertaken. Although the post was to be a generic neurology post, there was a move towards developing the post along similar lines to that of the MS social worker within the Leeds team. Networking with the post-holder in Leeds gave insight into how the post facilitated good links between health and social services. The publication of the NICE guidelines for MS, *Multiple Sclerosis: Management in Primary and Secondary Care* (2003), also added impetus to the development of the post, as the need for the post-holder to have some dedicated time to work within the MS service was recognized. The post was set up, with the current post-holder working as an integrated member of both the neuroscience team and social services.

Partly as a result of the research by Ford et al (2000), a clinic was set up in the rehabilitation unit where people with MS could self-refer to the MS nurse for information, symptom management and advice. This was to make a more effective use of the MS nurse's time, plus enable people with MS (who did not attend the specialist MS clinic) to have access to the MS nurse. This type of service was suggested as an effective way of meeting the needs of people with MS in research carried out by the MS Society (Robinson et al, 1996). Unfortunately, to date, in Leeds this clinic has not been well attended. This could partly be a result of the fact that possible service users have specific needs and are not aware that the clinic could meet their needs. Therefore, a further attempt to advertise and promote the service has been carried out, detailing possible reasons why people might want to attend. A new leaflet about the clinic has been created and includes this information. Currently, an audit is being undertaken to ascertain whether or not to continue with this service.

The MS service in York identified a possible need for people to have access to an MS nurse outside of the department's normal working hours. This perceived need stemmed from the observations that some people attending nurse-led clinics had problems being released from work, childcare was an issue or they wished to attend with a partner or friend who had difficulty taking time from work. A provisional plan was arranged to provide a nurse-led evening clinic between 6–9 pm one evening a month. Appointment within these clinics would be arranged at the request of the service user.

Before the clinics were set up, a questionnaire was distributed to 50 people who attended the MS clinic. The questions were designed to ascertain whether or not the 'out-of-hours' clinic would be used. Over 70% of the respondents suggested that they would not access the MS nurse clinic on an evening despite experiencing some of the difficulties attending during the day. There were comments from several people, suggesting that to attend in an evening would encroach on their own 'home' time, and they preferred not to do this. As the result, the clinic was not instigated.

There appears to be a difference between how professionals and people with MS view information giving. For people with MS, information has to be seen in a personal perspective, not just as an educational activity, replacing 'correct' or evidence-based information for 'incorrect' or non-evidence-based facts. It has to be appropriate to the individual (Robinson et al, 1996; Ford et al, 2000; Hepworth et al, 2002). The NSF (DoH, 2005) recognizes the importance for people to have the information they need, to enable them to make informed decisions about their care and disease management.

People with MS access information from a variety of sources, and there is a need for a 'one-stop' point where all the information can be obtained (Robinson et al, 1996; Hepworth et al, 2002). The NSF (DoH, 2005) states that:

'Information works best when it is in a range of different formats for people with long-term neurological conditions and their carers.'

Advances in technology are changing the way health care and information are being provided, as well as benefiting health professionals (DoH, 1999) and service users/patients (McIver and Brocklehurst, 1999; Powell et al, 2003).

Alternatives to leaflets to meet the educational needs of people with MS

One of the main roles of the MS nurse is to provide education to people with MS, their significant others and to other health and social-care professionals. While doing this, MS nurses work to empower people with MS, encouraging them to participate in planning and decision-making, enabling them to take control of their own lives and not to be controlled by others (Porter, 2001; UKMSSNA et al, 2001). One of the recommendations in the DoH's White Paper, *The Expert Patient* (2001), is to:

'*...promote awareness and create an expectation that patient expertise is a central component in the delivery of care to people with chronic disease.*'

There is also a recommendation in the NICE guidelines (2003) for MS that:

'*People with MS should be enabled to play an active part in making informed decisions in all aspects of their MS health care by being given relevant and accurate information about each choice and decision.*'

As well as involving service users in the development of services, much can be learnt from different centres and colleagues around the country. The cities of York and Leeds are only 20 miles apart, and there is a history of close collaboration and networking between staff in the two hospitals and university sites. This has enabled the MS nurses to develop joint working initiatives and peer group support systems.

Neuro Education is a non-profit-making organization that aims to provide education and information to people with neurological conditions and also to those who may be involved in the care and support of people with neurological conditions. The education and information is provided in many different settings and via different media (www.neuroeducation.org.uk).

A Neuro Education system to provide internet-based information about neurological conditions is currently in use at York. The 'NeuroNet' system aims to provide high-quality information from the internet within a protected environment. Access to information is made using a specially designed software programme that restricts the internet sites that can be displayed. In this way people can access information, safe in the knowledge that it is coming from a recognized, 'genuine' source. The system is designed to be used both by people with neurological conditions and professionals.

An accessible computer point has been designed and installed within the waiting area of the neurosciences outpatient department in York. This computer point is used on a daily basis by people who are waiting for appointments or who wish to search for information after an appointment in the department. Feedback from users has been positive (*Table 21.3*). In addition, the same software can be taken home to be installed on the person's own computer, allowing the same safe internet environment to be replicated for use in the person's own home.

Table 21.3: 'Neuro Net' family information point feedback — summary of initial feedback (*n*=31)

Question	Yes	No	Not answered
Was the information point easy to access?	27 (87%)	2 (6.5%)	2 (6.5%)
Did you find the information you were looking for?	All of it: 19 (61.3%) Some of it: 10 (32.2%)	None of it: 1 (3.2%)	1 (3.2%)
Was the information in clear and understandable language?	28 (90.3%)	0	3 (9.7%)
Did you find the information	Very useful: 14 (45.2%) Useful: 13 (42%) Little use: 1 (3.2%)	No use: 1 (3.2%)	2 (6.4%)
Do you think the information will help your understanding and/or your management of your condition?	A great deal: 20 (64.6%) A little: 5 (16.1%)	Not at all: 1 (3.2%) It has made things worse: 1 (3.2%)	4 (12.9%)

The NeuroNet system incorporates information about MS that has recently been reviewed and rewritten by the MS nurses in Leeds and York. Neuro Education also provides online lectures with audio presentations available via the internet. These online lectures are designed to provide an alternative source of information to all persons involved in specific neurological conditions. The MS nurses are currently involved in the development of a series of lectures about MS that will be available via the internet and via the NeuroNet information points. These online lectures will provide a further alternative and easily accessible media by which information about MS can be provided, as recommended in the NSF (DoH, 2005).

In Leeds, the neurology service is currently situated between two hospital sites (Leeds General Infirmary and St James' University Hospital). The service is to amalgamate shortly, when the service will be centred in Leeds General Infirmary. This is an ideal time to improve on the service already offered by making a new information resource facility available to service users. Service users will be involved in setting up this facility and possibly involved in its maintenance and development. Applications are being made for funding a wheelchair-accessible computer with internet access, similar to the one currently in use in York, to enable service users to access information they want via linked internet sites. A supply of current leaflets and books on MS will also be available, plus CD-ROMs and DVDs.

Future evaluation/developments

Once the information resource centre is set up in Leeds, an audit will be carried out to ascertain whether it meets the needs of service users. This will be supported by audits in both Leeds and York, looking into the usage and usefulness of the Neuro Education programmes for the service users with MS. Any further developments will be dependent on these audits/evaluations.

Conclusion

The MS nurse is at the forefront of responding to the information needs of people with MS. It is imperative that the information given must be appropriate, up to date and delivered in an acceptable format to the person with MS and/or their significant others. Involving service users, exchanging ideas and learning from the experiences of colleagues in other centres can enrich and enhance the knowledge and learning from evidence-based research.

References

Burgess M (2002) Types of MS. In: Burgess M. *Multiple Sclerosis, Theory and Practice for Nurses*. Whurr, London

Campion K (1996) Meeting multiple needs. *Nurs Times* **92**(24): 28–30

Compston A, Coles A (2002) Multiple sclerosis. *Lancet* **359**: 1221–31

De Broe S, Christopher F, Waugh N (2001) The role of specialist nurses in multiple sclerosis: a rapid and systematic review. *Health Technol Assess* **5**(17): 1–47

Department of Health (1999) *The Expert Patient: A New Approach to Chronic Disease Management for the 21st Century*. DoH, London

Department of Health (2001) *The Expert Patient: A New Approach to Chronic Disease Management for the 21st Century*. DoH, London

Department of Health (2005) *The National Service Framework for Long-term Conditions*. DoH, London

Ebers G (1999) Natural history of multiple sclerosis. In: Compston A, Ebers G, McDonald I, Matthews B, Wekerle H, eds. *McAlpine's Multiple Sclerosis*, 3rd edn. Churchill Livingstone, London

Embrey N, Lowndes C, Warner R (2003) Benchmarking best practice in relapse management of multiple sclerosis. *Nurs Stand* **17**(22): 38–42

Ford H, Gerry E, Johnson M, Williams R (2000) *Health Needs Assessment in a Population-Based Cohort of People with Multiple Sclerosis Living in Leeds*. Nuffield Institute for Health, Leeds

Hepworth M, Harrison J, James N (2002) *The Information Needs of People with Multiple Sclerosis*. Department of Information Science, Loughborough University, Loughborough

Johnson J, Smith P, Goldstone L (2001) *Evaluation of MS Specialist Nurses: A Review and Development of the Role*. *Report for the MS Trust*. South Bank University, London

Jones C (2004) Multiple sclerosis update. *Primary Health Care* **14**(2): 26–32

Joyce L (1999) Development of practice. In: Hamer S, Collinson G, eds. *Achieving Evidence-Based Practice*. Harcourt, London

Kirker SGB, Young E, Warlow CP (1995) An evaluation of a multiple sclerosis liaison nurse. *Clin Rehabil* **9**: 219–26

McDonald WI, Ron MA (1999) Multiple sclerosis: the disease and its manifestations. *Phil Trans R Soc Lond B Biol Sci* **354**: 1615–22

McIver S, Brocklehurst N (1999) Public involvement: working for better health. *Nurs Stand* **14**(1): 46–52

Multiple Sclerosis Society (2004) *What is MS? A Guide to Multiple Sclerosis*. MS Society, London

Multiple Sclerosis Society, United Kingdom Multiple Sclerosis Specialist Nurse Association, NHNN, ABN (2004) *Helping You Explain MS: A Teaching Resource for Healthcare Professionals*. MS Society, London

Multiple Sclerosis Trust (2004) *Multiple Sclerosis Information for Health and Social Care Professionals*. MS Trust, Letchworth

National Institute for Clinical Excellence (2003) *Multiple Sclerosis: Management in Primary and Secondary Care*. The National Collaborating Centre for Chronic Conditions, London

Porter B (2001) The MS specialist nurse in the UK. *Int MS J* **9**(2): 59–63

Powell JA, Darvell M, Gray JA (2003) The doctor, the patient and the world-wide web: how the internet is changing health care. *J Roy Soc Med* **96**(2): 74–6

Robinson I, Hunter M, Neilson S (1996) *A Dispatch from the Frontline: The Views of People with Multiple Sclerosis about their Needs. A Qualitative Approach*. MS Society, London

Thompson AJ (2003) Treatment of progressive multiple sclerosis. In: McDonald WI, Noseworthy JH, eds. *Multiple Sclerosis 2*. Butterworth-Heinemann, Philadelphia

United Kingdom Multiple Sclerosis Specialist Nurse Association, Royal College of Nursing, Multiple Sclerosis Research Trust (2001) *The Key Elements for Developing MS Specialist Nurse Services in the UK*. MS Research Trust, Letchworth

United Kingdom Multiple Sclerosis Specialist Nurse Association, Royal College of Nursing, Multiple Sclerosis Research Trust (2003) *Competencies for MS Specialist Nurses*. MS Research Trust, Letchworth

United Kingdom Multiple Sclerosis Specialist Nurse Association, Serono (2003) *The United Kingdom Multiple Sclerosis Clinical Symposia International Management Manual: Care Across the Disease Trajectory*. UKMSSNA and Serono Symposia International (place of publication unknown)

United Kingdom Multiple Sclerosis Specialist Nurse Association, Teva Aventis (2004) Slide library for UKMSSNA members

Ward N, Embrey N, Lowndes C, Vernon K (2002) Specialist nurse network improves MS practice. *Nurs Times* **98**(30): 34–6

Chapter 22

Information for young people when multiple sclerosis enters the family

Kerry Mutch

Multiple sclerosis (MS) is the most common cause of neurological disability for young adults (Burgess, 2002), and often causes financial and socioeconomic difficulties, as many sufferers have to stop working or reduce their working hours (Graham, 1998). MS can cause role changes within the family unit and therefore must also have an impact on children within the family. However, little work has been done to help children adapt and cope when living with MS in their family.

MS is an autoimmune condition affecting the central nervous system. By its very nature there are no set patterns, with each individual being affected differently and even similar symptoms being perceived differently (Burgess, 2002). Each person travels through their own MS pathway, and treatment will depend on the individual's symptoms. Living a life with MS brings uncertainty, unpredictability and worry for the future (Graham, 1998). Much support is given to the person affected by MS at each different stage or new development via newly diagnosed groups, MS specialist nurses and charities, such as the MS Society and MS Trust. The impact of MS on partners is also largely recognized (Robinson et al, 2000), and they are now often included in education programmes.

Background

The National Institute for Clinical Excellence (NICE) guidelines (2003) for the care of people with multiple sclerosis and the *National Service Framework (NSF) for Long-term Conditions* (Department of Health (DoH), 2005) have recognized that support for family and carers is essential. They recommend that:

> '...all carers of people with long-term neurological conditions are to be assessed to receive appropriate support and services that recognize their needs as a carer and as an individual in their own right.'

A definition by the Department of Health (2004a) for a young carer is:

'*...a young person who looks after, or helps to look after, a family member who has a physical disability, learning disability, long-term illness, mental health or drug/alcohol abuse problem.*'

For the young people who fit this definition, young carer groups such as Barnardos and the Princess Royal Trust for Young Carers are extremely beneficial as they provide social and emotional support and often have links to a child psychologist. The key message of the *NSF for Children, Young People and Maternity Services* (DoH, 2004a) is:

'*...every child matters.*'

However, the framework is aimed at people who have a chronic illness or physical disability and their parents/carers. The main problem with some care groups is that they assume that all carers do physical care, and do not accept the underlying worry and anxiety that comes with the long-term condition or the unpredictability of future care. Thus, many children lose out when a parent has MS, and often neither parents nor society see the children as formal carers (Yahav et al, 2005).

The book *Multiple Sclerosis: A Guide for Families* (Kalb, 1998) addresses the viewpoint of the parent with MS, examining how, for example, they could conserve energy, which may help them to be a more effective parent. Regularly, young people who have MS in their family do more in their homes and families than their 'normal'counterparts, although this is not classed as formal caring. The child may be relied on for extra jobs in the house, such as cleaning and shopping, or just being alone in the house with a disabled parent rather than physically 'caring'. Those with increased disabilities will often have a good package of care, with formal carers carrying out physical activities, such as washing, dressing and toileting. However, this will still leave several hours in the day when they are unattended.

Despite not being a formal carer, the teenager will have anxieties that are not addressed by the uncertainty caused by living with MS, such as: 'will mum/dad be all right?'; 'what will happen in the future?'; 'what will I do if something happens to them?'; or 'what if they fall when I go out?'. Also, little is done to address the extra workload they may do in the home, or hidden concerns the young people may have (Segal and Simkins, 1996). Worse is the burden of worry young people carry even if their parent is relatively well, as acknowledged by Cross and Rintell (1999). The national strategy for carers, *Caring for the Carers* (DoH, 2004b), offers practical help in ways that are needed. The strategy promises that carers will have better information and be better supported.

MS in the family

When a person is newly diagnosed with MS or develops new symptoms, they are given education and information to help them cope better on a daily basis. Over recent years, the importance of including partners within this information process has also been acknowledged (Burgess, 2002). However, Kalb (1998) acknowledges that parents will frequently try to protect their children by not telling them anything, especially if there are few physical symptoms evident, believing their own worries and anxieties do not show. There is often a belief that by not talking about MS, it will go away.

MS is an insidious disease with gradual changes occurring over a period of time, and family members may not notice the changes (Koch and Kralik, 2001); therefore, discussing the effects of MS is often not addressed. It is also difficult to talk about symptoms that are not so obvious, as with fatigue, where mum/dad always appear tired, or memory problems, which can become irritating for young people.

Young people often feel isolated in such situations. They are aware that something is wrong with mum/dad and often have a fear of the unknown. This can cause a major barrier, which results in them not wanting to discuss their worries at home as it may make the parent worse. Young people do not know who to go to or what questions to ask. They are reluctant to talk about their worries at school and feel they are probably the only person in the school who has a parent with MS. This anxiety and uncertainty can bring resentment and anger resulting from their lack of sense of control and can have an impact on their schoolwork, attitudes and behaviour, including being the victim of bullying or becoming the bully (Kalb, 1998).

While MS societies in America and Canada have good networks and interactions for young people who have parents with MS, in Britain there is no such structure, apart from a few information booklets aimed at younger children, printed by the MS Society and the MS Trust.

Setting up the workshop

The initiative to develop the workshop came following contact with two parents who were worried about the behavioural problems of their teenage daughters. Neither parent thought that MS was an issue as they were both well with their MS, working part-time and on disease-modifying treatment (DMT). The aim of DMT is to reduce the frequency and severity of relapses over a period of time and consequently the amount of disability.

The daughters knew their mums had MS, but didn't know what it was or what it could do. One daughter was particularly worried that mum must be really ill as she had injections in the fridge that 'were keeping mum alive'. Mum was surprised to find out that the one treatment that she believed was keeping her so well was actually the most worrying to her daughter. This supports the theory of Segal and Simkins (1993), who identified that most teenagers are aware when there is a health problem with a parent and, if no explanation is given, they use their imagination to conjure an explanation themselves. Kalb (1998) agreed with this notion and felt that children will often misinterpret silence as an indication that the problem is so terrible that it cannot be discussed, and therefore are often relieved to hear the truth.

The encounter with the two teenage girls identified the isolation and worry that can be felt, and they agreed an educational workshop for similar teenagers would be beneficial. Identifying key people to help organize the day was essential, and a meeting was arranged with a child psychologist, a child psychiatrist and a Barnardos

Table 22.1: 'Multiple sclerosis in the family' workshop

- Give information regarding multiple sclerosis (MS) in a practical, interactive way

- Meet other young people who have a parent with MS

- Identify others to share their worries or concerns with

- To enjoy the day and have some fun

support worker, who were extremely supportive and inspirational in setting up the workshop. The aim of the day was to cover educational, social and psychological aspects relating solely to living with MS, ensuring the day was practical, interactive and fun (*Table 22.1*).

The location of the day is also important, as hospitals are often frightening places owing to the fear that is associated when a parent goes into hospital. Venues such as a local community centre are often better alternatives. Schools will probably allocate the workshop day as educational and give children an authorized absence. It is also easier to enlist the assistance of others on weekdays. All helpers must be police checked and it is useful to have local young carer groups to help, particularly concerning psychological issues. Costs of hiring the venue, food and refreshments must be considered. It was also felt that the young people should not have to pay anything, and in order to assist with the overall costing, grants may be available from the MS Society or children's charities.

MS in the family workshop

The workshop is for any young person aged 9–14 years who has a parent with MS, regardless of the type, length of duration or the amount of physical disability. The emphasis of the day is to show young people that MS is individual and different for every person affected by it, and that nobody has all the symptoms. Success depends on reducing the isolation felt by young people as they meet others who also have a parent with MS.

The morning sessions explain MS in an interactive way, and involve the young people in practical activities, such as the young person acting at being part of a nerve pathway. The game demonstrates that MS is simply a series of mixed-up messages and, depending on the message that is interpreted by the person with MS, each will have different symptoms. Other activities simulate different symptoms to enhance the young person's understanding about the variable condition of MS, including a three-legged course that shows the difficulty with balance problems. There are also word finding and memory games to show the various types of memory that are used in daily life. Another activity involves wearing glasses that distort vision and then trying to perform tasks,

Table 22.2: Any questions?

- Can I catch it?
- Will mum/dad die?
- How do you get multiple sclerosis (MS)?
- What happens when you get MS?
- What can MS do?
- If dad falls, how do I pick him up?
- Does stress make MS worse?
- Will MS get better?
- Do people with MS need more sleep?
- Is there any cure for MS?
- What are the types of MS?
- Will dad soon be in a wheelchair?
- Does marijuana help?
- What can I do to help?
- Are mood swings part of MS?
- Does MS shorten your life?

Table 22.3: Multiple sclerosis affects me because

- My mum gets upset, which makes me upset
- It sometimes makes me worry
- My dad can never come out with us
- My mum spends a lot of time in hospital
- My mum is different from my friend's mum
- You can't just go out, it depends how mum's feeling
- My mum never sleeps and sometimes her personality changes
- It is hard to plan things
- Everything takes so long
- I don't mind my dad having MS
- My dad can't drive, so we never go anywhere
- Mum is always tired
- Mum is always forgetting things — is this normal?

which show the effects that double or blurred vision can have on a person.

Throughout the day young people are encouraged to ask questions by writing on stickers and applying them to blank posters (*Tables 22.2–22.3*).

The afternoon sessions are more personal and, with the assistance of psychologists and young carer groups, the effects of MS on the family are discussed, reviewing the needs, emotions and thoughts of the young person, the parent with MS and the other parent.

Benefits of attending the workshop

The main benefit of the workshop is that young people meet others who are in similar situations to themselves. They leave feeling less isolated as they have the opportunity to ask questions that may have worried them in the past, which they may have been hesitant to ask their parents for fear of upsetting them. They are also given contact numbers for support groups, and the participants can exchange contact information. The young people tend to worry less as they are reassured there is little chance of them either getting MS or their parents dying from it.

They develop a greater understanding about the symptoms of MS, especially the 'silent' ones, such as fatigue, memory difficulties and poor concentration. The hope is that they will have more patience with their parent as they begin to appreciate that the fatigue is real and not that their parent is lazy or not interested in them.

The feelings of young people, such as anger, resentment, worry and isolation, are acknowledged so they do not feel so alone. Although this does not stop the hurt and confusion sometimes felt by young people when they are the target of their parents frustration, it can help them identify the cause.

Parents' feedback and benefits

One of the biggest barriers when setting up the 'MS in the family' workshop is the parent's attitude and viewpoint that their MS does not affect their children. Parents worry that by giving information to their children they will frighten the children and worry them even more.

Initially, one must go through the parents when sending out information about the workshop. If the parent continues to feel this way, they simply do not give the young people the opportunity of going. However, once the children have attended the day, the feedback from parents has been positive as they find MS is no longer a secret within the family and some of the pressure from trying to be 'normal' all the time is reduced. The parents feel that the young people show some understanding and patience with their parent's MS symptoms and during a relapse where extra help may be required.

Discussion

MS changes many things in family life. It can change the way people feel about themselves and each other. Often there are role changes within the family, depending on physical, social and financial influences. MS has a roller-coaster effect on the whole family, therefore it is essential to include everybody in education, information and support. Despite parents' views that MS does not affect their children, their hidden concerns often cause more distress and worry than the truth. If parents do not talk about MS, the children often misinterpret silence as an indication that the problem is so terrible that it cannot be discussed (Segal and Simkins, 1993).

Rehm and Catarizaro (1998) found that children generally cope relatively well with the stresses of MS in the family, particularly with physical disability. However, the emotional sides of coping with parents' mood swings, increased irritability and yelling, as well as changes in family activities caused by lower income were acknowledged. These emotions were also found during the 'MS in the family' workshop. Lachey and Gates (2001), in their study of experiences by young people living with chronic illness in their family, concluded that family life, school and social areas were all affected. Youngsters need to be informed about the illness, have adequate support systems and still have time to be a child. The 'MS in the family' workshop gave the opportunity to do this.

Implications for specialist nurses

There are approximately 200 MS specialist nurses in Britain (http://www.mstrust.org.uk/default.jsp). Breaking the silence by talking openly with young people about MS helps relieve anxiety about their parent's health and their own security and wellbeing. Specialist nurses can ease the isolation and should not be worried about the consequences of giving out too much information. The nurse may be surprised to find that MS is not an issue; the young person has lived with it all his or her life and has adapted well.

The minimum the specialist nurse should do for young people is to provide access to information regarding the condition. Both American and Canadian MS societies have excellent websites aimed at a variety of age groups. The MS Society also has linked with the Princess Royal Trust for Young Carers, which has chat lines and discussion boards for young carers to access.

As a consequence of the workshop, the author has worked closely with the MS Society in Britain to produce a facilitator pack, which will guide specialist nurses through the process of organizing workshops similar to 'MS in the family'. Also, a further information pack is available for attendees to the workshop.

Another result is that the author is currently working with the MS Trust to produce a guide for young people who have parents with MS, which should soon be available.

References

Burgess M (2002) *Multiple Sclerosis. Theory and Practice for Nurses*. Whurr Publishers, London

Cross T, Rintell D (1999) Children's perceptions of parental multiple sclerosis. *Psychol Health Med* **4**(4): 335–60

DoH (2004a) *National Service Framework for Children, Young People and Maternity Services*. DoH, London

DoH (2004b) *Caring for the Carers*. DoH, London

DoH (2005) *National Service Framework for Long-term Conditions*. Department of Health, London

Graham J (1998) *A Self-Help Guide*. Harper Collins, London

Kalb R (1998) *Multiple Sclerosis: A Guide for Families*. Demos Vermande, New York

Koch T, Kralik (2001) Chronic illness: reflections on a community-based action research programme. *J Adv Nurs* **36**(1): 23–31

Lachey N, Gates M (2001) Adults recollections of their experiences as young caregivers of family members with chronic physical illness. *J Adv Nurs* **34**(3): 320–8

National Institute for Clinical Excellence (2003) *Multiple Sclerosis*. NICE. London

Rehm R, Catarizaro M (1998) 'It's just a fact if life'. Family members perceptions of parental chronic illness. *J Fam Nurs* **4**(1): 21–40

Robinson I, Neilson S, Rose F (2000) *Multiple Sclerosis at Your Fingertips*. Class Publishing, London

Segal J, Simkins J (1993) *My Mum Needs Me. Helping Children with Ill or Disabled Parents*. Penguin Books, London

Segal J, Simkins J (1996) *Helping Children with Ill or Disabled Parents: A Guide for Professionals*. Jessica Kingsley, London

Yahav R, Vosburgh J, Miller A (2005) Emotional responses of children and adolescents to parents with multiple sclerosis. *Mult Scler* **11**: 464–8

Useful information

- Barnardos: www.barnardos.org.uk
- Canadian MS Society: www.mssociety.ca
- MS Society: www.mssociety.org.uk
- MS Trust: www.mstrust.org.uk
- National MS Society: www.nmss.org
- Princess Royal Trust for Carers: www.youngcarers.net

Chapter 23

Nursing role in the multidisciplinary management of motor neurone disease

Jane Skelton

Motor neurone disease (MND) is the name given to a group of related diseases, characterized by progressive degeneration of motor neurones of the brain and spinal cord. Disease types include amyotrophic lateral sclerosis (ALS) (affecting 65% of MND patients) and progressive bulbar palsy (PBP), where speech and swallowing is affected (25%). The less common types are progressive muscular atrophy (PMA) (up to 10%) and primary lateral sclerosis (PLS) (about 2%) (Skelton, 1996a; Motor Neurone Disease (MND) Association, 2003). Upper and lower motor neurones are involved in MND to varying degrees (*Figure 23.1*).

MND is a terminal disease of a steadily progressive nature. The disease has an incidence rate of approximately two per 100 000 and a prevalence in the population of about seven per 100 000. The number of people affected in the UK is estimated to be up to 5000 (MND Association, 2003). Onset of the disease is insidious and mimics other neurological conditions, such as multiple sclerosis and myasthenia gravis (i.e. muscle dysfunction and abnormal fatigability of the muscles), neuropathies and trapped nerves, thus making diagnosis difficult. It is eventually diagnosed by eliminating other possibilities and performing a variety of tests (*Table 23.1*).

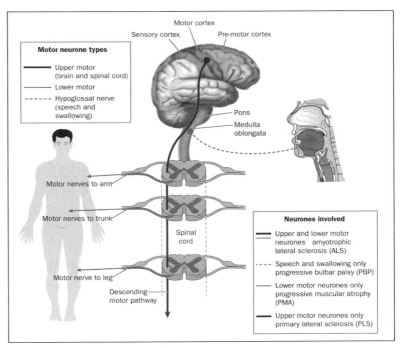

Figure 23.1: The various presentations of motor neurone disease and the neurones involved

Table 23.1: Tests carried out to diagnose motor neurone disease

- Magnetic resonance imaging (MRI) or computerized tomography (CT) to eliminate other possible diagnoses

- Electromyography (EMG) at 3–6-monthly intervals to test electrical activity of the muscle

- Blood tests (creatinine kinase is sometimes raised in motor neurone disease)

- Lumbar puncture to eliminate other possibilities

- Muscle biopsy

The speed and pattern of progression vary widely between individuals, and the progressing muscle weakness can affect the limbs, trunk, neck, speech and swallowing. The latter are the bulbar areas where the muscles involved in speech and swallowing are served by the upper and lower motor neurones that are at the base of the brain. The progressive muscle weakness results in wasting or loss of function of affected muscles and total dependence on others for care (Thomas, 1993). Speech and swallowing may become increasingly impaired, often resulting in total loss of function. Muscles involved in the voluntary control of respiration will ultimately be affected and occasionally may be the presenting symptom (Leigh et al, 2003).

The three cranial nerves that control movement of the eyes and lower sacral segments of the spinal cord are spared, as are the sensory nerves and the autonomic nervous system. Intellect, memory and continence remain intact in most cases (Skelton, 1996a). There may occasionally be involvement of other areas in the central nervous system (CNS) (Leigh et al, 2003). MND and dementia sometimes occur.

Multidisciplinary approach to care

As soon as a diagnosis of MND is made, it is essential that the district nurse becomes involved in the patient's management so that there is time to establish a therapeutic relationship with the person with MND. This rapport must be established with the patient before communication becomes difficult. The main roles of the district nurse in relation to caring for patients with MND are described in *Table 23.2*.

Table 23.2: Role and skills needed by the nurse

- Offering emotional support to the patient and family as they come to terms with a terminal disease

- Monitoring of patients' deterioration

- Advising and liaising with the GP on symptom control

- Referring to Macmillan colleagues

- Use of suction

- Management of percutaneous endoscopic gastrostomy (PEG)

- Bowel management (as abdominal muscles and diaphragm weaken)

- Respiratory management

- Syringe driver may be used to manage symptoms

The rate from diagnosis to death depends on how rapidly the motor neurones die and how well healthy motor neurones compensate for those that are lost. The other variable is the type of MND. The following survival timescales are relevant from the onset of symptoms and not from the time of diagnosis, which may be several years after the first symptoms:

- ALS: 2–5 years
- PBP: 6 months–2 years
- PMA: 5 years+
- PLS: 10 years or more (MND Association, 2003).

The nurse's immediate role will be to monitor the patient and provide emotional and psychological support for both patient and carer, while working with the GP to help provide symptom control. Time should be allowed for those living with MND to discuss the prognosis and its implications, especially once there are signs of respiratory problems. Most patients become highly dependent and develop communication difficulties (Leigh et al, 2003). Aspects of care such as positioning, transferring, feeding, oral hygiene and communication require great attention to detail and are time-consuming for the healthcare professionals involved.

It is equally important that a coordinated multidisciplinary approach is adopted, as the problems encountered by someone with MND are varied, complex and often overwhelming (Corr et al, 1998; Miller et al,1999; Leigh et al, 2003). A multidisciplinary team should incorporate the patient's own GP and practice team, clinical nurse specialists, occupational therapists, speech therapists and dietitians, along with social workers and palliative care specialists (Howard and Orrell, 2002; Leigh et al, 2003). Most patients with MND will remain at home, but this requires close cooperation and integrated care provision by health and social services, the palliative care team and, in some areas, the Marie Curie nursing services to ensure the patient's needs are met (Skelton, 1996a).

A dietitian will have to be involved to assess nutritional intake and the patient's weight, especially if swallowing is compromised by bulbar involvement (Leigh et al, 2003). Physiotherapists can help maintain maximum limb function and joint flexibility by instructing on gait, exercise and compensatory movements as well as helping delay the onset of respiratory problems and assisting with cough techniques. Respiratory difficulties can be delayed, as breathing exercises have the potential to increase lung capacity and cough techniques lessen the risk of chest infections (Bach, 1993).

Occupational therapists have a vital role in maintaining independence and relieving the strain for the carer by providing aids for daily living as well as environmental controls and call systems, e.g. Possum, which can be operated with a head movement. Occupational therapists will also coordinate the provision of wheelchairs, sticks and walking frames. Social workers will need to provide a package of care in the community, including financial benefits and other practical measures; although ultimately this may become a health responsibility as MND is terminal and the patient will at some point meet the continuing care criteria. It will then be the nurse's role to assess for continuing care needs (Beresford, 1997; Howard and Orrell, 2002).

All disciplines need to work closely together to provide regular assessments of need and to adjust provision accordingly. Fast tracking for provision is usually required because of the rapid progression of the disease (Leigh et al, 2003). It is also important to anticipate future needs and plan ahead so as to provide for them in a timely fashion. Ideally, the multidisciplinary team needs a coordinator as a single point of contact through which all the care needs of the individual can be channelled (Leigh et al, 2003).

The patient's desire for control of his or her care is often overlooked, and this can lead to a further sense of frustration among patients who have no way of preventing their MND from progressing, but feel they need to be allowed some autonomy (Skelton, 1996a).

The MND Association is keen to promote the importance of teamwork and has published a personal guide to MND, which includes communication pages where the patient is able to record his or her needs, wishes and plans for the future. Professionals are encouraged to record their own input at each visit (MND Association, 2002). In 10 of the 11 quality requirements in the National Service Frameworks for Long-term Conditions (MND Association, 2005) there is a separate section on special needs of those with a rapidly progressive condition, e.g. MND (see MND Association, 2005, for examples of good practice and further reading).

Communications issues

Most MND patients experience communication problems. This is owing to the weakening and wasting of tongue, lips and facial muscles, and the pharynx and larynx. This causes progressive difficulty with articulation, slurred speech, a weak voice and may result in anarthria (the loss of power to articulate words). As a result the patient may become withdrawn, isolated and frustrated (as will the relatives, who may feel inadequate as they find it increasingly difficult to understand their loved one). Nurses can also feel inadequate when they try to communicate with the person. It is important therefore to do so in a relaxed atmosphere and when the nurse has time.

In the author's experience the low self-esteem of people with MND often results from not being involved in conversations/decisions, and other people presuming their intellect is affected. They also feel a loss of control with fear and anxiety, as they are increasingly less able to express their fears, anxieties and wishes for their future.

A speech and language therapist should be made available as soon as any changes in voice or articulation are identified to advise on strategies for communication and arrange for assessment and provision of communication aids (Beresford, 1997). Voice amplifiers may only be helpful for patients with good articulation but a weak voice. Other speech aids and various writing devices are available, such as the Lightwriter using a keyboard. which is available through the MND Association. These devices employ sensitive switches that respond to the slightest muscle movement of the user (Leigh et al, 2003), and scanning devices.

Nutritional support

Referral to a speech therapist should be made at the first sign of alterations in speech or swallowing ability. The speech therapist will advise on strategies to ensure a safe swallow. Swallow assessment involves a speech therapist observing a patient eating a meal/swallowing water. A barium swallow may also be carried out. It is important that patients have their chin down when they swallow to block off the airway. In addition, a double or triple swallow may be needed to ensure all traces of food are dislodged from pockets within the throat, otherwise they may dislodge later and cause choking/inhalation of food particles, leading to inhalation pneumonia. The double or triple swallow involves the holding of breath while swallowing (Skelton, 1996b). The speech therapist can also advise on food and liquid consistencies and will liaise with the dietitian.

Dysphagia (difficulty in swallowing) and dysarthria (difficulty articulating words as a result of disease of the CNS) usually occur at the same time. This is owing to weakness of glossopharyngeal, vagus, accessory and hypoglossal nerves. This may result in problems chewing, propelling food with the tongue, forming a bolus, poor or absent lip seal and swallow reflex, failure to close airway, and muscle spasm. Drooling may result, which is a distressing symptom. Aspiration and impaired respiratory function are serious consequences, along with weight loss and dehydration (Howard and Orrell, 2002; Lechtzin et al, 2002).

Efforts to maximize nutrition are critical and are usually accomplished by the placement of a percutaneous endoscopic gastrostomy (PEG) tube into the stomach through the abdominal wall (*Figure 23.2*). PEG feeds are prescribed by a GP. The type used depends on GP preference and on advice from the dietitian. They can be bolus, drip or pump fed. Liquidized food can then be passed through the tube. The decision for a PEG placement should be made before the patient suffers considerable weight loss and before aspiration of food may lead to a chest infection. The nurse should involve the patient in early discussions about the possible need for PEG assistance. The dietitian, speech and language therapist, doctor and nurse should help in decision making (Howard and Orrell, 2002). With the exception of nutrition nurse specialists, nurses are not experts in this field and should reinforce advice given by nutrition experts. (See *Nuritional Management Guidelines* available from the MND Association.)

Plenty of time is needed to come to terms with a PEG and to accept its benefits. Many patients refuse it because they fear it will interfere with their present enjoyment of food. They understandably

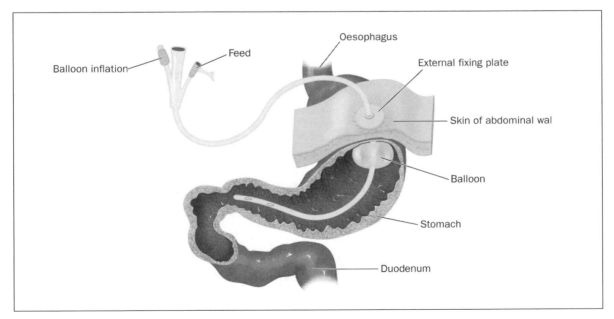

Figure 23.2: Percutaneous endoscopic gastrostomy (PEG)

wish to be able to swallow for as long as possible, and are afraid of any intervention that they think will interfere with this process. It important to explain to patients that this is not the case, and they can continue to swallow for as long as it is safe for them to do so. Acceptance may be aided by the introduction to someone who is already using a PEG successfully.

PEGs are primarily undertaken to improve quality of life, and an extension of life for a few months may result. It is worth noting, however, that a PEG insertion may lead to exacerbation of breathing problems in patients who have severe respiratory impairment, when forced vital capacity (FVC) is less than 50% predicted (Lechtzin et al, 2002). This occurs because the insertion of a PEG is a surgical procedure leading to a sore wound that is made less uncomfortable by not breathing deeply. In addition, sedation used during the procedure may depress respirations (Lechtzin et al, 2002; Leigh et al, 2003; Mitsumoto et al, 2003). This is why some experts report that PEG should be carried out in the earlier rather than later stages of the disease, as breathing problems, in most cases, occur later in the disease process (Mitsumoto et al, 2003).

An alternative to the PEG tube is a radiologically inserted gastrostomy (RIG) tube. This involves air insufflation into the stomach via a nasogastric tube and X-ray-guided insertion of a gastrostomy tube. Its main advantages are that it is tolerated by patients whose FVC is below 50%, and it avoids sedation and the need to swallow an endoscopic tube (Leigh et al, 2003). Chio et al (2004) found that RIG extended survival when compared to PEG, but other studies found there was no significant difference between the two procedures (Thornton et al, 2002; Desport et al, 2003).

The nurse will need to train and support people with MND and their carers on the care of the PEG, as well as in relation to the cleaning and inspection of the PEG site and rotation of the tube as required for the first few weeks. Before discharge home, all patients should be aware of how to obtain feeds and syringes and know who can be contacted in the event of feeding rate problems, blocked feeding tubes or other related emergencies. Possible complications of PEG placement are listed in *Table 23.3*.

Table 23.3: Possible complications of percutaneous endoscopic gastrostomy

- Transient laryngeal spasm (7.2%)
- Localized infection (6.6%)
- Gastric haemorrhage (1–4%)
- Failure as a result of technical difficulties (1–9%)
- Death as a result of respiratory arrest (1.9%)

From Miller et al (1999)

Management of bulbar weakness

Excessive saliva (pseudoptyalism) is a common problem when the bulbar area is involved. Suction can be effective, especially when the saliva is not thick. Anticholinergic drugs that have a side-effect of drying saliva, such as hyoscine, atropine or glycopyrrolate, can be used (Miller et al, 1999). However, there is a danger of causing the production of thick, tenacious saliva by overuse of these medications. In addition, difficulty in swallowing liquids and mouth breathing as a result of weak bulbar muscles exacerbate the problem (Howard and Orrell, 2002).

Nebulization with saline solution or a mucolytic such as Mucodyne (carbocisteine) as well as some natural products can help loosen tenacious saliva (Howard and Orrell, 2002). The MND Association supplies suction units, which are available on loan to patients. Alternatively, patients and carers can be taught effective coughing techniques either manually or mechanically (Leigh et al, 2003). Physiotherapists can teach the 'assisted cough' technique. An insufflator/exsufflator is sometimes appropriate with physiotherapy supervision. This machine can be very effective in removing secretions from the airways when coughing is ineffective. This prevents pneumonia and emergency hospital admission for acute exacerbations. Thus prolonging life and improving it's quality.

Respiratory support

In most cases of MND, respiration is eventually affected. The diaphragm is the main muscle of respiration and it gradually weakens together with the intercostal and abdominal muscles (Howard and Orrell, 2002). (See *Understanding How MND Might Affect my Breathing* from the MND Association.)

The nurse should be alert for the signs of impending respiratory problems. These include daytime somnolence, morning headaches, lethargy and poor concentration as a result of nocturnal hypoventilation (Howard and Orrell, 2002). The nurse should also be aware of the various tests and treatment options. FVC reflects respiratory muscle strength, and serial measurements performed at planned intervals, such as 6-weekly, to monitor respiratory function may be useful in predicting the onset of respiratory failure. Some protocols in the USA recommend initiating non-invasive ventilation when FVC is less than 50% of predicted (Howard and Orrell, 2002). Early discussions of this with the patient and carer, plus the long-term implications of non-invasive pulmonary ventilation (see below), are vital so that informed decisions can be made before a crisis occurs.

Discussion of fear of dying helps patients cope with the knowledge that they are terminally ill. This inevitability cannot be prevented, but patients can be helped to cope with it by discussing their fears and anxieties. In addition, they may have ungrounded fears such as choking or suffocating (Syrett and Taylor, 2003).

The MND Association has produced a 'Breathing Space Kit' for the emergency treatment of the acute episodes of respiratory distress. It is supplied on a named-patient basis to the patient's GP. It helps to address the fears and anxieties a patient may have in relation to 'suffocating' and provides practical help if breathing problems do occur. The GP is also sent the MND leaflets *Death and Dying* and *How Will I Die?*, so that he or she or the district nurse is encouraged to discuss these issues with the patient.

The medication suggested within the kit includes buccal lorazepam (1 mg–2 mg sublingually) or a diazepam (5 mg–10 mg) enema, which the carer may administer. This will relax the muscles in the chest or throat that are in spasm and that cause the feeling of choking. If this does not relieve the symptoms, the GP or nurse can give midazolam 5–10 mg, hyoscine 400–600 mcg and diamorphine 5 mg–10 mg intramuscularly as one injection or individually. These medications will further relax the throat or chest muscles and calm the patient, dry up secretions that may be exacerbating or may have caused the problems, and numb the painful memory of the situation.

A less obvious sign of respiratory failure is a poor night's sleep as a result of a weakened diaphragm, which causes the patient to wake at night aware that he or she has not been breathing properly. This may lead to increasing periods of wakefulness owing to poor breathing, a fear of going to sleep and nightmares. Patients complain of morning headaches and sometimes confusion. This is all because of poor gas exchange and hypercapnia (a build-up of carbon dioxide). A poor night's sleep may also be due to discomfort and/or fear and anxiety. This should be treated with medication to control symptoms, not night sedation. In addition the occupational therapist and physiotherapist can look at positioning in bed. The patient may need to sit up to breathe and may need bed elevation or a profiling bed. Muscle relaxants such as Zanaflex or baclofen can be prescribed for spasm. Pressure sores are rare.

Respiratory weakness can benefit from non-invasive positive pressure ventilation (NIV). It is more likely to be successful in patients with mild or no bulbar symptoms (presenting as speech and swallowing problems) (Aboussouan et al, 1997) or if the disease is progressing slowly. This is because patients with adequate bulbar muscle function are able to use a mouthpiece and nasal NIV to assist breathing, and can use mechanically-assisted coughing aids to prevent airway obstruction (Arroliga, 2001; Bach, 2002). In cases of bulbar dysfunction a PEG is usually performed to prevent aspiration of food particles when using NIV. 'Cough assist' or 'insufflator/exsufflator' can be very effective in removing secretions from the airways when coughing is ineffective. This prevents pneumonia and emergency hospital admission for acute exacerbations thus prolonging life and improving its quality (Bourke et al, 2003; Vianello et al, 2005).

The community nurse can address some practical problems caused by NIV such as ulceration of the bridge of the nose, by using hydrocolloid dressings and alternating face and nasal masks. However, the local respiratory centre where the patient will have been for the respiratory assessment tests may need to be consulted for other problems, such as ill-fitting masks, alternative masks, air leaks and pressure volumes needing adjustment. There are now cushioned face masks that can be adjusted to relieve pressure from the bridge of the nose. Acceptance of NIV often depends on correct choice of interface, e.g. type of mask or nasal cushion. In addition modern machines are quiet and will automatically adjust to the patient's breathing pattern. 'Smart' technology enables monitoring to be done at home. (See *Understanding How MND Might Affect My Breathing, Ventilation; Respiratory Problems Reading List; Clinical Guidelines in Nutritional Management in MND/ALS* available from MND Association.)

As respiratory muscles weaken, the patient uses NIV for longer periods, eventually possibly for 24 hours. Survival may be prolonged by a few months (Polkey et al, 1999). There is also strong evidence that it can reverse respiratory failure (Leigh et al, 2003). Bach (2002) has shown that patients using NIV along with mechanically-assisted coughing can prolong survival and delay the need for tracheostomy by up to a year. However, NIV does not alter the progression of MND. At some point the breathing will no longer be helped by NIV. As with a PEG, the aim is to improve quality of life. In MND that does not involve severe bulbar dysfunction NIV improves survival with maintenance or an improvement in quality of life (Bourke et al, 2006).

Several clinical studies have shown that NIV improves both quality of life (Lyall et al, 2001; Lechtzin et al, 2002; Butz et al, 2003) and survival rate (Aboussouan et al, 1997; Lechtzin et al, 2002; Butz et al, 2003). They also show a need for more support for carers when potentially life-prolonging treatments such as NIV are offered, as they are having to care for an increasingly dependent relative and will need to come to terms with the fact that the patient will die soon. They may also need to consider invasive ventilation, which will impose a heavy burden of care on them.

Invasive ventilation and palliative care options involve symptom control so that death is peaceful. These issues should be discussed with the patient as early as possible and throughout the progression of the disease, to ensure informed decisions are made (Miller et al, 1999). There is a need to be aware of the locked in syndrome.

Invasive ventilatory support may be an option when patients need more assistance than NIV or if excessive secretions preclude use of non-invasive ventilatory support. Usually a mechanical ventilator is connected to the trachea through a tracheostomy. The biggest problem for a person on a ventilator is keeping the airway clear of natural secretions such as saliva and mucus. If not cleared, these secretions can be aspirated and cause problems such as infections and pneumonia (Moss et al, 1993).

A respiratory physiotherapist can help prevent aspiration by regular suctioning and chest percussion. These secretion management techniques can be learnt by caregivers and home health carers. Only a small minority of patients choose to receive invasive ventilatory support because of the need for 24-hour care and poor quality of life (Moss et al, 1993). Many instead decide to let nature take its course and die peacefully. However, some patients on long-term invasive positive pressure ventilation have reported meaningful quality of lives (Moss et al, 1993). Even so, this intervention is seldom used in the UK because of funding, quality-of-life issues and the danger of burden on the whole family (Moss et al, 1993).

Death usually occurs as a result of ventilatory failure. This could be caused by bronchopneumonia following upper respiratory tract infection. Often the deterioration is gradual — the patient becomes drowsy during the day and drifts into a coma (O'Brien et al, 1992). Any distress caused by breathlessness can be treated by medications listed within the Breathing Space Kit (Oliver et al, 2000) and *A Problem-Solving Approach* published by the MND Association.

End-of-life issues

The management of MND has evolved rapidly over the past two decades. Although incurable, the effects of MND can be managed, and treatments and interventions have been developed to promote the best possible quality of life. These treatments do not, however, arrest progression or reverse weakness. Hence, they raise difficult practical and ethical questions about quality of life, choice and end-of-life decisions.

Prognosis and treatment options should be openly discussed with the patient and his or her relatives. Adequate assistance and palliative treatment in the terminal phase are of paramount importance (Leigh et al, 2003).

In the author's experience, the patient usually initiates the discussion of, and a request for, assisted suicide or euthanasia in the early stages of the disease. However, the author has found that once the patient is made aware of the existence of effective palliative care then this is no longer an issue. Usually as MND progresses patients accept their increasing dependency. Maintaining communication is essential to autonomy, and hence quality of life (Leigh et al, 2003). It is important that time is given to listen to concerns, issues and fears. For some patients with MND, their quality of life will always be unacceptable and they do not want to endure the physical and psychological burden of being dependant and waiting to die, for example Diane Pretty (who actually died peacefully). The patient's right to choose when to withdraw life-prolonging treatments has been the subject of High Court rulings in the UK (e.g. Burke *vs* General Medical Council (2004)).

Collaboration with hospices and completion of living wills, also known as advance directives, can be made available. The passing of the Mental Capacity Bill means living wills will be legally binding, as long as the intention is for symptom control and not end of life. A living will is an option so that all are aware of the wishes of the person with MND. It will allow the patient to give instructions about any possible medical treatment or intervention, should there be a time when the patient is unable to express his or her own decisions. A proforma for such a will is available from the MND Association. These should be reviewed regularly with the person with MND.

Psychological and spiritual care of patients and families are also important. This is aimed at supporting those making end-of-life decisions and would by provided by hospices or community nurses. Further information on end-of-life decisions is available from the MND Association.

Conclusion

Good management of patients with MND involves a multidisciplinary team based in the hospital and community. The essence of care is good symptomatic management, including nutritional support with percutaneous endoscopic gastrostomy, and ventilatory support with non-invasive ventilation. Palliative care should be introduced before the terminal stages after careful discussion with the patient and carers. It should be stressed that death caused by choking attacks is rare and that the final stages of MND are usually peaceful and dignified.

Knowledge of this condition has grown dramatically recently with a parallel improvement in treatment and ability to deal with the most troublesome symptoms (Corr et al, 1998; Miller et al, 1999; Howard and Orrell, 2002). As educators, nurses can provide patients and families with information, supporting them and helping them plan so that they obtain their wishes for living and dying. They can also liaise with other health and social care professionals to this end.

References

Aboussouan LS, Khan SU, Meeker DP, Stelmach K, Mitsumoto H (1997) Effect of non-invasive positive-pressure ventilation on survival in amyotrophic lateral sclerosis. *Ann Intern Med* **127**(6): 450–53

Arroliga AC (2001) Non-invasive positive pressure ventilation in acute respiratory failure: does it improve outcomes? *Cleve Clin J Med* **68**(8): 677–80

Bach JR (1993) Mechanical insufflation-exsufflation: comparison of peak expiratory flows with manually assisted and unassisted coughing techniques. *Chest* **104**(5): 1553–62

Bach JR (2002) Amyotrophic lateral sclerosis: prolongation of life by noninvasive respiratory AIDS. *Chest* **122**: 92–8

Beresford SA (1997) Communication aids for people with degenerative neurological conditions. *Br J Ther Rehabil* **4**(1): 8–13

Bourke SC, Bullock RE, Williams TL, Shaw PJ, Gibson GJ (2003) Noninvasive ventilation in ALS: Indications and effect on quality of life. *Neurology* **61**: 171–7.

Bourke SC, Tomlinson M, Williams TL, et al (2006) Effects of non-invasive ventilation on survival and quality of life in patients with amyotrophic lateral sclerosis: A randomised controlled trial. *Lancet Neurol* **5**: 140–7

Burke *vs* General Medical Council (2004) EWHC 1879 (Admin) (http://www.courtservice.gov.uk/judgmentsfiles/j2775/burke-v-gmc.htm) (last accessed 1 December 2004)

Butz M, Wollinsky KH, Wiedemuth-Catrinescu U et al (2003) Longitudinal effects of noninvasive positive-pressure ventilation in patients with amyotrophic lateral sclerosis. *Am J Phys Med Rehabil* **82**(8): 597–604

Chio A, Galletti R, Finocchiaro CA et al (2004) Percutaneous radiological gastrostomy: a safe and effective method of nutritional tube placement in advanced ALS. *J Neurol Neurosurg Psych* **75**(4): 645–7

Corr B, Frost E, Traynor B, Hardiman O (1998) Service provision for patients with ALS/MND. A cost-effective, multidisciplinary approach. *J Neurol Sci* **160**(Suppl 1): S141–5

Desport JC, Bouillet B, Preux PM, Makabakayele K, Mabrouk T, Couratier P (2003) Radiologically inserted gastrostomy is as safe as percutaneous endoscopic technique in ALS patients. Report from the 14th International Symposium on ALS/MND, 17-19 November, Milan, Italy. *Amyotroph Lateral Scler Other Motor Neuron Disord* **4**(Suppl 1): 71–5

Howard RS, Orrell RW (2002) Management of motor neurone disease. *Postgrad Med J* **78**: 736–41

Lechtzin N, Rothstein J, Clawson L, Diette GB, Wiener CM (2002) Amyotrophic lateral sclerosis: evaluation and treatment of respiratory impairment. *Amyotroph Lateral Scler Other Motor Neuron Disord* **3**: 5–13

Leigh PN, Abrahams S, Al-Chalabi A J et al (2003) The management of motor neurone disease. *J Neurol Neurosurg Psych* **74**(Suppl IV): iv32–47

Lyall RA, Donaldson N, Fleming T et al (2001) A prospective study of quality of life in ALS patients treated with noninvasive ventilation. *Neurology* **57**(1): 153-6

Miller RG, Rosenberg JA, Gelinas DF et al (1999) Practice parameter: the care of the patient with amyotrophic lateral sclerosis (an evidence-based review). *Neurology* **52**: 1311–23

Mitsumoto H, Davidson M, Moore D et al (2003) Percutaneous endoscopic gastrostomy (PEG) in patients with ALS and bulbar dysfunction. *Amyotroph Lateral Scler Other Motor Neuron Disord* **3**: 177–85

MND Association (2002) *Your Personal Guide to Motor Neurone Disease*. Motor Neurone Disease (MND) Association, Northampton

MND Association (2003) *A Problem-solving Approach*. 2nd edn. Motor Neurone Disease Association, Northampton

MND Association (2005) *National Service Frameworks for Long-Term Conditions*. Motor Neurone Disease (MND) Association, Northampton

Moss AH, Casey P, Stocking CB, Roos RP, Brooks BR, Siegler M (1993) Home ventilation for amyotrophic lateral sclerosis patients: outcomes, costs and patient, family and physician attitudes. *Neurology* **43**(2): 438–43

O'Brien T, Kelly M, Saunders C (1992) Motor neurone disease: a hospice perspective. *Br Med J* **304**: 471–3

Oliver D, Boarasio G, Walsh D (2000) *Palliative Care in Amyotrophic Lateral Sclerosis*. Oxford Press, Oxford

Polkey MI, Lyall RA, Davidson AC, Leigh PN, Moxham J (1999) Ethical and clinical issues in the use of home non-invasive mechanical ventilation for the palliation of breathlessness in motor neurone disease. *Thorax* **54**: 367–71

Skelton J (1996a) Caring for patients with motor neurone disease. *Nurs Stand* **10**(32): 33–6

Skelton J (1996b) Dysphagia in motor neurone disease. *Nurs Stand* **10**(33): 49–53

Syrett E, Taylor J (2003) Non-pharmological management of breathlessness: a collaborative approach. *Int J Palliat Nurs* **9**(4): 150–6

Thomas S (1993) Support that prolongs life. *Prof Nurse* **8**(10): 656–9

Thornton FJ, Fotherington T, Alexander M, Hardiman O, McGrath FP, Lee MJ (2002) Amyotrophic lateral sclerosis: enteral nutrition provision — endoscopic or radiological gastrostomy? *Radiology* **224**(3): 713–17

Vianello A, Corrado A, Arcaro G, Gallan F, Ori C, Minuzzo M, Bevilacqua M (2005) Mechanical insufflation-exsufflation improves outcomes for neuromuscular disease patients with respiratory tract infections. *Am J Phys Med Rehabil* **84**(2): 83–8

The Motor Neurone Disease (MND) Association

The MND Association is a registered charity that aims to improve quality of life for those living with MND and funds research into causes and cure for MND. The Association's services include information, a telephone helpline, equipment loan, financial support and regional care advisers across the country. There are also local support groups, trained visitors and a network of MND care centres.

Education, training and support for health and social care professionals, plus extensive written information for patients, carers and professionals are available. There is also information about living wills, pseudoptyalism, percutaneous endoscopic gastrostomy (PEG), radiologically inserted gastrostomy (RIG) procedures and saliva control. There is also a new revised professional resource file and a publications list is available.

For more information contact the MND Association on 01604 611870, email helpline@mndassociation.org or visit www.mndassociation.org.

Publications available from the Association include:

Clinical Guidelines in Nutritional Management in MND/ALS.

Clinical Guidelines in Respiratory Management in MND/ALS.

Making and Communicating the Diagnosis in MND.

Medical Guidelines: What they mean for people with MND.

Reading List on Respiratory Problems.

Chapter 24

Information-seeking behaviour among people with motor neurone disease

Mary R O'Brien

Motor neurone disease (MND) is a progressive degenerative disease of the nervous system. Average survival time from diagnosis has been estimated at just 14 months (Green, 2003). It is a relatively uncommon illness; there are approximately 6000 people with MND in the UK at any one time (Thomas, 1993). Most individuals diagnosed with MND experience a combination of upper and lower motor neurone degeneration, which can result in progressive weakness of bulbar (related to speech and swallowing), limb, thoracic and abdominal muscles, leading to the development of a number of distressing and disabling symptoms (Leigh and Ray-Chaudhuri, 1994). Sensation, bladder and bowel function are usually unaffected and intellectual function is usually preserved as dementia affects less than 5% of those diagnosed with MND (Shaw, 2000). The majority of people with MND are, therefore, fully aware of their predicament and the inexorable progression of their disability.

Introduction

Studies have shown that the majority of people, even if suffering from an illness that will ultimately result in their death, want to have information about their condition; otherwise the stress they encounter as a result of any ambiguity can actually be in excess of that generated by knowing that they are going to die (Silverstein et al, 1991; Benson and Britten, 1996; Meredith et al, 1996; Ley, 1998). The vast majority (98.2%) of respondents in one study actively wanted to be informed about any changes in the status of their disease, highlighting that having a terminal illness does not preclude a person from needing information about his or her condition (Kutner et al, 1999).

Conflicts can exist, however, between wanting more information and not wanting bad news. People can adopt a variety of different coping strategies to help them come to terms with issues relating to their illness, ranging from denial to obtaining relevant information about the situation (Taylor, 1986). People's attitudes to their illness and the coping strategies that they adopt can restrict their desire for information and interrupt individual efforts to obtain it. Leydon et al (2000) identified that patients with cancer halted their information seeking at different stages of their illness in an effort to maintain hope in the light of concern over negative information. In order to avoid exposure to information that might shatter their hope, patients also used the services of 'proxy informants', who were usually friends or family, to investigate new information on their behalf, which was then avoided if it was felt to be too fearful (Leydon et al, 2000).

Problems with sensational media coverage can render avoidance almost impossible and threaten to destroy hope for some people. Silverstein et al (1991), in a prospective survey of 38 people with MND attending the University of Chicago MND clinic, sought to identify patients' desire for information. This was part of a study investigating preferences for information and participation in decision-making about life-sustaining treatment over a 6-month period. They reported that 30 (81%) participants wanted as much information about MND as possible, whether it was good or bad, and suggested that the gradual progression of the illness allows patients and their families time to seek information with which to answer their questions. That finding does not reflect the author's clinical experience based on personal contact with hundreds of individuals with MND over a period of 8 years as an MND nurse specialist. Many patients experience a rapid progression of their symptoms, which effectively means that they have little time to come to terms with their current level of disability or seek information about existing problems before their physical condition deteriorates further.

If information does help to alleviate feelings of fear, anxiety and uncertainty associated with malignant terminal illness, there is a need to identify if it has similar properties for people with MND. Luker et al (1995) highlight that while nurses have traditionally assumed the role of patient educator, they have tended to focus more on the process of teaching to the detriment of the subject matter. There has been an assumption that nurses instinctively understand what patients want to know and have the required information to pass on to them. In order to ensure that patients are offered information appropriate to their needs, it is important to understand the ways in which individuals with MND obtain their information and to identify reasons why they resist further information or choose not to seek information about their illness.

The only previous work in this area adopted a positivist approach using standardized questionnaires and structured interviews with statistical analysis measuring relationships between variables and agreement between views expressed at interviews 6 months apart (Silverstein et al, 1991). Within health research generally, studies investigating information needs and information-seeking behaviour have mainly tended to adopt such quantitative methodologies with the aim of assigning a statistical validity to a causal relationship. Researchers within social, behavioural and biomedical sciences have conducted studies investigating information needs among individuals with terminal illnesses other than MND, utilizing sense-making, stress and coping style theories to explain information-seeking behaviour (Baker, 1995; Van der Molen, 1999; Bennenbroek et al, 2002). However, there has been an increasing trend over recent years in cancer-related studies to concentrate on the personal experiences of those affected by the illness, in an attempt to understand information requirements and approaches to obtaining or avoiding information from the personal perspective of those involved (Rose, 1999; Leydon et al, 2000).

Study aim

The aim of this study was to investigate the views of people at different stages in the progression of MND concerning their desire for information about their illness and to identify whether there was any pattern to information seeking among people with MND. A lack of literature on the subject would indicate that the study should be exploratory in nature (Crookes and Davies, 1998), with the intention of building on the limited available knowledge. Exploring the individual experiences of participants demands a sympathetic approach, which is capable of interpreting the phenomenon from the perspective of the individual who is experiencing it. Qualitative research, which is truly exploratory, aims to develop concepts that will help us towards this understanding of social phenomena within their naturally occurring setting, with an emphasis on the feelings, meanings and subjective experience of the participants. This work adds to the existing literature on information seeking in terminal illness as it complements other studies and addresses the area of information seeking in non-malignant terminal illness, for which there is a paucity of research. Previous studies have not sought an indepth exploration of the personal experiences of information seeking by people with MND. With such a focus, this study opens the way for further work using qualitative approaches.

Method

Participants

Participants were sought from patients under review at a nurse-led UK MND clinic. Qualitative researchers usually adopt non-probability techniques for sampling, as the sample is selected to provide 'information-rich' cases and not because it aims to be representative of the specific population being studied. Sample sizes, therefore, tend to be much smaller than for quantitative studies (Grbich, 1999). That was the case with this study, where participants were recruited because they had been diagnosed with MND for varying lengths of time and were willing to be interviewed about their experiences in obtaining information about their illness. Approval was obtained from the local research ethics committee.

Details of the study participants are shown in *Table 24.1*. Of the seven, three were men and four were women. Three participants had bulbar-onset and four had limb-onset disease. The

Table 24.1: Details of study participants

Participant (pseudonym)	Sex (m/f)	Age (years)	Onset type	Time from diagnosis to interview (months)
Alan	m	67	Limb	17
Bob	m	57	Limb	27
Cath	f	74	Bulbar	8
Dorothy	f	75	Limb	50
Elsie	f	60	Limb	3
Fred	m	64	Bulbar	4
Gwen	f	65	Bulbar	10

average age of participants was 66 years (range 57–75 years), with an average time from diagnosis to interview of 17 months (range 3–50 months).

It is recognized that the sample did not contain younger people with MND, who may behave in a different manner. However, the phenomenological nature of this study did not seek to obtain objective facts applicable to the MND population as a whole, but sought to explore facets of the lived experiences of the participants from their own internal frame of reference.

Materials

A semistructured interview schedule was developed, which enabled each participant to be questioned about the same topics, but was flexible enough to allow for indepth exploration of themes raised by participants in each interview. Each participant consented to having the interview audiotaped for later transcription. All interviews took place in the participant's own home, and participants were free to have someone else in attendance if they so wished. All interviews were conducted by the author and lasted between 45–90 minutes, allowing for rest periods as required. Each participant was asked questions about the topics listed in *Table 24.2*.

Table 24.2: Topics covered with participants in the interview

---

- Their understanding of motor neurone disease (MND)
- When they first sought information about MND
- Their experiences when they were given their diagnosis
- The source of any information they had received, its clarity and usefulness
- Whether their current information needs were being met
- Factors affecting their desire to seek information
- The impact of information about MND on their lives in general
- The effect of exposure to information available in the media

---

Analysis

The principles of interpretative phenomenological analysis (IPA) were adopted (Smith et al, 1999), with the aim of exploring the participant's own view of information-seeking behaviour in MND. The focus of IPA is on revealing the minutiae of a participant's experiences while attempting to understand how those affected make sense of their experiences (Shaw, 2000). This concern with the individual's personal account of his or her experiences site the approach firmly within phenomenology (Smith et al, 1999). IPA adopts an idiopathic case study approach that involves a detailed systematic analysis of a single case as a study in its own right, or as a starting point before similarly detailed analyses of further cases (Smith et al, 1999).

In order to determine whether themes existed within the interviews, each one was transcribed verbatim, with the aim of identifying and subsequently exploring shared experiences. The first transcript was read through a number of times, taking note of any comments of interest; the process was then repeated for the second and third transcripts in order to develop an overall impression of the content and note any areas of commonality as potential themes. The remaining interviews were treated in an identical manner, focusing on the developing themes from the first three interviews. As the purpose of the study was to generate theory about information-seeking behaviour, potential concepts and categories were developed during the interview process. Any emerging themes were incorporated into subsequent interviews to clarify their relevance to other participants. This process continued until a theoretical saturation point was reached and no new themes on the subject were forthcoming (Bowling, 1997).

After identification of shared themes, each transcript was re-read and relevant extracts supporting the theme were identified. Further analysis of the extracts was undertaken to see whether they could be grouped together in any meaningful way that might provide the basis of an understanding of why people with MND seek information and react to it in the way they do. Participants were approached after their interview to clarify their own contribution and discuss the emerging themes, while two independent sources reviewed the transcripts and the emerging themes to ensure accuracy and validity of the analysed data.

Results

When asked about their perception of what MND was, six of the respondents had at least a basic understanding of nerve damage resulting in muscle weakness. All participants had asked questions about their illness and all had read information about aspects of the disease. Information needs increased and decreased for individual participants over time and, like people with cancer, they appeared to base their information-seeking behaviour on their attitude to the management of their illness at that particular time (Leydon et al, 2000). All participants knew where to obtain information if they required it, but some would only encounter information after a third party had screened its content. Systematic analysis of the accounts of the personal experiences of the participants revealed three broad information-seeking categories, membership of which may or may not have remained constant throughout the duration of the illness.

These categories are described as:

- Active seekers
- Selective seekers
- Information avoiders.

Characteristics of these categories are described with direct quotations from the participants labelled with pseudonyms to ensure anonymity.

Active seekers

Active seekers often started acquiring information about MND early in the course of the illness. They sought information from a variety of sources, including verbal, written, visual and electronic material and were active personally in acquiring the information, not relying on others to screen material for suitability:

> *'We got all the books we could get…we got a videotape and went on the internet…to see what they had to say…I wanted to know everything'* (Elsie).

> *'I read whatever I could…and talked with my friends about it'* (Dorothy).

Active seekers display similar properties to people with multiple sclerosis (MS) categorized as 'monitors' (Baker, 1994, 1995, 1998) and those with Parkinson's disease (PD) classified as 'seekers' (Pinder, 1990), who when faced with an adverse event or threat sought information about it to help them cope with it. They can, however, eventually reach an information saturation point, where they stop actively seeking detailed and varied information:

> *'I felt that I'd reached a cut-off point where I didn't want to look for more information, I'd rather just plod along I suppose'* (Dorothy).

> *'I think you get the general what have you and that's enough, I don't want to keep getting information'* (Elsie).

Active seekers who reached this saturation point often resumed information seeking later on in their illness as new problems arose; however, they did not necessarily return to being active seekers. Participants did show evidence of moving between the categories depending on their individual needs at the time.

Selective seekers

Selective seekers did not want to have a full understanding of the potential implications of the illness at the time of their diagnosis. They invariably had access to written and verbal information but did not always use it personally. They often relied on 'buffers' to acquire information for them, which allowed for screening of the information in order to filter out unsuitable material that could be upsetting. This mirrors periods of 'self-censorship' (Leydon et al, 2000) adopted by people with cancer, who maintain hope by avoiding negative information about their illness. Selective seekers purposefully gathered information, seeking details about issues that concerned them at that particular time. They did not seek information about potential problems or general information about MND itself:

> *'If I want it [information] I can ask for it…I only ask relevant things…I don't ask what's going to happen'* (Bob).

These individuals coped on a day-to-day basis, feeling that it would be detrimental to them to have more detailed information about the illness. They saw it as anticipating future problems that might never occur, but the mere anticipation could have an adverse effect on them:

'I think it would frighten you the more you know...I was frightened of seeing other people a lot worse than me...I just think about now' (Bob).

Selective seekers, like 'weavers' with PD (Pinder, 1990), controlled their exposure to information, and if they had questions they knew where they could obtain answers. They often had willing accomplices who would provide those answers.

Information avoiders

Information avoiders did not actively seek information; however, they were not entirely ignorant about their illness. Like selective seekers, they might avoid information because of the fear of encountering details about aspects of the disease not currently affecting them. They often felt that problems described by others with the illness and documented in the literature would automatically affect them at some stage, which restricted their desire for information:

'I didn't want to know right at the beginning...I didn't want to know for the first year because there was nothing wrong with me apart from a foot drop' (Bob).

Information avoiders felt that anticipating future disability would not help their current situation. Having such information about potential problems will not prevent them from happening. This behaviour is similar to that of 'blunters' with MS (Baker, 1994, 1995, 1998) and 'avoiders' with PD (Pinder, 1990), who attempted to cope with their illness by rejecting information about it. Information avoiders always used a 'buffer' to screen information to which they were exposed and were extremely unlikely to encounter information unless it had been buffered. Buffering was more extreme than for selective seekers:

'She [his partner] generally tells me if I need to know something...she can protect me from it' (Fred).

This technique is also employed by people with cancer who often enlist the help of 'proxy informants' to seek out information on their behalf (Leydon et al, 2000).
Information avoiders were anxious about exposure to information about MND:

'I've been frightened of asking...it's been something that I haven't wanted to hear...I have found it completely shattering...literally mentioning it [MND] just blows me away' (Alan).

'If you get too much information, you start worrying, waiting for it to happen...I don't want information...it would make me depressed' (Gwen).

Some information avoiders may change their information-seeking behaviour during the course of their illness, but usually only to ask limited, specific questions about particular problems that they are encountering at that time.

Baker (1995) states that a person's information-seeking behaviour can be affected by internally and externally generated barriers. Internal barriers include fear, uncertainty and denial that there may be further interruptions to their lives as a result of a worsening of their condition. These barriers appear to be equally as important for people with MND, regardless of which information-seeking category they occupy.

Media coverage and unscreened information

It is likely that unsolicited information, often in the form of media coverage, will always have a negative effect on people with MND, regardless of their information-seeking characteristics, as there is a much increased likelihood of encountering details about someone with more advanced disease. One participant, who had previously actively sought information about the illness, was distressed at reading a newspaper article about a local man with MND because she felt that the story had invaded her personal space in a threatening way:

'It did upset me, because the man had been a big strapping man…and not long after he had been diagnosed with MND he died…when it's staring you in the face…I don't like that' (Elsie).

Although she avoided exposure to MND-related issues within some elements of the media, Dorothy did read some articles about MND in magazines as she came across them. However, she came to realize that it was not beneficial to her situation to continue to read them:

'It just seemed to frighten me reading them in the end because there is always an unhappy ending' (Dorothy).

One participant was badly affected after he read a leaflet intended for his wife, his 'buffer', which stated that the average life expectancy in MND was 2–5 years:

'It's a bit of a shock when you see [statistics] in black and white…that set me thinking…it had an adverse effect on me…definitely' (Bob).

Anticipation of exposure to unwanted information can shape behaviour. Participants reported avoiding newspaper and magazine articles as well as television coverage:

'If I read in the paper that someone with MND had their story, I wouldn't want to see it…most definitely wouldn't want to see it' (Elsie).

'I just turn it off, I don't want to know, I don't want worrying…it brings you down' (Gwen).

MND-related media campaigns can seek to advance the cause of particular individuals, raise awareness of the illness and its management or highlight attempts to identify the cause and potential treatments for this distressing disease. While it is recognized that media campaigns also have the potential to generate fear among people with MND (Green, 2003), they have not previously been approached for their views on the effect of their exposure to such campaigns. Fred had been diagnosed with MND when the Diane Pretty case was at its height in the UK and was unable to avoid exposure to information about the illness because of the media campaign associated with the case:

> *'All I knew about it [MND] was what I'd seen of that woman [Diane Pretty] on the television that wanted to die and that was really frightening'* (Fred).

Diane Pretty, a 42-year-old woman with MND, undertook the first legal challenge to the British law on assisted suicide in 2001, in an attempt to protect her husband from prosecution if he were to aid her death. The campaign associated with the case attracted national media coverage and brought the fate of people with MND into the public domain. It stressed the terminal nature of the illness, but also highlighted elements of suffering that most people with MND would not experience (Wilson, 2001).

Even if the person is unaffected by such unsolicited information, he or she can recognize that others could be:

> *'That lady [Diane Pretty] would do a lot of damage to people with MND in its early stages…because they could see what they may come to'* (Cath).

These findings are similar to other work (Leydon et al, 2000), which found that people with cancer could have difficulty avoiding information, particularly when faced with emotive media coverage and attention-grabbing headlines.

Conclusion

The participants in this study had similar characteristics and displayed similar attitudes to information seeking and avoidance as others with neurological illness, such as MS and PD, as well as those with malignant terminal illness. They displayed characteristics of information avoiders, reluctant to seek information about their condition out of fear for what it may mean to their future, or active seekers of information, determined to know what lies ahead in an effort to prepare for future problems. Selective seekers of information can have a foot in both camps. As was the case with people with PD (Pinder, 1990), while three distinct categories emerged, they were not static; respondents moved between categories over the duration of their illness, depending on their personal circumstances at the time.

These findings would indicate a need for nurses to identify the information requirements of individual patients at the time of their diagnosis, to enable them to be offered sufficient appropriate information at that time. There is also a need to check routinely which of the three information-seeking modes a person is situated in at any given time so that they may be appropriately supported. It is also important for any health or social care professional involved in the provision of care or services for people with MND to recognize that they may differ from each other in the type and amount of information that they require at different stages of the illness — they do not always want detailed information about their illness and they may even want to be protected from it. When they require information, however, it should be made available, but the appropriateness and suitability should always be checked after information has been given.

This study recognizes the contribution of 'buffers' who screen information on behalf of the person with MND. Most significantly, it draws attention to the importance of recognizing the effects of unsolicited information on people with MND, an area not previously studied. It has implications for those using the media when striving to increase publicity for their cause or raise awareness of the effects of the disease as, paradoxically, they may be adversely affecting the very people they are trying to help. The study also raises important questions about the promotion and preservation of autonomy and informed decision-making among people with MND.

The author would like to acknowledge the study participants and the neuroscience directorate at the Royal Preston Hospital where she was employed when the study was undertaken.

References

Baker L (1994) Monitors and blunters: patient health information seeking from a different perspective. *Bibliotheca Medica Canadiana* **16**: 60–3

Baker L (1995) A new method for studying patient information needs and information-seeking behaviour. *Top Health Inf Manage* **16**(2): 19–28

Baker L (1998) Sense making in multiple sclerosis: the information needs of people during an acute exacerbation. *Qual Health Res* **8**(1): 106–20

Bennenbroek F, Buunk B, van der Zee K, Grol B (2002) Social comparison and patient information: what do cancer patients want? *Patient Educ Couns* **47**: 5–12

Benson J, Britten N (1996) Respecting the autonomy of cancer patients when talking with their families: qualitative analysis of semistructured interviews with patients. *Br Med J* **313**: 729–31

Bowling A (1997) *Research Methods in Health: Investigating Health and Health Services*. Oxford University Press, London

Crookes P, Davies S (1998) *Research into Practice*. Ballière Tindall, London

Grbich C (1999) *Qualitative Research in Health: An Introduction*. Sage, London

Green R (2003) People with motor neurone disease not helped by media. *Br J Nurs* **12**: 341

Kutner JS, Steiner JF, Corbett KK, Jahnigen DW, Barton PL (1999) Information needs in terminal illness. *Soc Sci Med* **48**: 1341–52

Leigh PN, Ray-Chaudhuri K (1994) Motor neuron disease. *J Neurol Neurosurg Psychiatry* **57**: 886–96

Ley P (1998) *Communication with Patients: Improving Communication, Satisfaction and Compliance*. Croom Helm, London

Leydon G, Boulton M, Moynihan C et al (2000) Cancer patients' information needs and information-seeking behaviour: in-depth interview study. *Br Med J* **320**: 909–13

Luker K, Beaver K, Leinster S, Owens R, Degner L, Sloan J (1995) The information needs of women newly diagnosed with breast cancer. *J Adv Nurs* **22**: 134–41

Meredith C, Symonds P, Webster L et al (1996) Information needs of cancer patients in west Scotland: cross-sectional survey of patients' views. *Br Med J* **313**: 724–6

Pinder R (1990) *The Management of Chronic Illness: Patient and Doctor Perspectives on Parkinson's Disease*. Macmillan Press, Basingstoke

Rose K (1999) A qualitative analysis of the information needs of informal carers of terminally ill cancer patients. *J Clin Nurs* **8**: 81–8

Shaw C (2000) Amyotrophic lateral sclerosis/motor neurone disease: clinical neurology and neurobiology. In: Oliver, D, Borasio GD, Walsh D, eds. *Palliative Care in Amyotrophic Lateral Sclerosis*. OUP, Oxford

Silverstein MD, Stocking CB, Antel JP, Beckwith J, Roos RP, Siegler M (1991) Amyotrophic lateral sclerosis and life-sustaining therapy: patients' desires for information, participation in decision-making and life-sustaining therapy. *Mayo Clin Proc* **66:** 906–13

Smith J, Jarman M, Osborn M (1999) Doing interpretative phenomenological analysis. In: Murray M, Chamberlain K, eds. *Qualitative Health Psychology: Theories and Methods*. Sage, London: 218–40

Taylor S (1986) *Health Psychology*. 1st edn. Random House, New York

Thomas S (1993) Motor neurone disease: a progressive disease requiring a coordinated approach. *Prof Nurs* **8**(9): 583–85

Van der Molen B (1999) Relating information needs to the cancer experience: 1. Information as a key coping strategy. *Eur J Cancer Care* **8:** 238–44

Wilson J (2001) Terminally ill woman fights for right to die. *The Guardian* **21 August**

Chapter 25

Healthcare professionals' knowledge of motor neurone disease

Mary R O'Brien

Motor neurone disease (MND) is a progressive degenerative disease of the nervous system. Average survival time from diagnosis has been estimated at just 14 months (Green, 2003). It is a relatively uncommon illness; there are approximately 6000 people with MND in the UK at any one time (Thomas, 1993). Most individuals diagnosed with MND experience a combination of upper and lower motor neurone degeneration, which can result in progressive weakness of bulbar (related to speech and swallowing), limb, thoracic and abdominal muscles, leading to the development of a number of distressing and disabling symptoms (Leigh and Ray-Chaudhuri, 1994). Sensation, bladder and bowel function are usually unaffected and intellectual function is usually preserved as dementia affects less than 5% of those diagnosed with MND (Shaw, 2000). This results in the majority of people with MND being fully aware of their predicament and the inexorable progression of their disability. The management of MND focuses primarily on symptomatic relief and should involve a range of healthcare professionals within a multidisciplinary team (Howard and Orrell, 2002).

Nurses must base their professional practice on the *Code of Professional Conduct* (Nursing and Midwifery Council (NMC), 2002), which emphasizes their responsibility for ensuring that patients have access to information about their condition that is appropriate to their needs. Similarly, healthcare professionals have a professional obligation to ensure that patients' needs for information about their condition are addressed (Moody, 2003). In order to function effectively within their professional roles and to address patient-related problems, healthcare professionals need to be knowledgeable about the conditions that patients are experiencing (Baker, 1995). Yet as Coulter et al (1999) highlight, patients may not receive sufficient appropriate information about their illness because healthcare professionals themselves may be poorly informed about the condition. Continuing professional development should be undertaken to ensure that healthcare professionals keep themselves updated and informed. This is particularly pertinent when they are involved with a patient whose medical condition is uncommon.

Healthcare professionals may be approached by people diagnosed with MND for information about their illness and for answers to questions about their condition. As MND is a relatively rare condition, healthcare professionals with irregular involvement with the illness may not feel sufficiently informed or experienced about it themselves to address the concerns of patients and their families. It was seen as vital to assess the knowledge of healthcare professionals who are likely to be involved in providing services for people with MND, in order to ensure that they are fully informed regarding the disease and its management, so that they may provide appropriate and effective assistance to patients following diagnosis. No previous work has been undertaken to assess the specific information needs and information-seeking behaviour of healthcare professionals in relation to MND. This study set out to address this gap in the literature by investigating the level of knowledge and understanding about MND among a group of healthcare professionals who were at the time, or had recently been, involved in the management of a person with MND.

Method

Participants

Healthcare professionals who were currently providing, or had recently provided, services for people with MND were identified from care plans at a nurse-led UK MND clinic. A self-administered postal questionnaire was sent to a random cross-section of 100 of these healthcare professionals. Ethical approval for the study was obtained from the local research ethics committee before administering the questionnaire. As the management of MND crosses primary and secondary care boundaries, healthcare professionals in both health sectors were approached. Fifty-eight questionnaires sent out were to community-based healthcare professionals. A pre-paid reply envelope was included to encourage response, and participants were requested to return the questionnaire within 3 weeks to avoid delays in analysis. Returned questionnaires bore no identifying marks to ensure participants' anonymity. The overall response rate of 65% was composed of 41 (63%) community-based respondents, 22 (34%) hospital-based respondents and 2 (3%) respondents who split their time equally between hospital and community (*Table 25.1*).

Table 25.1: Response rate by professional group and location

Profession	Hospital	Community	50–50 split	Total sample	
GP (*n*=20)	0	12	0	12	19%
Nurse (*n*=14)	3	6	0	9	14%
SLT (*n*=18)	11	2	1	14	22%
OT (*n*=24)	4	13	0	17	26%
Physiotherapist (*n*=10)	1	5	0	6	9%
Dietitian (*n*=14)	3	3	1	7	11%
Total (n=100)	22 (34%)	41 (63%)	2 (3%)	65	

Number of questionnaires sent out in brackets
SLT=speech and language therapist; OT=occupational therapist

The total sample targeted (*n*=100) comprised 20 GPs, 14 nurses, 18 speech and language therapists, 24 occupational therapists, 10 physiotherapists and 14 dietitians. Within each professional group the response rate was as follows: 12 (60%) GPs, nine (64%) nurses, 14 (78%) speech and language therapists, 17 (71%) occupational therapists, six (60%) physiotherapists, and seven (50%) dietitians.

Measures

The questionnaire was developed in consultation with a university-based academic and healthcare professionals with an understanding of the topic in an attempt to ensure face and content validity. Questionnaire responses were discussed with healthcare professionals within the target sample in an effort to assure the validity of the findings. The questionnaire consisted mostly of closed questions with precoded response categories for ease of analysis. Five-point Likert scales were incorporated into the questionnaire for ease of analysis, administration and interpretation (Bowling, 1997). Self-administered questionnaires should ideally be restricted to closed questions, as it is felt that many respondents would not take the time to write their own replies to a series of open questions that may not be self-explanatory, with the result that response rates may be adversely affected (Bourque and Fielder, 1995).

Participants were initially asked to indicate their professional orientation and to state whether they were hospital or community based. This was in order to determine if the respondents were representative of the population of healthcare professionals who would be expected to be involved in the provision of care for people with MND. Respondents were then asked to rate their knowledge of the disease processes in MND and their profession's contribution to the management of MND. In an attempt to identify the most valuable sources of information for these professional groups, participants were asked to indicate from where they had obtained information and to identify which information source was most useful to them. Finally, respondents were asked to rate if they felt that their overall knowledge of MND was adequate. It is recognized, particularly when asking people about their knowledge, that open-ended questions are preferable in order to gain the individual's specific perspective and for probing topics in more depth for explanation and clarification (Bowling, 1997). Space was therefore included for open text for respondents to elaborate and provide individual comments about the subject if they wished.

Analysis

Data obtained from the returned questionnaires were subject to analysis using the Statistical Package for the Social Sciences (SPSS). Descriptive statistics were obtained to describe the frequency with which findings occurred. All responses were initially analysed to describe the features of the group as a whole. Each professional group's responses were then subjected to descriptive analysis and the output organized by variable. The responses to each question were examined to identify if any patterns existed among the professional groups regarding their information seeking and the adequacy of the participants' knowledge of MND.

Results

The results are presented as a percentage response rate for the sample as a whole; however, when reference is made to individual professional group preferences, the actual number of respondents is shown, as these subsample sizes were too small to be subjected to statistical analysis.

Over 89% of all respondents rated their knowledge of the disease processes in MND as average or above. Seven respondents (11%) (three GPs, three nurses and one dietitian) rated their personal knowledge of MND as poor (*Figure 25.1*).

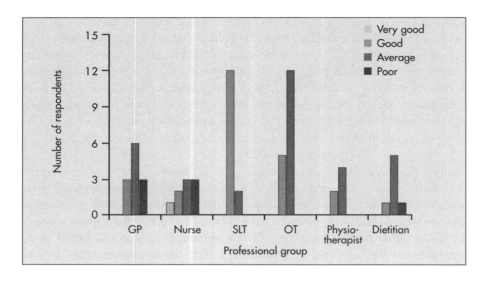

Figure 25.1: Current knowledge of disease processes in motor neurone disease by professional group. SLT=speech and language therapist; OT=occupational therapist

When asked to rate their knowledge of their own profession's contribution to the management of MND, 94% of respondents rated it as average or above. Three GPs and one dietitian admitted to having a poor understanding of their profession's role in the management of MND (*Figure 25.2*).

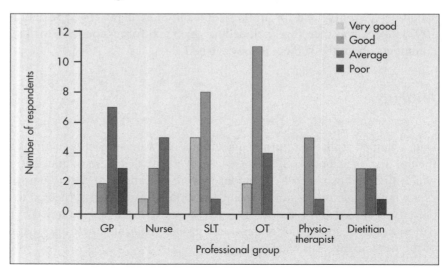

Figure 25.2: Knowledge of own profession's contribution to MND by professional group. SLT=speech and language therapist; OT=occupational therapist

Almost all participants (97%) had actively sought information about MND; the two respondents who had not sought information about the illness were both GPs. Participants in this study had accessed information about MND from a variety of sources (*Figure 25.3*).

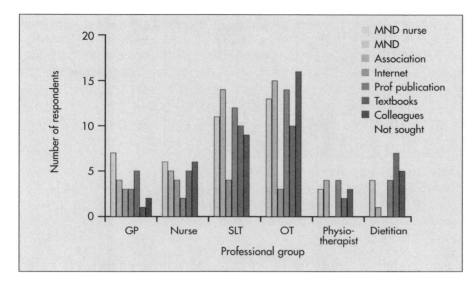

Figure 25.3: Sources of information used by professional group. SLT=speech and language therapist; OT=occupational therapist; MND=motor neurone disease; Prof=professional

Just over 67% of all respondents had obtained information about the illness from a local MND nurse specialist, with most respondents from all but one of the individual professional groups (50% physiotherapists) using this source of information. Many respondents (66%) had sought information from the Motor Neurone Disease Association (the national charity for MND in England, Wales and Northern Ireland). All speech and language therapists and a majority of occupational therapists, physiotherapists and nurses had sought information from the Motor Neurone Disease Association, while just four GPs and one dietitian had done so.

Most respondents (60%) had acquired information about MND from professional publications; however, only three GPs and two nurses had done so. Textbooks were also used as a source of information by 60% of respondents. All dietitians used textbooks for information about MND, while less than half of the GPs, occupational therapists and physiotherapists had used them. Other professional colleagues had been approached for details about MND by 62% of respondents. Within individual professional groups, a majority of dietitians, occupational therapists and nurses plus half of the speech and language therapists and physiotherapists and one GP had approached a colleague for information about the illness. Despite the prominence of the internet in everyday and professional life, electronic information was sought by just 22% of respondents, with no physiotherapists or dietitians reporting use of the internet for details about MND.

Most respondents (45%) rated the Motor Neurone Disease Association as the most useful source of information. A majority of speech and language therapists, occupational therapists and nurses, plus half of the physiotherapists and two GPs rated it so; however, none of the dietitians felt that the Motor Neurone Disease Association was the most useful source of information for them. The MND nurse specialist was rated as the most useful source of information by 26% of respondents, which included a majority of dietitians (*Figure 25.4*).

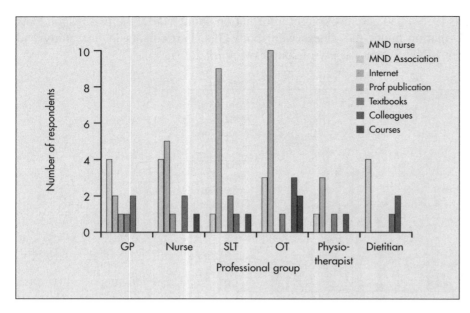

Figure 25.4: Most useful source of information by professional group. SLT=speech and language therapist; OT=occupational therapist; MND=motor neurone disease; Prof=professional

When asked to state their preferred format for information, 55% of respondents favoured written material, followed by 28% who preferred seminars as a means of obtaining information. Only four respondents rated electronic information as the most useful format.

A majority (57%) of all respondents rated their current level of overall knowledge about MND as inadequate. When broken down by individual professional groups, a majority of GPs, nurses, occupational therapists and dietitians felt this way, while a majority of speech and language therapists and physiotherapists regarded their level of knowledge as adequate (*Figure 25.5*).

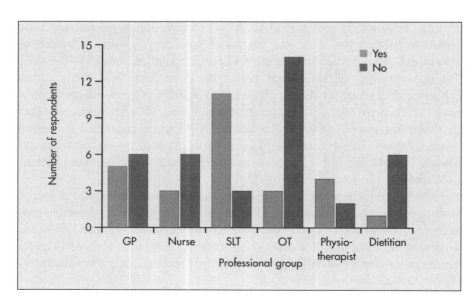

Figure 25.5: Is current level of overall knowledge of motor neurone disease (MND) adequate by professional group? SLT=speech and language therapist; OT=occupational therapist

Discussion

MND is an extremely variable disease, both in its presentation and progression. Thomas (1993) emphasizes the highly specialized nature of the management of the disease, which requires a multidisciplinary approach including input from GPs, nurses, speech and language therapists, occupational therapists, physiotherapists and dietitians, among others. Yet MND is a relatively rare illness with many healthcare professionals never encountering the illness professionally and the average GP only coming across one case during their professional career (Cochrane, 1987). When people with MND do consult healthcare professionals, it is likely to be for advice, support and information about their illness and ways to cope with the resultant disabilities.

This study found that many healthcare professionals were very knowledgeable, not only about the disease processes in MND but also about their own profession's role in the management of the illness. It is interesting to note, however, that while a GP is likely to be the first point of contact within the health service for a person developing MND, four of the 12 GPs who responded regarded their knowledge of the disease processes and their profession's contribution to MND management as poor.

Healthcare professionals in this study sought information from a broad range of sources. The MND nurse specialist was the most accessed source of information, emphasizing the importance of the role and the accessibility of the service. GPs accessed information from the MND nurse specialist more than any other source of information, which echoes Snelgrove and Hughes' (2000) findings of a blunting of the traditional demarcation lines between the professions, where nurses are highly experienced within specialized areas of practice.

The Motor Neurone Disease Association was accessed for information by all professional groups, but especially so by speech and language therapists and occupational therapists. It is important that all professional groups are aware of and access the MND Association, as it produces comprehensive written and visual information as well as funding a range of items used in the management of MND.

Baker (1995) claims that doctors are most likely to seek information from another colleague, while also accessing textbooks, journals and electronic material. This study does not entirely reflect her findings in that only one GP sought information from a colleague, although generally GPs did access textbooks, professional publications and the internet. Nurses in this study adopted similar information-seeking approaches to doctors with the exception of the use of professional publications, which supports Baker's (1995) findings for nurses. Although Baker's (1995) study did not investigate the information-seeking behaviour of other professional groups, in this work it broadly reflects that of doctors.

In order to function effectively within their roles, healthcare professionals require a certain level of knowledge and have a professional duty to ensure that they have acquired an appropriate level of understanding and awareness about illnesses they will encounter in their professional capacity. Healthcare professionals have limited time in which to update their knowledge and pursue professional development. Whatever efforts are made to acquire relevant knowledge should be focused on the sources of information that have been found to be the most useful. Although 62% of respondents in this study had approached a colleague for information about MND, only 9% rated this as the most useful source of information.

Textbooks and professional publications were used by 60% of respondents, yet only 9% and 8%, respectively, regarded them as the most useful source of information. All dietitians accessed information from textbooks, yet only one rated them as the most useful source of information.

Despite their information-seeking activity, 57% of respondents felt that their current level of overall knowledge about MND was inadequate. These findings would suggest that, although the vast majority of the healthcare professionals in this study had actively sought information about MND from a variety of sources, the value of some of the information they acquire is questionable. This has obvious implications for the care provided for people with MND.

This study highlights the need for relevant, specialized, easily accessible information for healthcare professionals on the management of MND. Healthcare professionals with limited time for professional updating about MND should seek information from the sources that were identified in the study as being the most useful, i.e. the Motor Neurone Disease Association and MND nurse specialists, where available.

Nurses have a duty to provide appropriate information to address the needs of their patients (NMC, 2002). Provision of high-quality, reliable information has been shown to have a beneficial effect not only on patients' decision-making and empowerment, but also on their psychological and physical status (Moody, 2003). This is perhaps particularly so when patients are affected by a rare illness, such as MND. People with MND require support, education and information in order to come to terms with the effects of the illness (Thomas, 2001), and often approach nursing staff for answers to their questions. MND nurse specialists can help to meet these needs by ensuring that their knowledge and understanding of the illness is kept up to date in order to provide advice, information and support for patients and their families throughout the course of the illness. Nurse specialists also have a responsibility to ensure that their specialist knowledge is made available to others who may encounter MND infrequently. One example of this is the disease management paradigm produced by an MND nurse working group, which identified key stages in the management of the disease for use by health professionals not familiar with the disease (Royal College of Nursing, 2001).

Limitations

It is recognized that this study has limitations. While the professional groups do broadly reflect the professional involvement that would be expected with MND, the individual subsample sizes were too small to subject to meaningful statistical analysis. The overall response rate of 65% was good for a postal questionnaire, but as respondents had present or previous experience of managing a patient with MND and may have attended special interest groups or multidisciplinary meetings on the subject, the sample may be skewed towards professionals who were more actively involved in acquiring information about the disease. However, as all had or were involved in managing someone with MND, it might be expected that they should be knowledgeable about the disease and their role in its management.

Conclusion

Most healthcare professionals in this study had a good understanding of the disease processes in MND and their professional role in the management of the condition. They sought information from a variety of sources, although in this work the sources used did not entirely reflect the findings from other published work. Although they obtained information from numerous sources, they did not rate much of it as being very useful. With limited time and resources available for healthcare professionals to keep themselves up to date, it is vital that their enquiries are directed to an appropriate source of relevant, useful information.

It would appear that when seeking information about infrequently occurring illnesses, such as MND, that healthcare professionals would gain most from accessing specialist sources of information such as the Motor Neurone Disease Association and MND nurse specialists. Individual MND nurse specialists and the Motor Neurone Disease Association host a number of educational study days and special interest groups for healthcare professionals; attendance at these would provide an ideal opportunity to acquire up-to-date information regarding the illness and the input required by the multidisciplinary team.

References

Baker L (1995) A new method for studying patient information needs and information-seeking patterns. *Top Health Inf Manage* **16**(2): 19–28

Bourque L, Fielder E (1995) *How to Conduct Self-administered and Mail Surveys*. Sage, London

Bowling A (1997) *Research Methods in Health: Investigating Health and Health Services*. Open University Press, Buckingham

Cochrane GM (1987) *The Management of Motor Neurone Disease*. Churchill Livingstone, London

Coulter A, Entwistle V, Gilbert D (1999) Sharing decisions with patients: is the information good enough? *Br Med J* **318**: 318–22

Green R (2003) People with motor neurone disease not helped by media. *Br J Nurs* **12**: 341

Howard RS, Orrell RW (2002) Management of motor neurone disease. *Postgrad Med J* **78**: 736–41

Leigh PN, Ray-Chaudhuri K (1994) Motor neurone disease. *J Neurol Neurosurg Psychiatry* **57**: 886–96

Moody R (2003) Overcoming barriers to delivering information to cancer patients. *Br J Nurs* **12**: 1281–7

Nursing and Midwifery Council (2002) *Code of Professional Conduct*. NMC, London

Royal College of Nursing (2001) *MND Nurse Working Group. A Paradigm for Disease Management in Motor Neurone Disease*. RCN, London

Shaw C (2000) Amyotrophic lateral sclerosis/motor neurone disease: clinical neurology and neurobiology. In: Oliver D, Borasio GD, Walsh D, eds. *Palliative Care in Amyotrophic Lateral Sclerosis*. Oxford University Press, Oxford: 1–19

Snelgrove S, Hughes D (2000) Interprofessional relations between doctors and nurses: perspectives from South Wales. *J Adv Nurs* **31**: 661–7

Thomas S (1993) Motor neurone disease: a progressive disease requiring a coordinated approach. *Prof Nurs* **8**: 583–5

Thomas S (2001) Caring for people with motor neurone disease. *Primary Health Care* **11**(6): 27–30

Useful information

Motor Neurone Disease Association
www.mndassociation.org
Helpline: 08457 626262

Scottish Motor Neurone Disease Association
www.scotmnd.org.uk
Tel: 0141 945 1077

UK MND Networking Group
c/o Jan Clarke, Box 125 National Hospital, Queen Square, London WC1N 3BG
Email: Jan.Clarke@uclh.org
Tel: 0207 676 2026

Chapter 26

Caring for patients with hemiplegia in an arm following a stroke

Rosie Goulding, Debbie Thompson, Chris Beech

The patient's arm affected by hemiplegia is a common problem following a stroke, and it has been estimated that 50–80% of stroke patients experience such a problem (Wade et al, 1985). Despite rehabilitation treatments to an affected arm, permanent and persistent disability may result. Care management of a patient with a hemiplegic arm following a stroke is not the prerogative of one specific discipline in one specific specialty. To provide effective care for such patients, there is a need to understand the problem in its entirety. This is because the term 'hemiplegia', which is defined in clinical practice as paralysis of one side of the body, is a limited physiological description of the effects of a stroke on a person's limb.

Any nurse involved in the care of a patient who has had a cerebrovascular accident (CVA) must possess essential knowledge of the stages, associated symptoms and impact of hemiplegia. Such knowledge ensures that nursing care addresses all the patient's needs, and unnecessary complications may be avoided.

Impaired motor function of an affected arm

A motor impairment to an arm following a stroke may be owing to either:

- Damage to the motor cortex of the brain
- Damage to the descending fibres of the corticospinal tract. If this neurological damage is above motor decussation, the signs and symptoms will be seen in the limb on the opposite side of the body (Carr and Kenny, 1992) (*Figure 26.1*).

The direct consequence of such neurological damage is the loss of motor function to some or all parts of an affected arm, thus causing disability. This loss of motor function may be devastating to a stroke patient, but to understand the potential severity of a patient's loss, the nurse must appreciate the ubiquity of arm function in everyday life. *Table 26.1* provides a general classification of arm function, and from this the effects of motor function loss on normal activities of living may be deduced.

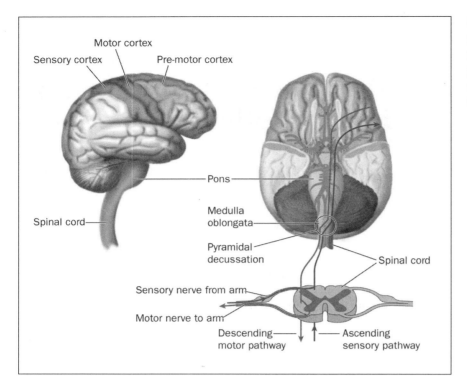

Figure 26.1: Diagrammatic representation of the motor and sensory pathways between the arm and the cerebral cortex

Table 26.1: Normal arm function

- Eating and drinking
- Communication including body language
- Sensory activity, such as touch, temperature changes and pain
- Manipulation
- Attending to personal hygiene
- Locomotion
- Defence and aggression
- Sexual activity

From Davies (1977), Beech (2003)

Stages of hemiplegia

Caillet (1980) suggests that hemiplegia may be a dynamic process in which motor dysfunction progresses in the following two stages:

- Decreased tone (hypotonicity)
- Increased tone (hypertonicity).

The duration and progression of each stage may vary in intensity and duration and an arm may fully or partially recover. Alternatively, following a period of recovery, the arm may again deteriorate. In clinical practice it may be observed that some stroke patients have both stages (increased and decreased tone) present at the same time in different parts of an affected arm.

While the stages of hemiplegia are not necessarily distinct, clinical objectives are aimed at restoring normal movement. The nurse and multidisciplinary team must discuss, advise and recommend possible treatment options with the patient. Then, with the patient's consent, plan care that addresses any abnormal tone that may be present and thus reduce joint misalignment and abnormal movement.

Decreased tone

Caillet (1980) describes decreased tone as the first stage of hemiplegia, which may last less than 24 hours or may continue for months. This stage is characterized by a total loss of deep tendon reflexes, a loss of muscle tone and an inability to initiate motor function. As recovery from the stroke evolves, motor return may occur, but this may not be uniform and the pattern of muscle control may be unbalanced. Any progression may be sudden or gradual and it is an important observation that should be documented in the nursing record. Indeed, as advocated within the *Guidelines for Records and Record Keeping* (Nursing and Midwifery Council, 2002), effective care planning may be impeded if the nursing documentation does not accurately reflect a patient's condition.

Increased tone

Gould and Barnes (2002) suggest that to understand increased tone, a stroke episode should be considered as an upper motor neurone event. This is biologically significant because the brain stem contains the flexor patterns of the arms, which are normally controlled by the premotor cortex. Following a stroke the control of the reflexes are interrupted, thus the flexor patterns may dominate and be observed in an affected arm (*Table 26.2*; see *Figure 26.1*).

Table 26.2: Flexor patterning of a hemiplegic arm

- Shoulder – depressed, protracted
- Humerus – adducted, internally rotated
- Elbow – flexed
- Forearm – pronated
- Wrist – flexed
- Fingers – flexed

From Gould and Barnes (2002)

During stroke recovery if muscle tone returns to the affected arm the hypertonicity present may progressively increase to the extent that it interferes with a person's ability to regain arm function. This is commonly described in clinical practice as spasticity, and because of its deleterious effects professional consensus advocates spasticity prevention through reflex-inhibiting positions of limbs (Carr and Kenny, 1992; Rowat, 2001).

Associated symptoms

Although the term 'hemiplegia' is commonly used in stroke literature to describe an affected arm (Adams et al, 1990; Carr and Kenny, 1992), motor impairment may not be the only physiological effect present in the limb (Gould and Barnes, 2002). A stroke lesion, depending on its location and extent, may also cause sensory deficits. This is because of damage to the somatic sensory cortex or ascending sensory pathways (see *Figure 26.1*). As a result, a patient may experience dysfunction in his or her sensory abilities, such as touch, pain, vibration, temperature and proprioception, which share the same sensory pathways (Gould and Barnes, 2002).

Some stroke patients may experience an unpleasant coldness in the affected arm but may rarely seek medical advice for the symptom (Wanklyn et al, 1995), and therefore it is unfamiliar to healthcare professionals. In a study to examine the symptom, it was postulated that this unfamiliarity among healthcare professionals was because the symptom tended to develop after discharge. This problem, despite its covert nature, may be clinically significant in regards to pressure ulcer risk and may contribute to pressure ulcer development in vulnerable areas of the affected arm. For example, such areas may include the palm of the hand and the axilla. Indeed, one study (Wanklyn et al, 1995) demonstrated that stroke patients with abnormal cold sensations have reduced blood flow and lower skin temperatures in their affected arm. These are recognized intrinsic risk factors for pressure ulcer development (National Institute for Clinical Excellence (NICE), 2003).

A stroke survivor may also experience attention deficits such as neglect (Bowen et al, 2002). Consequently, as a result of damage caused by the stroke lesion, the patient may behave as though everything to one side of a vertical mid-body line does not exist. Such a problem may expose the patient to complications of soft tissue injury, shoulder pain and joint injury. This is because a patient may not comprehend when his or her arm is unsupported. In such circumstances gravity and the arm's weight will have a deleterious effect on the unsupported glenohumeral joint (Joynt, 1992; Gould and Barnes, 2002).

Preventing complications in an affected arm

Table 26.3 lists some common complications that may arise in an affected arm. The aetiology of such complications is diverse and is best dealt with by adopting a multidisciplinary approach where different healthcare professions assist each other and the patient and family to ensure a complete treatment and management care plan.

Table 26.3: Complications that may arise in a hemiplegic arm

- Painful subluxation of the glenohumeral joint
- Pressure trauma
- Oedema
- Coldness
- Pain
- Trauma to the arm from external forces
- Shoulder hand syndrome pain

From Carr and Kenny (1992)

The *National Clinical Guidelines for Stroke* (Royal College of Physicians, 2000) suggest that a multidisciplinary assessment provides the framework for coordinated care. Any nurse providing care for stroke patients must be aware of possible complications arising, and take steps to reduce a patient's exposure to them by working with the patient, family and other healthcare professionals. This view is mirrored within the *National Service Framework for Older People* (Department of Health, 2001). Standard five of this framework is devoted to stroke, and it requires that stroke survivors should be able to participate in a multidisciplinary programme of secondary prevention and rehabilitation.

Nursing care to prevent complications must include pressure ulcer prevention (NICE, 2003). This will include performing frequent skin inspection of the arm to determine the patient's skin tolerance to pressure. A skin inspection will allow a repositioning schedule to be individualized to the patient and avoids ritualistic practice (NICE, 2003). To examine the skin on a patient's palm if the patient's fingers are permanently flexed, gently stroke the back of the affected hand to evoke a primitive hand reflex, which will cause the fingers to extend temporarily. This releases pressure on the palm caused by the fingers and nails and also allows hand hygiene to be performed (Beech, 2003).

Another major component of preventive care is to develop individualized safe-handling techniques of the affected limb. If the patient has hypersensitivity to touch and/or pain in the affected arm, the multidisciplinary team and patient must work together to determine which handling techniques allow the arm to be handled correctly and without discomfort to the patient. This is extremely important.

The Royal College of Physicians (2002) updated its *National Clinical Guidelines for Stroke* and suggested that incorrect handling was a contributing factor in development and/or exacerbation of shoulder pain in stroke patients. As shoulder pain is implicated in poor recovery for the stroke patient, it is an area of great importance for the patient and his or her carers.

The actual cause of shoulder pain is unclear, but it is a common problem following a stroke and may affect up to 80% of stroke survivors in the first 12 months of a stroke (Gould and Barnes, 2002). Although the aetiology of shoulder pain is poorly understood, historically it has been associated with subluxation of the glenohumeral joint. This association is not necessarily established and study findings are contradictory (Gould and Barnes, 2002). Nevertheless, regardless of the ambiguity, the importance of preventing both shoulder pain and subluxation cannot be underestimated. Pain is seen as a very important predictor of poor recovery and associated depression (Turner-Stokes and Jackson, 2002), while subluxation has been linked to poor functional recovery (Hanger et al, 2000). Subsequently, the presence of shoulder pain and subluxation will require ongoing clinical support from many healthcare professions following hospital discharge. Such far-reaching implications arising from pain and subluxation make preventive care strategies the ethical treatment option.

The *National Clinical Guidelines for Stroke* (Royal College of Physicians, 2000) advocated the interventions and strategies listed in *Table 26.4* to prevent shoulder pain arising in the first instance.

Table 26.4: Interventions and strategies to prevent shoulder pain arising

- Avoid the use of overhead arm slings
- Use foam supports
- Use shoulder strapping
- Educate healthcare professionals and family carers about the correct handling of an affected arm
- Develop local guidelines on the care of an affected shoulder

From Royal College of Physicians (2000)

Optimal positioning of an affected arm

Careful positioning of an affected arm is an important element of care for all stroke patients and pervades the stroke literature (Carr and Kenny, 1992; Rowat, 2001; Forster and Young, 2002). Despite the importance of positioning, studies that have specifically looked at the effects of positioning an affected arm have been inconclusive (Dean et al, 2000). (To address some of the ambiguity, funding for a 36-month study to examine the possible effects following treatment positioning of an affected arm was granted in 2001 by The Stroke Association.) *Figure 26.2* shows an unsupported arm and *Figure 26.3* shows incorrect handling — notice the lack of support of the glenohumeral joint (*Figure 26.4*).

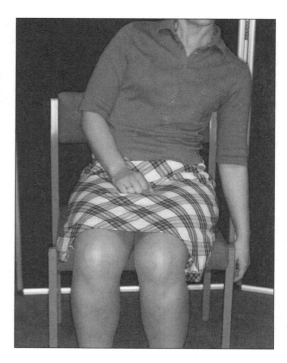

Figure 26.2: An unsupported arm

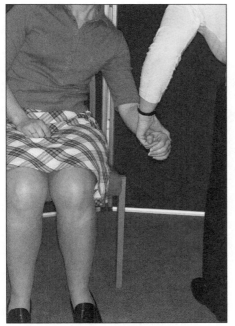

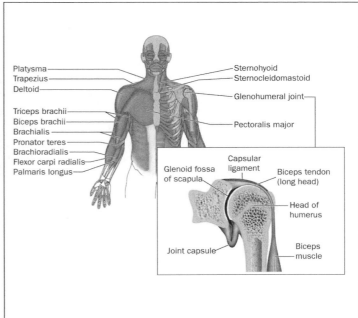

Figure 26.3: Incorrect handling; notice the lack of support of the glenohumeral joint

Figure 26.4: Muscles of the arm, neck and thorax with detail of the glenohumeral joint

There are different positions into which an arm may be placed. Such variation is not without its problems. In a literature review of stroke positioning (Carr and Kenny, 1992), it was identified that there was considerable uncertainty on positioning and also conflicting advice. In the intervening years since the review was published, clinical practice remains undefined and uncertain. In 2001, two studies were published illustrating variety in clinical practice. One study looked at nursing and therapy interventions in the prevention and treatment of post-stroke shoulder pain using a postal questionnaire (Pomeroy and Niven, 2001). The study showed that there were 175 different types of intervention used and a variation in use between different professions.

The second study looked at what nurses and therapists think about the positioning of stroke patients using a postal questionnaire (Rowat, 2001). The study showed a lack of consensus between nurses and therapists in patient positioning and observed that there was a lack of research to guide nursing practice.

Despite the lack of clinical definitions available there are limited studies that demonstrate the importance of correct handling and provide guidance to healthcare professionals. One particular study on handling the shoulder highlighted the importance of supporting the arm beneath the axilla to move the shoulder joint rather than producing the movement from the forearm (Tyson and Chissim, 2002). Another related study advocated the need to maintain external rotation in an affected shoulder if trauma was to be avoided (Zorowitz et al, 1996).

In reviews of stroke literature, the need to ensure the arm is continually supported was a main finding (Carr and Kenny, 1992; Rowat, 2001). This may be done by correctly aligning the glenohumeral joint and correctly positioning the humerus and ensuring the weight of the limb is supported by using appropriate equipment such as wheelchair arm supports (Carr and Kenny, 1992; Turner-Stokes and Jackson, 2002).

Figure 26.5 shows the correct handling — notice the glenohumeral joint is supported before repositioning. If the glenohumeral joint is to be protected throughout the patient's care episode, all members of the multidisciplinary team must possess the various clinical skills required to align and stabilize the glenohumeral joint. The simplest way of observing muscle wasting in the hemiplegic shoulder is to compare the affected side with the unaffected side. If there is any muscle wasting, the contours of the upper arm will be different with obvious decreased muscle bulk, particularly on the outer side (lateral deltoid) aspect of the shoulder. A shoulder exhibiting asymmetry may do so as a result of muscle wasting and from joint malalignment. In this case, the shoulder may look 'lower' on the affected side and may also have a palpable subluxation.

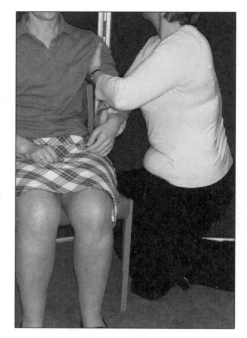

Figure 26.5: Correct handling; notice the glenohumeral joint is supported before repositioning

Tenderness in the hemiplegic shoulder may be present on handling and is particularly noticeable when assisting patients with activities, such as washing and dressing. It is during these activities that pain on movement and a decreased range of movement compared with the other shoulder may be observed. While handling the affected limb there may be a difference in skin temperature, alerting the clinician to a possible peripheral circulation problem.

In summary, many skills required to assess the stability of the shoulder, as summarized in *Table 26.5*, may be done by careful observation of the affected shoulder in relation to the unaffected side.

Table 26.5: Observational skills required to assess the stability of the shoulder

The nurse should be able to observe for:

- Muscle wasting
- Asymmetry
- Swelling and oedema
- Tenderness
- Pain with motion
- Decreased range of motion
- Decreased reflexes
- Peripheral circulation — pulse and skin temperature
- Observation should be bilateral and should include all aspects of the shoulder complex

From Gould and Barnes (2002)

Table 26.5 lists the observational skills and *Table 26.6* describes palpitation skills that the healthcare professional requires to ensure that glenohumeral joint stability is maintained throughout the patient's day according to best practice.

Table 26.6: Palpitation of the glenohumeral joint

- Palpitation should be bilateral
- Findings should be compared with the opposite shoulder
- Using finger breadth palpate the gap between the acromion and the head of humerus

From Gould and Barnes (2002)

Passive non-activity

Many nurses in clinical practice may observe improvement and recovery in stroke patients. This may be owing to a mixture of natural healing, therapy, and medical and nursing interventions. When considering recovery, the concept of rehabilitation is usually advocated. In any rehabilitation service provision the skills and competencies of the multidisciplinary team of healthcare professionals are important in care management programmes. However, predicting a patient's rehabilitation potential is extremely difficult and is limited by professional interpretation of what constitutes rehabilitation. Ideal therapeutic interventions are not yet established in clinical practice, and the measurement of objective patient outcomes on the benefits of rehabilitation is still evolving.

Within a rehabilitation environment it would be erroneous to state that patients will spend the majority of their day in 'intensive therapy' sessions. Indeed, studies have demonstrated that many stroke patients (including those in a rehabilitation environment) spend a large proportion of their recovery period in passive non-activity (Keith and Cowell, 1987; Tinson, 1989; Forster and Young, 2002). In examining non-activity in the context of a hemiplegic arm, one study's findings reported that stroke patients may spend 85% of the day with their affected arm down by their side (Ada et al, 1987).

A more recent study indicates that stroke patients continue to spend long periods in poor positions (Forester et al, 1999). Furthermore, nurses are more likely to adjust a patient's position for a specific nursing intervention, such as administration of medicine, than to review a patient's position and correct poor positioning (Dowsell et al, 2000). Such a position may indicate that the shoulder muscles are shortened and vulnerable to physiological changes that reduce function and recovery potential (Dean et al, 2000). Given the often scarcity of the therapy resource, it is essential that healthcare professionals from all disciplines work collaboratively to share and teach skills and knowledge to ensure that patients' needs are met.

For the stroke patient it is imperative that correct limb and body positioning is maintained 24 hours a day by all members of the multidisciplinary team. Thus, positioning and handling are essential skills that all healthcare professionals who care for stroke patients must have. The skills are particularly relevant to the nursing profession because in the initial period of stroke recovery it is the nursing profession that supports the patient 24 hours a day for 7 days a week. In all circumstances, therefore, it is important that care management plans should be multidisciplinary, and there should be shared learning within the multidisciplinary team of each profession's skills and knowledge. For example, the nursing profession must possess an essential knowledge on reflex-inhibiting limb positioning, and therapists must possess essential nursing knowledge such as pressure ulcer prevention.

It is also important that integrated care management continues in a wider context. Wanklyn et al (1996) reported that patients at home had an increase in shoulder pain in the first few weeks following discharge. Family carers looking after these patients admitted to pulling the hemiplegic arm despite being told not to do so. There is a need for good education for carers, but genuine teaching will only occur if healthcare professions are comfortable and competent with their own correct handling techniques before teaching carers.

Psychological adjustment to the consequences of stroke

The sudden loss of function following a stroke is a traumatic event commonly experienced by stroke patients, but successful recovery is not just about regaining limb function. Psychological adjustment to the consequences of a stroke is poorly understood and research in care interventions is rudimentary. Every person is unique and will react differently to the effects of a stroke, and a patient's reactions may vary over time.

In a recent 4-year study, stroke patients' outcomes were compared when two different therapy approaches were used in rehabilitation programmes (Langhammer and Stanghelle, 2003). Interestingly, the subjects in the study groups experienced similar deterioration in function and increasing dependency. Despite such deterioration, both groups reported experiencing improved quality of life, which is an interesting observation that health professionals need to consider. The study noted that most therapy occurred in the initial 12-month period of the stroke event. After that period, the therapy reduced and remained limited during the remaining study period of 3 years.

The improvement experienced may indicate that subjects had accepted their disability and adapted to their situation. This is an influential finding because it demonstrates that a patient needs to adjust to the impact of a stroke, and that this may occur over an extended period. Determining success in rehabilitation and recovery programmes needs to be considered from the patient's perspective and measured in the context of the patient's experiences and feelings of wellbeing.

Healthcare professionals need to acknowledge that the impact of stroke on a person's life is changeable. Care management must reflect this fact and the multidisciplinary team approach must encompass education on disability. This will ensure that a patient reaches his or her full potential whatever his or her functional outcome.

Conclusion

Arm function is ubiquitous in all aspects of a person's life, and thus a loss of arm function can be devastating to stroke patients. Ethical care of a stroke patient is not the prerogative of one discipline in a specific care environment. To help the stroke patient face the challenges of stroke recovery, all healthcare professionals from all disciplines must share knowledge and work together to ensure that the patient's care needs are met and the patient's quality of life is optimized.

References

Ada L, Ward D, Mackey F, Perrott R, Van Vliet P (1987) Analysis of secondary shoulder dysfunction following stroke. *Australian Synapse (Bulletin of the Australian Physiotherapy Association National Neurology Study Group)* **5:** 19–21

Adams RW, Gadevia SC, Skuse NF (1990) The distribution of muscle weakness in upper motorneuron lesions affecting the lower limb. *Brain* **113:** 1459–76

Beech C (2003) *The Impact of Disability.* Unpublished tutorial. Harvey Besterman Education Centre, Jersey

Bowen A, Lincoln N, Dewey M (2002) Spatial neglect: is rehabilitation effective? *Stroke* **33:** 2728–9

Caillet R (1980) *Shoulder Pain.* FA Davis Company, Philadelphia

Carr EK, Kenny FD (1992) Positioning of the stroke patient: a literature review. *Int J Nurs Stud* **29**(4): 355–70

Davies PR (1977) *Some Significant Aspects of Normal Upper Limb Functions: Joint Replacement in the Upper Limb.* Mechanical Engineering Publications, London

Dean C, Mackey FH, Katrak P (2000) Examination of shoulder positioning after stroke: a randomized controlled pilot trial. *Aust J Physiother* **46:** 35–46

Department of Health (2001) *National Service Framework for Older People.* Department of Health, London

Dowsell G, Dowsell T, Young J (2000) Adjusting stoke patients' poor position: an observational study. *J Adv Nurs* **32:** 286–91

Forester A, Dowsell G, Young J, Wright P, Bagley P (1999) Effect of a physiotherapist-led stroke training programme for nurses. *Age Ageing* **28:** 567–74

Forster A, Young J (2002) *The Clinical Cost Effectiveness of Physiotherapy in the Management of Elderly People Following a Stroke.* Chartered Society of Physiotherapy, London

Gould R, Barnes R (2002) Shoulder and Hemiplegia. emedicine. (http://www.emedicine.Com/Pmr/Topic132.htm) (accessed 16 April 2004)

Hanger HC, Whitewood P, Brown G, Ball MC, Harper J, Cox R, Sainsbury R (2000) A randomized controlled trial of strapping to prevent post-stroke shoulder pain. *Clin Rehabil* **14:** 370–80

Keith RA, Cowell KS (1987) Time use of stroke patients in three rehabilitation hospitals. *Soc Sci Med* **24**(6): 529–33

Langhammer B, Stanghelle JK (2003) Bobath or motor relearning programme? A follow-up one and 4 years post-stroke. *Clin Rehabil* **17:** 731–4

National Institute for Clinical Excellence (2003) *Clinical Practice Guideline for Pressure-Relieving Devices: the Use of Pressure-Relieving Devices (Beds, Mattresses and Overlays) for the Prevention of Pressure Ulcers in Primary and Secondary Care.* NICE, London

Nursing and Midwifery Council (2002) *Guidelines for Records and Record Keeping.* Nursing and Midwifery Council, London

Pomeroy VM, Niven DS (2001) Unpacking the black box of nursing and therapy practice for post-shoulder pain: a precursor to evaluation. *Clin Rehabil* **15:** 67–83

Rowat AM (2001) Issues and innovations in nursing practice: what do nurses and therapists think about the positioning of stroke patients? *J Adv Nurs* **34**(6): 795–803

Royal College of Physicians (2000) *The Intercollegiate Working Party for Stroke: National Clinical Guidelines for Stroke.* Royal College of Physicians, London

Royal College of Physicians (2002) *National Clinical Guidelines for Stroke: Stroke Update 2002*. Royal College of Physicians, London

Tinson DJ (1989) How stroke patients spend their days. *Int Disabil Stud* **11:** 45–9

Turner-Stokes L, Jackson D (2002) Shoulder pain after stroke: a review of the evidence base to inform the development of an integrated care pathway. *Clin Rehabil* **16:** 276–98

Tyson SF, Chissim C (2002) The immediate effect of handling technique on range of movement in the hemiplegic shoulder. *Clin Rehabil* **16:** 137–40

Wade DT, Langton Hewer R, Skilbeck CE, David RM (1985) S*troke: a Critical Approach to Diagnosis, Treatment and Management*. Chapman and Hall, London

Wanklyn P, Forster A, Young J, Mulley CP (1995) Prevalence and associated features of the cold hemiplegic arm. *Stroke* **26:** 1867–70

Wanklyn P, Young J, Forster A (1996) Hemiplegic shoulder pain: natural history and investigation of associated features. *Disabil Rehabil* **18:** 497–502

Zorowitz RD, Hughes MB, Idank D, Ikai T, Johnston MY (1996) Shoulder pain and subluxation after stroke: correlation or coincidence? *Am J Occup Ther* **50:** 194–201

Chapter 27

Thrombolysis for acute ischaemic stroke and the role of the nurse

Maria Fitzpatrick, Jonathan Birns

The importance of specialist management of stroke cannot be overstated. Stroke is common, affecting approximately 150 000 people every year in the UK alone. It is the third leading cause of death and the single largest cause of adult physical disability in the world (Bath and Lees, 2000). Few stroke survivors make a complete recovery: 12–18% are left with speech problems; 25% are unable to walk; 50% have residual weakness; and 24–53% remain dependent on carers for day-to-day activity (Sacco, 1997).

The diagnosis of stroke

Stroke has been defined as rapid onset of focal neurological deficit lasting more than 24 hours, with no apparent cause other than disruption of blood supply to the brain (World Health Organization (WHO), 1989). This clinical definition includes both haemorrhage and infarction and, although still robust, has been refined by the increasing use of neuroimaging in recent years.

Early brain scanning is needed to distinguish other pathology that may mimic stroke, exclude haemorrhage (especially if thrombolysis is being considered) and provide information on the type and location of stroke, all of which may influence early management decisions (Kidwell et al, 2000). Immediate scanning is mandatory if thrombolysis is being considered, not only to exclude cerebral haemorrhage, but also to exclude patients with large infarcts in whom the risk of intracranial haemorrhage increases six-fold if thrombolysed (National Institute of Neurological Disorders and Stroke (NINDS) and Tissue Plasminogen Activator (t-PA) Stroke Study Group, 1997; Larrue et al, 1997).

Early management of stroke

Until relatively recently, stroke was not considered to be a medical emergency and hospitalization was considered to be necessary only for nursing, physiotherapy or social care needs (Wade and Langton Hewer, 1985). This has been changed by evidence of the effectiveness of acute stroke care

(Hacke, 2000; Kalra et al, 2000) and thrombolysis for selected patients (Wardlaw et al, 2003). Management on a specialized acute stroke unit from the time of admission results in 19% more patients being alive and independent at 1 year compared with being managed on a general medical ward, even with specialist stroke team support (Kalra et al, 2000; Evans et al, 2001). Similarly, treatment with thrombolysis within 3 hours of stroke onset results in 30% more patients being alive and independent at 3 months (National Institute of Neurological Disorders and Stroke (NINDS) and Tissue Plasminogen Activator (t-PA) Stroke Study Group, 1995).

A total of 85% of strokes are ischaemic, in which the primary deficit is of impaired blood flow. Part of the blood supply to the brain is occluded either by *in-situ* thrombosis or by embolism from the heart or a more proximal artery. The aim of thrombolytic therapy is to break up the occluding thrombus or embolus and reduce the volume of brain tissue irreversibly damaged (Pereira et al, 2001).

Randomized controlled clinical studies have shown thrombolysis to reduce significantly the number of patients dead or dependent, from 58% in control patients to 53.3% in treated patients (Wardlaw et al, 2003). Thrombolysis within a 3-hour time window results in an additional 141 independent survivors and 130 fewer dependent survivors per 1000 patients treated. Recent evidence suggests that the benefit of tissue plasminogen activator (rt-PA) could extend beyond 3 hours to 6 hours, especially with the use of newer neuroimaging techniques (Schellinger et al, 2004). At present, the thrombolytic agent rt-PA is licensed for the treatment of acute ischaemic stroke within a 3-hour time window from symptom onset. However, the earlier thrombolytic therapy is started, the greater the benefit (Hacke et al, 2004) (*Figure 27.1*) .

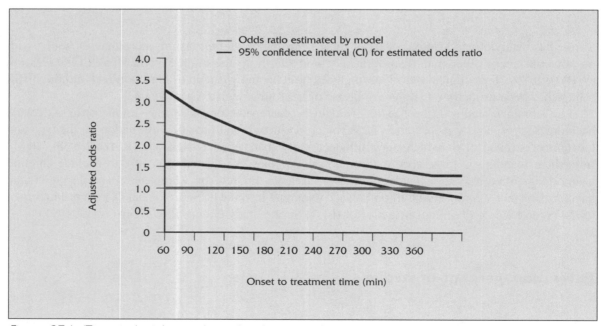

Figure 27.1: 'Time is brain' — relationship between the interval from stroke onset to start of tissue plasminogen activator (rt-PA) treatment with odds ratio for favourable 3-month outcome. From Hacke et al (2004)

Barriers to implementation of acute care

Despite increasing recognition of the importance of timely medical attention in acute stroke management, many stroke patients fail to receive optimal care (Stone, 2002). There is a perception that the vast majority of patients do not present to stroke services early enough to benefit from thrombolysis, mainly because of failure to recognize stroke or to treat it as an emergency (Kwan et al, 2004a).

That this was not true was suggested by a nationwide prospective study conducted in 22 centres across the UK, which showed that 37% of stroke patients presented to accident and emergency (A&E) departments within 3 hours of stroke onset and that 50% were already in the A&E department within 6 hours of stroke onset (Harraf et al, 2002).

However, medical evaluation was undertaken in only 38% of patients within 30 minutes of presentation (optimum time if thrombolysis is being considered) and in 65% of patients within 3 hours of presentation.

In contrast, a nursing evaluation had been completed in 93% of patients within 30 minutes of presentation (Harraf et al, 2002). This suggests that the main barriers to quality acute care were acute stroke not being marked as a priority in emergency departments and a lack of diagnostic facilities or staff trained in acute stroke management (Kwan et al, 2004a). However, the early assessment by nurses suggested that empowering nurses in the recognition and assessment of stroke patients may present an opportunity for implementing thrombolysis.

Optimal management of patients with a suspected stroke

The use of fast-track systems in A&E has been advocated as a method to evaluate rapidly patients presenting with suspected stroke (Kwan et al, 2004b). At King's College Hospital, London, a nurse-led fast-track system exists in the emergency department to identify acute stroke patients appropriately. Using the 'Face Arm Speech Test' stroke identification tool (*Figure 27.2*), nurses trained in acute stroke care examine for facial asymmetry, word-finding or other speech difficulties and limb weakness in order to identify suspected acute stroke (Harbison et al, 2003). This leads to patients being prioritized and a 'nurse's admission time' being communicated to the hospital site manager in order to organize the provision of an acute stroke unit bed.

The fast-track system not only aids speedy transfer to the acute stroke unit but also leads to the initiation of appropriate investigations within the emergency department. This is especially important for those patients who present within a timeframe for thrombolysis for whom a thrombolysis protocol is initiated. This involves emergency department nurses performing venesection, siting cannulae, organizing electrocardiogram (ECG) and computed tomography (CT) brain scanning and alerting the on-call specialist stroke registrar who is available 24 hours a day, 7 days a week. The stroke registrar assesses the patient for a clinical diagnosis of stroke in terms of a measurable acute neurological deficit of power, sensation, coordination, gaze, vision, neglect, inattention and/or language, and examines his or her brain imaging.

Fast-track stroke protocol

Name:_____ Hospital number:_____

Date:_____ DOB:_____ Time:_____

Must be over 18 years old

1. Airway, breathing and circulation assessed and managed appropriately

2. Baseline observations

T_____ P_____ RR_____ BP_____

BM_____ Sats_____ GCS_____

3. Glasgow coma score less than 8 contact A&E doctor immediately

4. Unequal smile/facial asymmetry

5. Weakness of one arm or leg

6. Word finding difficulties/speech problems

If yes to any of 4,5,6 and onset less than 6 hours

Contact stroke team via aircall

Time team called

Time team arrived

Initiate stroke protocol

7. Nurse admission time

8. ECG completed and checked

9. Venflon and bloods taken

FBC

U&E

Glucose

Clotting

10. CT ordered

CT done

11. Inform Acute Stroke Unit staff of admission and requirement for provision

12. Decision to admit time

13. TIA clinic ref

Nurse completing form   Signature

Figure 27.2: Fast-track stroke proforma used by nurses at King's College Hospital, London

In the absence of contraindications to thrombolysis (*Table 27.1*), rt-PA is infused over 1 hour at a dose of 0.9 mg/kg, with 10% of the total dose being given as a bolus over 2 minutes. The decision of whether to administer treatment is always taken for the best interests of the patient and, where possible, consent for treatment is obtained from the patient and assent is obtained from the next of kin.

Table 27.1: Contraindications to thrombolysis for stroke

- Symptoms rapidly improving
- History consistent with subarachnoid haemorrhage
- History of previous intracranial haemorrhage
- History of seizure at stroke onset
- History of arteriovenous malformation or aneurysm
- History of stroke or head injury in the past 3 months
- Major surgery or trauma in the past 14 days
- History of gastrointestinal bleeding, liver disease or varices
- Evidence of active internal bleeding
- Pregnancy
- Current pancreatitis
- Current post-myocardial infarction pericarditis
- Recent lumbar puncture
- Recent arterial puncture at a non-compressible site
- Systolic blood pressure consistently >185 mmHg
- Diastolic blood pressure consistently >110 mmHg
- Haemoglobin <10 g/dl
- Platelets <100x10^9/litre
- Internal normalized ratio (INR) >1.7
- Glucose <2.7 mmol/litre
- Evidence on brain scanning of: haemorrhage; 1/3 middle cerebral artery territory acute ischaemic change; extensive small vessel disease

---

Nursing guidelines have been developed for the assessment and management of acute stroke patients in areas proven to have a positive impact on outcome. These include swallowing, hydration, nutrition, glucose and temperature control, oxygenation, positioning and prevention of complications of bed rest (Royal College of Physicians, 2002). In addition, for those patients thrombolysed for acute ischaemic stroke, specific nursing guidelines exist with regard to blood pressure monitoring and control, neurological observations and identification of symptoms or signs of haemorrhage.

With regard to blood pressure (BP) monitoring, the local guidelines require BP to be measured every 15 minutes for the first 2 hours of treatment, then every 30 minutes for 6 hours and then every hour for 18 hours. If systolic BP is greater than 180 mmHg or diastolic BP is greater than 105 mmHg on two readings 5–10 minutes apart, the doctor is called to assess the need for antihypertensive therapy and the patient is observed every 15 minutes if on antihypertensive therapy. With regard to neurological observations, the guidelines require observations to be performed whenever BP is measured (Innes and International Stroke Trial (IST-3) Stroke Nurse Collaborative Group, 2003).

All patients given rt-PA have repeat brain scanning 24 hours after thrombolysis, and their outcome is assessed using the modified Rankin scoring system (internationally recognized tool for the assessment of disablity and dependence) (Rankin, 1957) at 1 day, 7 days and 3 months. Furthermore, in line with rt-PA licensing guidelines, these patients are all registered within SITS-MOST (Safe Implementation of Thrombolysis in Stroke MOnitoring STudy, 2004) — an observational study set up to monitor and ensure the safe implementation of thrombolysis for acute ischaemic stroke in clinical practice.

Neuroimaging plays a critical role in acute stroke management, aiding diagnosis and decisions on further investigations and therapy. At King's College Hospital, London, CT brain scanning is undertaken in all stroke patients. In patients in whom thrombolysis is clinically indicated, further perfusion scanning is undertaken to assist treatment decisions (*Figure 27.3a,b*).

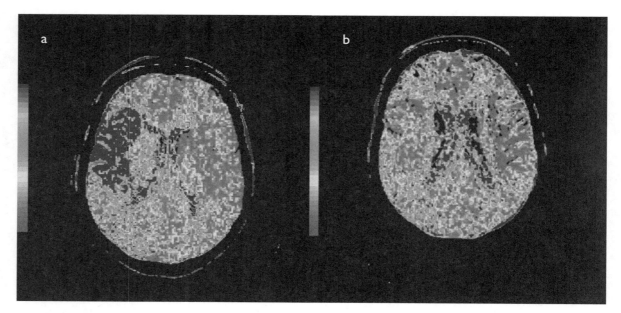

Figure 27.3: (a) Admission perfusion computed tomography (CT) brain scan demonstrating increased mean transit time for cerebral blood flow (blue) within the right middle cerebral artery territory compared with normal (red/orange) in a 65-year-old man presenting with acute onset of left-sided sensorimotor deficit, inattention and neglect. (b) Post-thrombolysis perfusion CT brain scanning demonstrating restoration of cerebral blood flow

The role of the specialist nurse in acute stroke care

Specialist nurses have a specific impact on the outcome of patients, playing a major role in patient education and management, and reducing length of stay (Armstrong, 1999). In aiming to ensure stroke as a clinical priority, the *National Service Framework for Older People* (Department of Health, 2001) and the Royal College of Physicians' (2002) *National Clinical Guidelines for Stroke* emphasize the need for specialist stroke services comprising staff with appropriate expertise and experience. Such initiatives promoted the introduction of clinical nurse specialists in stroke with crucial roles in ensuring service delivery.

Primary functions of the clinical nurse specialist in acute stroke care include those factors listed in *Table 27.2*.

Table 27.2: Primary functions of the clinical nurse specialist in acute stroke care

---

- Development and implementation of local protocols for acute care and secondary prevention in response to national guidelines
- Directing patient care
- Providing expert consultation
- Acting as a role model, communicator, educator, patient advocate and support mechanism for relatives and carers
- Promoting stroke service user involvement
- Leading a nurse-led follow-up clinic
- Acting on and assessing competencies in stroke care delivery
- Participating in clinical audit locally and nationally

In addition to these responsibilities, the clinical nurse specialist in stroke is crucial to the development of a fast-track service for patients with acute stroke. Fast-track services have been shown to be successful in optimizing the management of acute myocardial infarction and fractured neck of femur in A&E departments (De Bono and Hopkins, 1994; Dinah, 2003). There is a similar need for fast tracking of patients with acute stroke as described above, particularly in view of the potential benefits from thrombolytic treatment for acute ischaemic stroke.

Recognizing this need and development of an evidence-based proposal applicable locally is central to the successful implementation of an efficient stroke thrombolysis service. Developing this service involves meeting with the relevant stakeholders including A&E, neurology and neuroradiology departments, all nursing teams delivering acute stroke care, site and bed management teams and the trust directorate. Identifying logistical barriers to the development of a thrombolysis service is important so that strategies to overcome each problem may be formulated between the stakeholders. Reservations among stakeholders about the introduction of a thrombolysis service in terms of an increase in emergency costs and use of diagnostic facilities need to be weighed up against the potential for reductions in lengths of stay and improvements in clinical outcome with rt-PA.

Stressing the benefits of developing a thrombolysis service in A&E is important not only to patient outcome but also in terms of staff satisfaction and morale, and hospital profile. The clinical nurse specialist is responsible for educating emergency department staff, identifying the stroke nurse champions in acute care settings and liaising between the stakeholders to facilitate the successful implementation of thrombolysis for acute ischaemic stroke. This practice needs to be supported by ongoing educational programmes and assessment of competencies for all staff concerned (Carroll, 2002). Introducing thrombolysis into an existing service may prove challenging, but sustaining people's interest may prove more difficult. Maintaining the initial momentum can be achieved by ongoing publicity of the results of the service and feedback to all staff involved in addition to the continuing educational programmes.

Thrombolysis services at King's College Hospital, London

Thirty patients with acute ischaemic stroke have been thrombolysed with rt-PA at King's College Hospital; 14 of whom in the past 12 months. Of these 14, nine were male, the mean age was 73 years (standard deviation 9 years) and the median premorbid modified Rankin score was 1. The time intervals between these patients' stroke onset, presentation to hospital and subsequent investigation and thrombolytic treatment are shown in *Table 27.3*.

Table 27.3: Time intervals between stroke presentation, investigation and treatment

Interval between	Median time/minutes
Stroke onset and arrival at hospital	58
Stroke onset and brain scanning	145
Stroke onset and tissue plasminogen activator (rt-PA)	203
Arrival in hospital and brain scanning	71
Arrival in hospital and rt-PA	114
Brain scan and rt-PA	38

Some patients were thrombolysed beyond 3 hours after stroke onset on the basis of perfusion mismatch demonstrated by perfusion CT scanning. Using the SITS-MOST global outcome scoring system to assess outcome after rt-PA (1=dead, 2=much worse, 3=worse, 4=unchanged, 5=better, 6=much better), median outcome scores at 1 and 7 days were both 6. No intracerebral haemorrhages occurred, but superficial bleeding or bruising occurred in four individuals. No patient died as a result of rt-PA therapy, but two of the aforementioned patients died within 2 weeks of stroke onset from causes related to stroke severity.

Despite the existence of fast-track systems, audit has shown that a small proportion of patients who may have benefited from thrombolysis are not identified, and there are avoidable delays between presentation of patients and thrombolysis. If the standard is to thrombolyse within 30 minutes of presentation on the assumption that 'time is brain', there is considerable room for improvement in the existing fast-track system, which can be achieved by improving communication, simplifying procedures and empowering frontline staff. The stroke specialist nurse has an important role to play in many of these initiatives.

Conclusions

Thrombolysis is a highly effective treatment for acute ischaemic stroke, but patients need to be identified early and selected carefully. This requires the involvement of several professionals in different clinical, laboratory and imaging settings working within strict time restraints. Organization and coordination of various processes is crucial to the provision of this treatment, and nurses trained in stroke, including the specialist stroke nurse, play a pivotal role in ensuring the time frames are met and services are delivered.

Figure 27.1 *is reprinted from Hacke et al (2004), with permission from Elsevier.*

References

Armstrong P (1999) The role of the clinical nurse specialist. *Nurs Stand* **13**(16): 40–2

Bath PMW, Lees KR (2000) ABC of arterial and venous disease. Acute stroke. *Br Med J* **320**: 920–3

Carroll M (2002) Advance nursing practice. *Nurs Stand* **16**(29): 33–5

De Bono DP, Hopkins A (1994) The management of acute myocardial infarction: guidelines and audit standards. Report of a workshop of the Joint Audit Committee of the British Cardiac Society and the Royal College of Physicians. *J R Coll Physicians Lond* **28**: 312–17

Department of Health (2001) *National Service Framework for Older People*. Department of Health, London

Dinah AF (2003) Reduction of waiting times in A&E following introduction of 'fast-track' scheme for elderly patients with hip fractures. *Injury* **34**: 839–41

Evans A, Perez I, Harraf F, Melbourn A, Steadman J, Donaldson N, Kalra L (2001) Can differences in management processes explain different outcomes between stroke unit and stroke-team care? *Lancet* **358**: 1586–92

Hacke W (2000) A late step in the right direction of stroke care. *Lancet* **356**: 869–70

Hacke W, Donnan G, Fieschi C et al (2004) Association of outcome with early stroke treatment: pooled analysis of ATLANTIS, ECASS and NINDS rt-PA stroke trials. *Lancet* **363**: 768–74

Harbison J, Hossain O, Jenkinson D, Davis J, Louw SJ, Ford GA (2003) Diagnostic accuracy of stroke referrals from primary care, emergency room physicians and ambulance staff using the face arm speech test. *Stroke* **34**: 71–6

Harraf F, Sharma AK, Brown MM, Lees KR, Vass RI, Kalra L (2002) A multicentre observational study of presentation and early assessment of acute stroke. *Br Med J* **325**: 17

Innes K, International Stroke Trial (IST-3) Stroke Nurse Collaborative Group (2003) Thrombolysis for acute ischaemic stroke: core nursing requirements. *Br J Nurs* **12**: 416–24

Kalra L, Evans A, Perez I, Knapp M, Donaldson N, Swift CG (2000) Alternative strategies for stroke care: a prospective randomised controlled trial. *Lancet* **356**: 894–9

Kidwell CS, Villablanca JP, Saver JL (2000) Advances in neuroimaging of acute stroke. *Curr Atheroscler Rep* **2**: 126–35

Kwan J, Hand P, Sandercock P (2004a) A systematic review of barriers to delivery of thrombolysis for acute stroke. *Age Ageing* **33**(2): 116–21

Kwan J, Hand P, Sandercock P (2004b) Improving the efficiency of delivery of thrombolysis for acute stroke: a systematic review. *Q J Med* **97**: 273–9

Larrue V, von Kummer R, del Zoppo G, Bluhmki E (1997) Hemorrhagic transformation in acute ischemic stroke. Potential contributing factors in the European Cooperative Acute Stroke Study. *Stroke* **28**(5): 957–60

National Institute of Neurological Disorders and Stroke (NINDS) and Tissue Plasminogen Activator (t-PA) Stroke Study Group (1995) Tissue plasminogen activator for acute stroke. *N Engl J Med* **333**(24): 1581–7

National Institute of Neurological Disorders and Stroke (NINDS) and Tissue Plasminogen Activator (t-PA) Stroke Study Group (1997) Intracerebral hemorrhage after intravenous t-PA therapy for ischemic stroke. *Stroke* **28**: 2109–18

Pereira AC, Martin PJ, Warburton EA (2001) Thrombolysis in acute ischaemic stroke. *Postgrad Med J* **77**: 166–71

Rankin J (1957) Cerebral vascular accidents in patients over the age of 60: II. Prognosis. *Scott Med J* **2**: 200–15

Royal College of Physicians (2002) *National Clinical Guidelines for Stroke*. Royal College of Physicians, London

Sacco RL (1997) Risk factors, outcomes and stroke subtypes for ischemic stroke. *Neurology* **49**(5 Suppl 4): S39–44

Safe Implementation of Thrombolysis in Stroke Monitoring Study (2004) *Stroke Trials*. The Internet Stroke Center, The Stroke Research Unit, Stockholm, Sweden (http://www.strokecenter.org/trials/TrialDetail.asp?ref=296&browse=acute) (accessed 26 October 2004)

Schellinger PD, Kaste M, Hacke W (2004) An update on thrombolytic therapy for acute stroke. *Curr Opin Neurol* **17**(1): 69–77

Stone S (2002) Stroke units. *Br Med J* **325**: 291–2

Wade DT, Langton Hewer R (1985) Hospital admission for acute stroke: who, for how long and to what effect? *J Epidemiol Commun Health* **39**(4): 347–52

Wardlaw JM, Sandercock PA, Berge E (2003) Thrombolytic therapy with recombinant tissue plasminogen activator for acute ischemic stroke: where do we go from here? A cumulative meta-analysis. *Stroke* **34**(6): 1437–42

World Health Organization (1989) Special report. Stroke — 1989: recommendations on stroke prevention, diagnosis and therapy. *Stroke* **20**: 1407–31

Chapter 28

The use of practice guidelines for urinary incontinence following stroke

Wendy Brooks

Urinary incontinence (UI) is common following stroke. Brittain et al (1999) undertook a review of the literature and reported that 32–79% of hospitalized patients suffered with UI. This is a wide range that may be caused by differences in defining UI and when incontinence is measured (e.g. at admission, at 72 hours or at 1 week). More recently the *National Sentinel Stroke Audit (2001/2002)* reported that 44% of patients who are hospitalized following stroke suffer with UI at 1 week post-event (Intercollegiate Stroke Working Party, 2002).

The impact of UI for patients and their carers is significant and has been shown to have an adverse affect on stroke survival, disability and institutionalization rates (Patel et al, 2001). UI is linked with stroke severity (Burney et al, 1996), and this may explain why it is often associated with poor prognosis. There are also psychological implications for sufferers, and depression is twice as likely in stroke survivors who are incontinent compared with those who are not (Brittain, 1998).

Studies documenting recovery post-stroke report that 25–50% of patients are still suffering from UI on discharge (Ween et al, 1996; Barratt, 2001; Patel et al, 2001); however, little information was given in these studies on the interventions used to promote continence, and this may, in part, account for the variation in the number of patients reported to have regained continence. Gelber et al (1993) investigated causes of UI post-stroke and identified three mechanisms (*Table 28.1*).

Although the causes of incontinence post-stroke are identified, there is currently little stroke-specific research looking at the effectiveness of treatments/interventions; in the absence of such data, it is necessary to draw on the evidence that is available for the treatment of UI generally. Bladder hyperreflexia will cause patients to have urgency/frequency of micturition, and recent reviews indicate that bladder training may be a useful intervention (Roe et al, 2003).

Table 28.1: Causes of urinary incontinence after a stroke

- Disruption of the neuromicturition pathways resulting in bladder hyperreflexia
- Incontinence caused by stroke-related cognitive, language or mobility deficits
- Concurrent neuropathy or medication use resulting in bladder hyporeflexia

From Gelber et al (1993)

Incontinence related to cognitive, language or mobility deficits is often called 'functional incontinence', and strategies such as prompted voiding (Eustice et al, 2003), provision of hand-held urinals (male and female) and advising patients on easy-to-remove clothing (e.g. velcro fly fastenings, loose jogging trousers) may help reduce/eliminate episodes of incontinence.

Bladder hyporeflexia can cause urinary retention and incomplete bladder emptying. Intermittent catheterization is the method of choice for managing unobstructed incomplete bladder emptying, because the common problems associated with long-term indwelling catheters, such as infection, are greatly reduced (Hunt and Whitacker, 1984; Barton, 2000).

Stress incontinence does not occur as a direct consequence of stroke; however, it is fairly common in the elderly female population (Gorton and Stanton, 1998). Weakness of the pelvic floor muscles (or prostatectomy in some men) can result in urine leakage on exertion (standing, coughing, sneezing). Stroke may exacerbate any existing stress incontinence owing to increased weakness, reduced muscle tone and additional mobility problems that may increase the amount of exertion required to move. Pelvic floor exercises have proven beneficial in the treatment of stress incontinence (Bo, 1999). However, a randomized, controlled trial evaluating the effectiveness of a 12-week programme of standardized pelvic floor muscle training in a stroke population failed to demonstrate a significant difference (Tibaek et al, 2004). The lack of significance in this particular study may be related to its small size (n=26).

The *National Clinical Guidelines for Stroke* (Intercollegiate Stroke Working Party, 2004a) specify that all wards and stroke units should have established assessment and management protocols for UI and that there should be active bowel and bladder management from admission. The guidelines do not provide detail on the protocols or treatments to be provided.

The latest *National Sentinel Stroke Organizational Audit* (Intercollegiate Stroke Working Party, 2004b) included all hospitals treating patients with stroke. With a 100% response rate (256 hospitals), results showed that practice guidelines for continence were not available in 19% of stroke units, 29% of rehabilitation units and 55% of all other wards. Where guidelines were available, it is not known what information they contained or how actively they were implemented. This is a cause for concern considering the high incidence of UI post-stroke and the impact that it has both physically and psychologically on sufferers.

This chapter describes how the use of audit and the introduction of practice guidelines improved continence care for stroke patients.

Stroke and incontinence audit

An audit was undertaken in 2001 to ascertain the standard of care for patients with UI following stroke. In the absence of a published, validated audit tool, the literature was reviewed and an audit tool developed locally to compare practice with best evidence. The case notes of 39 consecutively admitted stroke patients were reviewed, and 19 patients (49%) were found to be incontinent.

At this time there was no stroke unit and patients were admitted to various wards. None of the patients audited had documented evidence of a full assessment of their incontinence. There were no care plans for promoting continence (the only care plans available were for catheter care). Eighty-nine per cent of the incontinent patients had an indwelling catheter at some point during their hospital stay. Of the incontinent group, 10 (53%) survived to be discharged from hospital, and three (30%) of these patients regained continence before discharge.

The audit identified that changes were required, and an ideal opportunity to improve care for stroke patients arose with the opening of a stroke rehabilitation unit in 2002. This meant that guidelines (*Figures 28.1–5*) could be implemented and monitored within a focused area.

Nursing intervention	Rationale
All patients admitted to the stroke unit will receive a basic nursing assessment within 24 hours of admission	To identify patients who are incontinent of urine
All patients will have their urine tested with Nephur 6 dipstix within 24 hours of admission	To identify positive reaction to leucocytes, nitrites and protein which indicate a urinary tract infection
Where there are positive findings for leucocytes, nitrites and protein, a midstream specimen of urine will be sent to the laboratory	To identify appropriate antibiotic treatment
If there are other abnormal findings (e.g. glucose) refer to medical team	Other disease processes may be present
For all patients with urinary incontinence 48-hour monitoring of frequency of fluid intake, fluid output and volumes voided each time will be conducted during the first week (following admission to unit or from onset of urinary incontinence)	To assess the maximum and minimum bladder volumes and maximum and minimum length of time the patient is able to hold on to urine in the bladder during both day and night time. This information will: Affect the timing of bladder training Show if particular times are problematic (e.g. dry during the day but wet at night time) Identify the number of drinks taken
Full assessment of urinary incontinence will be undertaken within a week (following admission to unit or from onset of urinary incontinence)	To identify problems caused by or contributing to urinary incontinence To identify the type of incontinence so that appropriate treatment and management can be initiated
Treatment options will be discussed and agreed with the patient or relevant other person	To promote patient-centred care and reduce anxiety for patient/carer
A plan of care for the treatment and management of urinary incontinence will be documented in the patient's notes within 7 days of admission	To promote continuity of care

Figure 28.1: Urinary incontinence guidelines

Nursing intervention	Rationale
Start bladder retraining at a length of time the patient can manage (based on the frequency volume chart)	This intervention may be useful for urge incontinence (Roe et al, 2003). It encourages the bladder to progressively hold more and more urine until a normal time interval is reached
Body worn pads of appropriate size if required (bearing in mind that this may compound the problem by slowing down access to the toilet/bedpan/bottle)	To provide confidence and comfort until continent
Exclude or reduce caffeine (tea, coffee, Coca-Cola, chocolate) and citrus fruits (oranges, lemons and limes) from the patient's diet (following the explanation and agreement with the patient or relevant other)	These substances may exacerbate symptoms
If the patient reaches a plateau with the bladder retraining programme, discuss with medical staff regarding drugs for urinary frequency (oxybutynin, tolterodine etc.)	This may help the patient to progress further with bladder training

Figure 28.2: Detrusor instability (urge incontinence) guidelines

Nursing intervention	Rationale
Ensure all aids to communication are employed. Nurse call bell within easy reach, printed picture/text cards at bedside if required	To help the patient express elimination needs
Body worn pads and pants of appropriate size if required (bearing in mind that this can sometimes compound the problem if the problem is poor manual dexterity)	To provide confidence and comfort until continent
Hand held urinals (with absorbent gel if required)	Can be used in a bed or chair, may help prevent episodes of incontinence owing to poor mobility. Absorbent gels help to prevent spills
Advice to patient or relevant other on adapted or easy to remove clothing (loose jogging trousers, velcro fly fastening, hold up stockings, wrap around skirts)	To provide quick, easy access to toileting
Frequency volume chart to monitor episodes of incontinence	To monitor progress and aid planning of treatment (patient may be consistently wet at lunch time when staff are giving out meals. Taking the patient to the toilet prior to lunch may solve the problem)
Regular toileting regime, based on results of 48-hour monitoring	Ensures that the patient is given the opportunity to use the toilet on a regular basis

Figure 28.3: Functional incontinence guidelines

Nursing intervention	Rationale
During the acute period, encourage regular toileting. Offer absorbent pads if appropriate	Although the appropriate intervention for stress incontinence is pelvic floor education, the exercises involved require concentration, effort and persistence, as well as the expertise that needs to be learnt by the patient. This would be best initiated after the acute period when some recovery has taken place. Regular toileting will help ensure that the bladder does not become too full, which may make the problem worse
Following the acute period the patient should be assessed for ability to undertake pelvic floor education. If patient is considered able they should be referred to continence adviser for pelvic floor education	Pelvic floor exercise has been shown to be effective in reducing the amount of leakage caused by stress incontinence and may cure this type of incontinence completely (Bo, 1999)
A patient diary recording episodes of wetness should be commenced	This will help monitor progress and highlight activities resulting in wetness

Figure 28.4: Stress incontinence guidelines

Nursing intervention	Rationale
Exclude faecal impaction	The bowel may be causing obstruction to the bladder
Consider drugs that the patient is taking	Some drugs may have an effect on bladder tone resulting in retention
Intermittent catheterization using polyvinyl chloride (PVC) disposable nelaton catheter 2 4 times a day. This may be undertaken by the patient, nurses or carer as appropriate	Less traumatic to urethra than an indwelling catheter Less risk of infection than with an indwelling catheter Preserves normal bladder function of filling/emptying Often acts as a treatment producing normal bladder emptying
In some cases (severe obstruction owing to enlarged prostate or urethral trauma, for example) intermittent catheterization may not be appropriate. In these cases refer to medical staff or appropriate person	An indwelling urethral catheter or suprapubic catheter may need to be inserted if intermittent catheterization cannot be used

Figure 28.5: Urinary retention (with or without overflow incontinence)

Nursing staff (qualified and unqualified) on the stroke unit were asked about their knowledge of urinary incontinence and their confidence in managing it. Many reported that they did not feel confident in assessing patients for UI and found the assessment form complicated and time-consuming. They also admitted a lack of knowledge about the treatments/ interventions for UI. Most of the nurses mentioned lack of time as a factor in preventing them from providing care for patients with UI.

Guidelines for the treatment and management of UI following stroke were developed locally using best evidence and expert opinion. A shorter more simplified continence assessment form was designed, and teaching sessions were provided for all stroke unit staff on incontinence following stroke and the new guidelines and documentation. The changes were well received and nurses found the new documentation easy to use. The continence status of patients was discussed at ward rounds and multidisciplinary team case conferences, with the aim of raising the profile of continence care and prompting assessment and care planning.

A re-audit was undertaken in 2003 to evaluate the effectiveness of the guideline implementation on the standard of care for incontinent stroke patients. Fifty-one casenotes were reviewed and 25 (49%) were found to be incontinent of urine. Non-stroke unit patients were included in the audit.

Sixteen (64%) of the incontinent patients were treated on the stroke unit, compared with nine (36%) on other wards. Eight (32%) patients had a full assessment for UI (all on the stroke unit), and 10 (40%) patients had a plan of care to promote UI (all stroke unit patients). The catheterization rate (indwelling) was 31% (5 out of 16) for the stroke unit and 78% (7 out of 9) on other wards.

Overall in total this means that 48% (12 out of 25) of patients were catheterized. Of the 11 surviving patients who stayed on the stroke unit, nine (82%) regained continence before discharge, and two (18%) patients remained incontinent. Of the four surviving non-stroke unit patients, the outcome of two was unknown (not documented) and two remained incontinent.

Discussion

The audit results indicate that patient care has improved following implementation of practice guidelines for the management and treatment of UI. In the re-audit there appears to be a difference in terms of process and outcome for patients treated on the stroke unit compared with other wards. However, the stroke rehabilitation unit uses specific criteria to select patients who will benefit most from rehabilitation. This means that patients with very mild stroke and transient ischaemic attacks may not stay on the stroke unit, but these patients are less likely to be suffering from UI.

Patients are also unlikely to be treated on the stroke rehabilitation unit if they are unconscious, severely cognitively impaired or unable to participate in active rehabilitation. These patients are most likely to be suffering from UI and are least likely to regain continence (Owen et al, 1995; Patel et al, 2001). Owing to the difference in case mix, it is not useful to make a direct comparison between stroke unit and non-stroke unit care.

It is, however, relevant to compare the 2001 audit with the 2003 audit as they both included consecutive stroke admissions admitted to any ward. The results indicate that improvements are demonstrated between the first and second audit. The overall catheterization rate (on the stroke unit and other wards) had almost halved, with a reduction from 89% to 48%. This can be viewed as a positive outcome.

Indwelling catheterization is the main cause of urinary tract infections (UTIs) (Pinkerman, 1994), the most common hospital-acquired infection, possibly accounting for up to 45% of all hospital-acquired infections (Winn, 1996). Platt et al (1982) identified a three-fold increase in mortality associated with catheter-related UTI. There was a reduction in mortality rate between the two samples from 47% to 40%; however, the sample was too small for this to be a significant finding.

The number of patients who were assessed and had a plan of care was significantly increased on the stroke unit compared with on other wards. This may have been influential in the increase in the percentage of patients regaining continence, which had doubled from 30% to 60%. This indicates that interventions for UI may be effective.

Conclusions and recommendations

The results of this small audit indicate that the implementation of guidelines for the treatment and management of UI post-stroke may be effective in terms of reducing mortality and promoting continence.

In the absence of detailed guidance in national stroke guidelines and a lack of stroke-specific research into treatment of UI post-stroke, practitioners must rely on information that is available generally. This is a time-consuming process and therefore sharing of this information is vital. The recent development of the National Stroke Nursing Forum (www.nationalstrokenursingforum.co.uk) has provided a much-needed resource to enable the sharing of best practice. The guidelines will be available for members to access on the website. Meanwhile, further research is required to investigate the effectiveness of individual treatments and interventions for UI in the stroke population.

References

Barratt JA (2001) Bladder and bowel problems after a stroke. *Rev Clin Gerontol* 12: 253–67

Barton R (2000) Intermittent self-catheterization. *Nurs Stand* 15(9): 47–52

Bo K (1999) Single blind, randomized controlled trial of pelvic floor exercises, electrical stimulation, vaginal cones and no treatment in the management of genuine stress incontinence in women. *Br Med J* 318: 487–93

Brittain K (1998) Urinary symptoms and depression in stroke survivors. *Age Ageing* 27(Suppl 1): 116–17

Brittain K, Peet SM, Potter JF, Castleden CM (1999) Prevalence and management of urinary incontinence in stroke survivors. *Age Ageing* 28(6): 509–11

Burney TL, Senapti M, Desai S, Choudary ST, Badlani GH (1996) Effects of cerebrovascular accident on micturition. *Urol Clin North Am* 23: 483–90

Eustice S, Roe B, Paterson J (2003) *Prompted Voiding for the Management of Urinary Incontinence in Adults*. Cochrane Review. The Cochrane Library 3, Oxford: update software CD002 113

Gelber DA, Good DC, Laven LJ, Verhulst SJ (1993) Causes of urinary incontinence after acute hemispheric stroke. *Stroke* 24(3): 378–82

Gorton E, Stanton S (1998) Urinary incontinence in elderly women. *Eur Urol* 33: 241–7

Hunt GM, Whitacker RH (1984) Intermittent self-catheterization in adults. *Br Med J* 289: 467–8

Intercollegiate Stroke Working Party (2002) *National Sentinel Stroke Audit (2001/2002)*. Royal College of Physicians, London

Intercollegiate Stroke Working Party (2004a) *National Clinical Guidelines for Stroke*. 2nd edn. Royal College of Physicians, London

Intercollegiate Stroke Working Party (2004b) *National Sentinel Stroke Organizational Audit*. Royal College of Physicians, London

Owen DC, Getz PA, Bulla S (1995) A comparison of characteristics of patients with completed stroke: those who achieve continence and those who do not. *Rehabilitation Nurse* **20**(4): 197–203

Patel M, Coshall C, Rudd AG, Wolfe CD (2001) Natural history and effects on 2-year outcomes of urinary incontinence after stroke. *Stroke* **32**(1): 122–7

Pinkerman ML (1994) Indwelling urinary catheters: reducing infection risks. *Nursing* **24**(9): 66

Platt R, Polk B, Murdock B, Rosner B (1982) Mortality associated with nosocomial urinary tract infection. *N Engl J Med* **307**: 367–42

Roe B, Williams K, Palmer M (2003) *Bladder Training for Urinary Incontinence in Adults*. Cochrane Review. The Cochrane Library 3, Oxford: update software

Tibaek S, Jensen R, Lindskov G, Jensen M (2004) Can quality of life be improved by pelvic floor muscle training in women with urinary incontinence after ischaemic stroke? A randomized, controlled and blinded study. *Int Urogynecol J Pelvic Floor Dysfunct* **15**(2): 117–23

Ween J, Alexander M, D'Esposito M, Roberts M (1996) Incontinence after stroke in a rehabilitation setting. *Neurology* **47**: 659–63

Winn C (1996) Catheterization: extending the scope of practice. *Nurs Stand* **10**(52): 49–54

Chapter 29

Patient–professional partnership in spinal cord injury rehabilitation

Glynis Collis Pellatt

Patient-centred care has been advocated by professionals and patients for some time, and this has added to the growing pressure to increase patient empowerment with greater patient involvement and representation in the delivery of health services (Dinsdale, 2002). This has led to policy initiatives such as *The NHS Plan*, which states that patients must have more say in their treatment and more influence over the way the NHS works (Department of Health (DoH), 2000), and a range of structures such as the *National Service Frameworks* and clinical governance have been set up to facilitate these initiatives (Tennant, 2001). The *National Service Framework for Long-Term Conditions* (Department of Health, 2005) is the most recent initiative relevant to spinal cord injury rehabilitation.

The NHS Executive (2000) aims to:

> '...promote patients' involvement in their own health care as active partners with professionals'.

This philosophy has been seen as fundamental to the aim and purpose of rehabilitation in recent years. However, it has been suggested that what limited involvement does occur is often tokenistic, with poor communication between professionals and patients (Nolan et al, 1997).

There are considerable gaps in knowledge about partnerships and empowerment of patients, and gaps in area of patients' experiences of team membership or involvement in decision-making in spinal cord injury rehabilitation. Accordingly, this study aimed to explore and describe patients' and professionals' perceptions and experience of patients' participation in team decision-making processes.

Literature review

A wide range of sources were consulted for the literature review, which spanned the past two decades (1980–2003) as rehabilitation became a specialty in its own right in the 1980s. CINAHL and Ovid were searched for their nursing and rehabilitation emphasis, Medline for medical coverage and EBSCOhost for medical, therapy and social science research. To prevent a North American bias,

British Nursing Index, AMED (Allied and Alternative Medicine Database) and Internurse databases were used. The DoH website (www.dh.gov.uk) was also visited. Key search terms used were 'rehabilitation', 'patient participation', 'partnership', 'involvement', 'power', 'empowerment', 'autonomy' and 'paternalism'.

In spinal cord injury rehabilitation, empowering the individual to direct and plan his or her own care has been advocated as an ultimate goal of successful rehabilitation (Sandstrom et al, 1998). It has been suggested that research on relationships between healthcare professionals and patients and chronic illness has shifted towards viewing the individual as empowered and capable of participating in healthcare decisions (Thorne and Patterson, 1999). However, what research is available comes mostly from other countries, such as the US, with different cultures and healthcare systems. Research into rehabilitation that has been undertaken has tended to focus on stroke care (Enderby, 2002; Gibbon et al, 2002) or the care of older people (Gair and Hartery, 2001; Hudson, 2002). Nolan et al (1997) undertook an extensive review of rehabilitation literature and most of the articles they retrieved were about stroke rehabilitation.

Although it has been proposed that patients should be regarded as co-workers whose contributions to health care are equally important as those of healthcare professionals, there are barriers such as lack of physical resources and funding that prevent this from happening (McLeod, 1995). Team members may carry out decision-making either individually or collectively (Ovretveit, 1995). The patient may or may not be involved in the decision-making process (Sainio and Lauri, 2003) and decision-making may take place on different levels (Roberts, 2002). It has been suggested that professionals may not be willing to facilitate shared decision-making. Suggested reasons for this are cited in *Table 29.1*.

Table 29.1: Possible reasons why health professionals do not facilitate shared decision making

- The balance of power in healthcare relationships is such that participation involves patients who generally have less skill and knowledge than the professionals responsible for making the decision

- Patients are less accountable for the outcome of the decision or have a more self-interested level of involvement than the professionals who carry ultimate responsibility for the decisions. This can create tensions for healthcare professionals

From McLeod (1995); Elwyn et al (1999)

Partnership is a key factor in patient participation (Barr and Threlkeld, 2000). A partnership can be defined as an alliance where people work together in mutual respect (Enehaug, 2000). However, changing to a more participative way of delivering health care requires a change of attitude by healthcare professionals. The paternalistic way in which health care is currently delivered can be accused of fostering passivity and dependence (Coulter, 2002).

The focus of work carried out into the patient's role in decision-making in spinal cord injury rehabilitation has been on the concept of goal planning (Kennedy et al, 1996; McLeod and McLeod, 1996; Foley, 1998; Duff et al, 1999). This is seen to enable patients to take part in rehabilitation planning, but goals may not necessarily be patient-directed (Playford et al, 2000).

Goal setting, however, is only one facet of a more complex issue of what constitutes the patient's role. What limited research has been carried out into patients' perceptions of their role has produced conflicting results, although this may relate to the type of rehabilitation studied — mostly stroke rehabilitation and the care of older people (Gair and Hartery, 2001; Enderby, 2002; Gibbon et al, 2002; Hudson, 2002). Some findings suggest that patients do not expect to be actively involved in the planning and implementation of rehabilitation (Sheppard, 1994; Abbott, 1999). Other work, however, suggests that patients do wish to be actively involved and that they recognize the importance of their input (David, 1995; Brillhart and Johnson, 1997).

The literature review has revealed considerable gaps in knowledge about the role of spinal cord-injured patients in the decision-making process in rehabilitation. The need for research into this issue at this time is twofold (*Table 29.2*). The findings discussed in this chapter constitute one area of a larger study designed to explore patients' and professionals' experience of decision-making by the spinal cord injury rehabilitation team (Pellatt, 2003a,b).

Table 29.2: Need for research

- Current policy initiatives emphasize the need for patient participation in decision-making about their care (DoH, 2000; NHS Executive, 2000). Research evidence is needed to improve ways of meeting policy requirements

- A *National Service Framework* for long-term chronic conditions that includes spinal cord injury has been developed (Department of Health, 2005). Research evidence is needed to inform the framework

---

Method

The study was qualitative as qualitative enquiry is concerned with real-world observations, dilemmas and questions that have emerged from the interplay of the researcher's direct experience, tacit theories and scholarly interests (Marshall and Rossman, 1995). Within this paradigm, an ethnographic approach was adopted. Ethnography is a way of accessing beliefs and practices surrounding the organization and delivery of health care and the experience of illness, allowing them to be viewed in the context in which they occurred (Savage, 2000). A strong autobiographical element drove the scholarly interest in that the researcher has many years' experience of working as a nurse in the specialty. A reflexive approach was taken to bridge the academic–practice gap by questioning the author's practice, values and preconceptions (Pellatt, 2003b). This ongoing critique and self-appraisal is a way of enhancing the rigour of qualitative research (Koch and Harrington, 1998).

Participant sampling

Purposive sampling was used to select key informants who would most facilitate the development of emerging theory (May, 1997). These informants had specific characteristics or knowledge that would add to emerging theory and, therefore, enhance the researcher's understanding of the setting.

Informants were recruited from healthcare professionals and patients in a spinal cord injury unit in the UK. All the professionals were at a level of seniority that involved them in decision-making about patient care, goal planning and discharge planning. *Table 29.3* lists characteristics of the informants.

Table 29.3: Characteristics of informants

- 14 nurses — all female, clinical grades from E grade to clinical nurse specialist
- Five doctors — one female and four male, grades from senior registrar to consultant
- Three occupational therapists — all female, grades from senior grade to superintendent
- Five physiotherapists — three female and two male, grades from senior grade to superintendent
- Two clinical psychologists — one male and one female
- One discharge planning coordinator — male
- Eight patients who had been injured for some years and who had been living at home since their initial injury or attended as outpatients regularly — five male and three female
- 12 patients who were recently injured and were still in their initial hospital inpatient phase — seven male and five female

---

Ethical issues

Ethical approval for the study was obtained from the local research ethics committee. Patients and staff were provided with an information leaflet about the research and a consent form to sign at least a week before the interview. Patients who were physically unable to sign the form gave verbal consent that was witnessed by someone not involved in the research, such as a relative or friend. Acutely ill patients were not approached as they might not have been well enough to give informed consent. Participants were able to withdraw from the study at any time and assured that refusal to participate would not affect their care in any way. All participants were guaranteed confidentiality (Nursing and Midwifery Council (NMC), 2002). For this reason each patient's level of spinal cord injury and professional's grade or gender is not specified in this chapter. For the same reason, the clinical psychologists and discharge planning coordinator are collectively referred to as allied health professionals.

Data collection

Data-collection techniques used were interviews, participant observation and a research diary; however, this chapter focuses on data collected from semistructured interviews. This ethnographic method has been described as 'adjectival ethnography' because it studies descriptive language (Gillibrand and Flynn, 2001). Fielding (2001) points out that ethnography involves a variety of methodological techniques, including formal interviewing. The aim of the interviews was to discover the structures that guided participants' world views (Marshall and Rossman, 1995) and described the cultural knowledge of the informant (Sorrell and Redmond, 1995).

Boyle (1994) suggests that with regard to interviews and observations most ethnographers have a preference for one over the other, and this epistemological preference influences both data collection and analysis. Semistructured interviews enabled issues of importance to the research question to be focused on, and comments made by participants could be probed and clarified. At the same time, participants were able to address issues that they felt to be important (Rose, 1994). The interviews ranged from 20 minutes to 1 hour in length, and all were tape-recorded with the participants' permission.

Data analysis

Data analysis was not a distinct phase of the research, rather the initial analytic process was embedded in the process of recording and analysing interviews (Hammersley and Atkinson, 1995). Each tape was listened to, transcribed *verbatim* in handwriting and then typed up by the researcher. Although a lengthy procedure, it was worthwhile as it facilitated considerable familiarization with the data. Analysis was conducted using 'Webb's osmosis method' (Webb, 1999), whereby conducting the analysis by hand gives a 'feel' for and intimacy with what participants have said and leads to an almost automatic process of analysis. To make the process manageable, files were created using Microsoft Word. Therefore, analysis was a combination of manually coding and storing the categories on computer files instead of paper files.

Analysis was an iterative process, which is an interpretive/interactive field-based approach (Grbich, 1999). It involved sorting through pieces of data to detect and interpret thematic categorizations (Thorne, 2000). The levels of analysis were as described in *Table 29.4*.

Table 29.4: The levels of analysis

- Ongoing preliminary analysis where data were critiqued as they came in to identify gaps in information, and concepts and frames were used to see if they shed any light on the issues in relation to the research question (Grbich, 1999). Hammersley and Atkinson (1995) suggest several readings of the data to become thoroughly familiar with them. This enabled the identification of patterns — anything that was surprising or puzzling, inconsistent or contradictory. For example, on the one hand participation was articulated as being a feature of the rehabilitation process, yet the way participants were saying it happened in practice contradicted the notion of participation that had been suggested in the literature and government policy

- Thematic analysis. Once the picture of the topic was complete, tentative themes were contextualized, examined for typologies and propositions generated (Patton, 1990). A typology that was constructed that represented distinct categories in naturally occurring variations in data (Marshall and Rossman, 1995) was the 'patient participation' typology

- Coding began the analysis and went on throughout it. Coding took place to develop a broad range of themes, typologies, propositions and concepts. Data were checked against these codes to see if they 'fitted' (Silverman, 1993). Care was taken not to force the data into predetermined frames and to ensure that the frames emerged from the data. There are two main types of code: descriptive codes and inferential (pattern) codes (Punch, 1998). The early labels were descriptive codes, which allowed a 'feel' for the data. Later codes were more interpretive and pulled data together into smaller and more meaningful units

---

The data were returned to again and again; as this was occurring simultaneously with data collection, although it was not a grounded theory study, it could be seen as a variant of the constant comparison method. Constant comparison is used by ethnographers to identify categories and instances within the data (Boyle, 1994). In constant comparison, the coded concepts are refined, extended and cross-referenced with the data as a whole and related to each other (Smith and Biley, 1997).

This study used the traditional approach to ethnographic data analysis where the researcher holds pre-existing theoretical interests (that have their origin in theory or research literature) and these interests guide the questions and observations (Boyle, 1994). A sensitizing concept in this study was 'patient participation'. Analysis involved switching backward and forward between the '*etic*' perspective (the researcher's assumptions, ideas, questions and explanations) and the '*emic*' point of view (data generated from participants), and testing the former against the latter (Boyle, 1994). At first the data appeared to indicate that patient participation was something that did or did not happen. However, as the former was tested against the latter, it emerged that there were different levels of patient participation. Participants perceived that participation was happening but they described different levels, ranging from no participation to active participation.

All research methods have their limitations, and in this study, in an attempt to improve the rigour of the research, interpretations of the research were discussed with four participants — two professionals and two patients chosen randomly (Appleton, 1995) who concurred with the researcher's interpretations.

Findings

The aim of this study was to describe and explore patients' and professionals' experience of patient participation in team decision-making processes. During the process of data analysis it emerged that the concept of participation was seen by professionals as implicit to their practice, and most of the professionals felt that they involved patients in decisions. However, the data also identified that there was some inconsistency in this perception of partnership.

Partnership in care is derived mostly from the perspective of healthcare professionals (Wade, 1995). Ikonomidis and Singer (1999) have distinguished between 'hard paternalism', which justifies imposition of values and judgments on people 'for their own good', and 'soft paternalism', which permits interference when individuals are unable to give voluntary consent.

The responses of some participants in this study suggest an open and obvious paternalism, mostly of the 'hard' category. The findings suggest there might be a third category in which both professionals and staff perceive that they are involved in a partnership with patients making the decisions, but in practice this is not actually the case. In this category, participation may in reality be paternalism dressed up like a 'wolf in sheep's clothing', i.e. what appears to be a partnership is actually a relationship in which professionals make decisions for patients.

Data analysis identified a typology of levels of participation that ranged from open paternalism to active participation, as outlined in *Table 29.5*.

Table 29.5: Levels of paternalism

- Open paternalism — power and control lies with professionals, no input by patients
- They tell me what they are doing — patients are told what the professionals have decided
- They can always say no — patients can agree or disagree with the decision
- Making the 'right choice' — patients steered towards the 'right' choice as identified by professionals
- Active participation — patient chooses the course of action

Open paternalism

In a paternalistic model of provider–patient relationships the locus of control is with the provider. The professional is seen as holding the knowledge of what is in the patient's best interest (Fosnaught, 1997). The relationship is a parent–child approach, with the professional taking on the role of guardian (Sabatini, 1998). An occupational therapist in this study observed:

> *'The medical model says that we're in control, we're the ones with the power…and we're the ones with the knowledge.'*

Patients in other studies have stated that they did not feel they were involved in decisions and that they were not asked or listened to with regard to their wishes before treatment decisions were made (Abbott, 1999; Nordgren and Fridlund, 2001); this finding was echoed by some participants in this study:

> *'Sometimes it might be a change of medication…but the first the patient knows is when they are given a different dose'* (Nurse).

> *'Oh, if they came in here and discussed it with me and I didn't agree I'd put my input in and perhaps persuade them otherwise. On ward round yesterday I'm laying practically on my face…and I hear them mumbling behind me and I can't hear them talking'* (Patient).

At this level patients are not involved in decisions; therefore, the power and control lies with the professionals.

They tell me what they are doing

Some patients felt that they were told about decisions that had been made. One patient remarked:

> *'I don't think that you necessarily feel it's being done behind your back.'*

Another patient felt she was told, but only if she asked for information:

'Whereas before I used to take it — that's what I was given, take it, but I'm more likely to ask now.'

The paternalistic approach may be taken because patients are not perceived as being ready or able to take on that decision-making role. One nurse said:

'I think it's difficult initially because they don't know what they need and they don't know what they want.'

The extent of involvement of patients may depend on professionals' perception of their own professional knowledge and their perception of the amount of knowledge patients possess (Mead, 2000). At this level patients have little or no input.

They can always say no

Some participants saw participation as being able to agree or disagree with a decision. This could be construed as some degree of participation; however, Ozer (1999) suggests this is the lowest level of participation, with only 20% patient contribution. One nurse commented:

'At the end of the day it's the patient and they fully have the right to refuse things.'

Patients who did say no felt they had to be assertive to overturn a decision, as one said:

'I'm quite forceful so if I don't want to have anything I don't have it.'

Professionals did not always perceive patients who said no in a positive light. As one allied health professional remarked:

'When a patient says they don't want this, the first thing we do is make judgments upon them.'

Professionals may find it difficult to 'let go' and grant patients autonomy, especially when they do not conform to what the professionals see as the correct course of action (Pill et al, 1999).

Making the 'right' choice

When giving patients information on which to make a decision, there is a danger that the alternatives might not be presented or it may be biased towards a particular option (Jewell, 1996; Holmes-Rovner et al, 2001). Doctors have acknowledged that they normally bias their presentation of facts in order to 'steer' patients into making the decision the doctor thought they ought to make (Elwyn et al, 1999). Findings in this study suggest that some patients are steered towards what the professionals thought was the 'right' choice. One patient recounted an example of this strategy:

'I'll give a little example where its decisions are made with my input, but sometimes they're steered. For example, my doctor looked at my pressure sore and said there might be a few complications in trying to close it surgically and it would be better to let nature take its course. I said fine, good, you're the doctor, you know, you've got years of experience with this. Then on the following visit while consulting with his fellow doctors he said, we're not going to close this surgically because I know [the patient] is very keen, very, very keen to let nature take its course.'

Several professionals recognized that patients might be steered towards certain options. A physiotherapist said:

'I think we have to steer them in a direction.'

One physiotherapist acknowledged the tensions between patient participation and professionals' wishes:

'They tend to be given options and then I suspect it's like a lot of things, we'd like to think we've truly given them options. Now whether they feel that they truly have a choice or whether the way we present the options to them is actually signalling what we would like them to choose, I'm not sure.'

Bottorff et al (2000) call this approach 'pseudochoices' or 'leading choices' that are phrased or offered in a way that supports the professional's agenda.

Active participation

Two patients felt that they had been fully involved in choosing the course of action to take:

'I was involved every step of the way...I was involved in the decision making as to what would happen and I made the choice there.'

'It was a matter of, well, those are the choices; you don't have to decide today, let me know what you think.'

Bottorff et al (2000) describe this approach as letting the patient 'set the pace'. This gives patients time to think about the alternatives and to determine priorities in relation to their individual setting. Braddock et al (1997) outline six criteria for informed decision making (*Table 29.6*). The two patients cited above appear to have experienced this approach to decision making.

Table 29.6: Criteria for informed decision making

- Description of the nature of the decision
- Discussion of alternatives
- Discussion of risks and benefits
- Discussion of related uncertainties
- Assessment of the patient's understanding
- Elicitation of the patient's preference

From Braddock et al (1997)

357

For some patients, active participation can depend on how well the patient is or his or her physical fitness. Being too ill is a reason cited by patients for not participating in decision making (Biley, 1992). An occupational therapist suggested that some patients needed to build up to that stage, whereas others were ready earlier:

'For various reasons it might be that a patient is just not ready to take on that role and needs alot more support and pushing, and some people just take it on automatically...they want to be in control and they want to be in charge.'

So, for some patients full participation might be something that happened immediately, for others it might be a more gradual process. A nurse, however, recognized that pressure from patients for full participation was inevitable:

'With people with more knowledge and more autonomy alot of it is patient-led. You find alot more patients are wanting to take over their own care...they want to get more involved and that's really developing.'

It has been suggested that some patients do not want to be active participants in their care and, therefore, do not want to be fully involved in decision making (Waterworth and Luker, 1990; Caress et al, 1998). In this study, patients did appear to want to have some input into the decision-making process, and professionals espoused a partnership with patients. There were, however, different levels of involvement. At most of the levels of participation, professionals had control over the decision-making process.

The patient as a team member

Unsworth (1996) suggests that the rehabilitation team consists of a wide range of healthcare professionals, and patients may also be included in the team. Participants in this study for the most part articulated the belief that patients are team members. Some patients who had lived with a spinal cord injury for many years felt that their participation as a team member had changed for two reasons:

- The concept of patient involvement in team processes had evolved over time
- They had gained confidence because of their experience of living with a spinal cord injury.

As a patient who had lived with spinal cord injury for 44 years said:

'The whole system seems to have changed and involve the patient much more.'

This sentiment was echoed by a patient with 30 years' experience of spinal cord injury:

'I do this time [feel part of the team] much more this time. I don't feel angry whereas last time I felt angry alot of the time.'

Another patient felt his years of experience enabled him to contribute to the team process:

'*I do feel part of the team. I do feel if I make a suggestion it's heeded. When I had the original injury I was a bit too gobsmacked to, but I've had 28 years of experience of it now. So I feel I am qualified enough to give some input.*'

Being newly injured or unwell is a factor that inhibits participation and team membership. As a patient pointed out:

'*If you're unwell then you can't partake as actively as you'd like to be. But once you've got over the hurdle then to be part of the team helps them to help you to get out again.*'

However, both patients and staff recognized that without the patient there would be no need for the team and therefore assumed that this was evidence for patient membership. One nurse said:

'*Well, an integral part I suppose because if they weren't there I don't suppose there'd be any point in us being here. I think they've got as much to offer as we have to offer.*'

A patient pointed out this fact:

'*Oh yes, well if I wasn't here they wouldn't have much to do would they?*'

There is a great deal in the professional literature about patient-centred care models (Ellis, 1999) and effective team interventions (Scott and Cowen, 1997; Watkins et al, 2001). What does not appear to have been recognized is the fact that if the patients were not there then the team would not be required. It could be argued that this is a fact that is obvious, but at the same time the disability movement is questioning whether there is a role for professionals in the management of disability (Oliver, 1999).

The implications of this reliance on patients for their existence tend not to be contemplated by professionals. It is interesting that in this study professionals and patients bluntly articulated this fact.

Discussion

This study has attempted to explore and describe patients' and professionals' experiences of patient participation in team decision-making processes in spinal cord injury rehabilitation.

Paterson (2001) has identified a type of paternalism where professionals think that patients are making decisions without noticing that all might not be quite as it appears. This research appears to highlight a similar contradiction in that patient participation in team decision-making processes is seen to be both desirable and, by most participants, as something that does happen. However, participation appears to happen rarely as part of an equal partnership.

In the decision-making process, what appears to be participation and partnership between patients and professionals may in reality be different levels of paternalism with professionals in control of the decision-making process at all but one level. However, under current legal and ethical principles, beneficence is no longer adequate — respect for autonomy is seen as vital and that requires patient participation (Deber, 1994).

In acute spinal cord injury care, professionals have more experience and knowledge of rehabilitation, and true equity may be difficult to achieve. When patients had many years experience of living with a spinal cord injury and could be considered as expert patients, their experience was of greater involvement as team members. However, participation still took place on different levels. The pressure for change with regard to patient partnership that is coming from government and patients requires healthcare professionals to consider carefully how they can address those pressures.

When patients are admitted to a spinal cord injury unit, they enter an environment of unequal power relationships, which impact on their rehabilitation. Generally, patients were positive about their experience of care and rehabilitation — some had expressed the relief they felt when they were admitted from a general hospital to the specialist unit where it was apparent that the staff had the expertise to manage their injury and rehabilitation.

In an earlier study of ex-patients of a spinal unit, the rehabilitation programme was seen to be too physicalist and inflexible (Oliver et al, 1988). This appears to have changed as patients and professionals talked about rehabilitation geared to patient goals. Despite this, there still appeared to be issues for some patients surrounding the extent to which they were actually involved in decision making.

The findings from this study suggest that practitioners should examine their own practice to ascertain if they work in an empowering way with patients. The development of a definition of participation would provide a philosophical focus for patients and professionals. This may involve a careful examination of values and beliefs that may be painful. There is scope for research in the form of an action research study to address this issue. Action research uses spiralling reflective cycles to identify a problem in practice and implement a research-based change (Cerinus, 1999). Patients and professionals could jointly identify ways of improving patient participation in the decision-making process, implement a change in practice and evaluate the outcome.

Conclusion

The impact of paternalism, whether overt or covert, can have a considerable impact on the rehabilitation experience for patients. Where the patient–professional relationship is supportive and empowering, it can be a positive experience. One patient described his experience when he was first admitted:

'You felt as though you'd suddenly become part of another family. Staff and the other patients were part of that family and everybody helped each other.'

However, where the relationship does not nurture partnership and equality, it can have a negative effect on the rehabilitation experience for patients. They need the expertise of professionals but may be aware that the ultimate sanction for rebelling or disagreeing with them may be the loss of that expertise. As another patient said:

'You've got to do what they say, you don't get the final decision even as far as going home. If you've had enough you can't just up and go because you don't know if they'll take you back again.'

Ethnography is a means of gaining access to the beliefs and practices of a culture. By exploring the experiences of patients and professionals, this research has provided an insight into current practice to enable values and preconceptions to be questioned. It has gone some way towards highlighting issues for professionals to consider when caring for patients with a spinal cord injury. Spinal cord injury rehabilitation is designed to prepare individuals to live in the community where they will need to make decisions about their health and welfare on a regular basis.

A patient who had sustained a spinal cord injury 30 years ago described leaving the spinal unit as 'like jumping off a cliff'. If a paternalistic approach to rehabilitation is taken by professionals, patients may not develop the problem-solving, decision-making skills that will enable them to survive that leap into the unknown.

References

Abbott S (1999) Planning and implementation of care: the patient's role. *Br J Ther Rehabil* **6**: 398–401

Appleton J (1995) Analysing qualitative interview data: addressing issues of validity and reliability. *J Adv Nurs* **22**: 993–7

Barr J, Threlkeld A (2000) Patient–practitioner collaboration in clinical decision-making. *Physiother Res Int* **59**(4): 254–60

Biley F (1992) Some determinants that affect patient participation in decision-making about nursing care. *J Adv Nurs* **17**: 414–21

Bottorff J, Steele R, Davies B, Porterfield P, Carossino S, Shaw M (2000) Facilitating day-to-day decision-making in palliative care. *Cancer Nurs* **23**(2): 141–50

Boyle J (1994) Styles of ethnography. In: Morse J, ed. *Critical Issues in Qualitative Research Methods*. Sage, Thousand Oaks: 159–85

Braddock C, Fihn S, Levinson W, Jonsen A, Pearlman R (1997) How doctors and patients discuss routine clinical decisions. *J Gen Intern Med* **12**(6): 339–45

Brillhart B, Johnson K (1997) Motivation and the coping process of adults with disabilities: a qualitative study. *Rehabil Nurs* **22**(5): 249–56

Caress A, Luker K, Ackrill P (1998) Patient-sensitive treatment decision-making? Preferences and perceptions in a sample of renal patients. *NT Research* **3**(6): 364–72

Cerinus M (1999) What price research? Good preparation contributes to good performance. *Nurs Stand* **13**(49): 32–7

Coulter A (2002) After Bristol: putting patients at the centre. *Br Med J* **326**: 648–51

David J (1995) Patients' views on rehabilitation. *J Cancer Care* **4**(2): 57–60

Deber R (1994) Physicians in healthcare management: 8. The patient–physician partnership: decision-making, problem solving and the desire to participate. *Can Med Assoc J* **151**(4): 423–7

Department of Health (2000) *The NHS Plan: A Plan for Investment, A Plan for Reform*. The Stationery Office, London

Department of Health (2005) *The National Service Framework for Long-Term Conditions*. DH Publications, London

Dinsdale P (2002) In on the Act. *Nurs Stand* **16**(41): 13

Duff J, Kennedy P, Swalwell E (1999) Clinical audit of physical rehabilitation: patients' views of goal planning. *Clin Psychol Forum* **129**(1): 34–9

Ellis S (1999) The patient-centred care model: holistic/multiprofessional/reflective. *Br J Nurs* **8**: 296–301

Elwyn G, Edwards A, Gwyn R, Grol R (1999) Towards a feasible model for shared decision-making: focus group study with general practice registrars. *Br Med J* **319**: 753–6

Enderby P (2002) Teamworking in community rehabilitation. *J Clin Nurs* **11**: 409–11

Enehaug I (2000) Patient participation requires a change of attitude in health care. *Int J Health Care Qual Assur* **13**(4): 178–81

Fielding N (2001) Ethnography. In: Gilbert N, ed. *Researching Social Life*. 2nd edn. Sage, London: 145–63

Foley A (1998) A review of goal planning in the rehabilitation of the spinal cord-injured person. *J Orthopaed Nurs* **2**(3): 148–52

Fosnaught M (1997) From paternalism to advocacy: patient empowerment. *PT — Magazine of Physical Therapy* **5**(11): 70–7

Gair G, Hartery T (2001) Medical dominance in multidisciplinary teamwork: a case study of discharge decision making in a geriatric assessment unit. *J Nurs Manag* **9**(1): 3–14

Gibbon B, Watkins C, Barer D et al (2002) Can staff attitudes to teamworking in stroke care be improved? *J Adv Nurs* **16**: 354–61

Gillibrand W, Flynn M (2001) Forced externalisation of control in people with diabetes: a qualitative exploratory study. *J Adv Nurs* **34**: 501–10

Grbich C (1999) *Qualitative Research in Health. An Introduction*. Sage, London

Hammersley M, Atkinson P (1995) *Ethnography: Principles in Practice*. 2nd edn. Routledge, London

Holmes-Rovner M, Llewellyn-Thomas H, Entwistle V, Coulter A, O'Connor A, Rovner D (2001) Patient choice modules for summary of clinical effectiveness: a proposal. *Br Med J* **322**: 664–7

Hudson B (2002) Interprofessionality in health and social care: the Achilles heel of partnership? *J Interprof Care* **16**(1): 7–17

Ikonomidis S, Singer P (1999) Autonomy, liberalism and advance care planning. *J Med Ethics* **25**(6): 522–7

Jewell S (1996) Elderly patients' participation in decision making: 1. *Br J Nurs* **5**: 914–32

Kennedy P, Henderson J, Gallagher S (1996) Improving goal attainment with spinal cord injury patients. *J Assoc Qual Health Care* **3**(4): 145–50

Koch T, Harrington A (1998) Reconceptualising rigour: the case for reflexivity. *J Adv Nurs* **4**: 882–90

McLeod E (1995) Patients in interprofessional practice. In: Soothill K, Mackay L, Webb C, eds. *Interprofessional Relations in Health Care*. Edward Arnold, London: 331–48

McLeod G, McLeod L (1996) Evaluation of client and staff satisfaction with a goal planning project implemented with people with spinal cord injuries. *Spinal Cord* **34**: 525–30

Marshall C, Rossman G (1995) *Designing Qualitative Research*. 2nd edn. Sage, Thousand Oaks

May T (1997) *Social Research: Issues, Methods and Process*. 2nd edn. Open University Press, Buckingham

Mead J (2000) Patient partnership. *Physiotherapy* **86**(6): 282–4

NHS Executive (2000) *Patient and Public Involvement in the New NHS*. The Stationery Office, London

Nolan M, Booth A, Nolan J (1997) *New Directions in Rehabilitation: Exploring the Nursing Contribution*. ENB, London

Nordgren S, Fridlund B (2001) Patients' perceptions of self-determination as expressed in the context of care. *J Adv Nurs* **35**: 117–25

Nursing and Midwifery Council (2002) *Code of Professional Conduct*. NMC, London

Oliver M (1999) The disability movement and the professions. *Br J Ther Rehabil* **6**: 377–9

Oliver M, Zarb G, Silver J, Moore M, Salisbury V (1988) *Walking into Darkness: The Experience of Spinal Cord Injury*. Macmillan, Basingstoke

Ovretveit J (1995) Team decision-making. *J Interprof Care* **9**(1): 41–51

Ozer M (1999) Patient participation in the management of stroke rehabilitation. *Topics Stroke Rehab* **6**(1): 43–59

Paterson B (2001) Myth of empowerment in chronic illness. *J Adv Nurs* **34**: 574–81

Patton M (1990) *Qualitative Evaluation and Research Methods*. 2nd edn. Sage, Newbury Park

Pellatt G (2003a) Perceptions of the nursing role in spinal cord injury rehabilitation. *Br J Nurs* **12**(5): 292–9

Pellatt G (2003b) Ethnography and reflexivity: emotions and feelings in fieldwork. *Nurse Res* **10**(3): 28–37

Pill R, Rees M, Stott N, Rollnick S (1999) Can nurses learn to let go? Issues arising from an intervention designed to improve patients' involvement in their own care. *J Adv Nurs* **29**: 1492–9

Playford E, Dawson L, Limbert V, Smith V, Ward C, Wells R (2000) Goal setting in rehabilitation: report of a workshop to explore professionals' perceptions of goal setting. *Clin Rehabil* **14**(5): 491–7

Punch K (1998) *Introduction to Social Research: Quantitative and Qualitative Approaches*. Sage, London

Roberts K (2002) Exploring participation: older people on discharge from hospital. *J Adv Nurs* **40**: 413–20

Rose K (1994) Unstructured and semi-structured interviewing. *Nurse Res* **1**(3): 23–32

Sabatini M (1998) Healthcare ethics: models of the provider–patient relationship. *Dermatol Nurs* **10**(3): 201–5

Sainio C, Lauri S (2003) Cancer patients' decision-making regarding treatment and nursing care. *J Adv Nurs* **41**: 250–60

Sandstrom R, Burgess A, Coffel M (1998) Measuring empowerment of individuals with spinal cord injury: preliminary results. *J Rehab Outcome Measures* **2**(5): 25–9

Savage J (2000) Ethnography and health care. *Br Med J* **321**: 1400–2

Scott E, Cowen B (1997) Multidisciplinary collaborative care planning. *Nurs Stand* **21**(1): 39–42

Sheppard B (1994) Patients' views of rehabilitation. *Nurs Stand* **9**(10): 27–30

Silverman D (1993) *Interpreting Qualitative Data*. Sage, London

Smith K, Biley F (1997) Understanding grounded theory: principles and evaluation. *Nurse Res* **4**(3): 17–29

Sorrell J, Redmond G (1995) Interviews in qualitative research: differing approaches for ethnographic and phenomenological studies. *J Adv Nurs* **21:** 1117–22

Tennant R (2001) The patient's voice in primary care. *Pract Nursing* **12**(4): 126–8

Thorne S (2000) Data analysis in qualitative research. *Evidence-Based Nursing* **3**(1): 68–70

Thorne S, Patterson B (1999) Review: research on chronic illness has shifted towards viewing the individual as empowered and a partner in the health management process. *Evidence-Based Nursing* **2**(1): 30

Unsworth C (1996) Team decision-making in rehabilitation: a commentary. *Am J Phys Med Rehabil* **75**(6): 483–6

Wade S (1995) Partnership in care: a critical review. *Nurs Stand* **9**(48): 29–32

Waterworth S, Luker K (1990) Reluctant collaborators: do patients want to be involved in decisions concerning care? *J Adv Nurs* **15:** 971–6

Watkins C, Gibbon B, Leathley M, Cooper H, Barer D (2001) Performing interprofessional research: the example of a team care project. *Nurse Res* **9**(2): 29–48

Webb C (1999) Analysing qualitative data: computerized and other approaches. *J Adv Nurs* **29:** 323–30

Chapter 30

Improving the continuing care for individuals with spinal cord injuries

Sue Williams

Each year in Britain it is estimated that more than 800 people will acquire a spinal cord injury (SCI) (Smith, 1999), indicating the total number of people living with SCI to be over 40 000 (Smith, 1999). The effects of a traumatic cord injury are variable and may be permanent; there is currently no cure, emphasizing the need for effective management to prevent potential complications.

Fifty years ago a diagnosis of SCI was akin to a death sentence. Today, as a result of increased awareness and better management of SCIs and their associated complications from an early stage, life expectancy of patients with SCIs can be equal to that of their fellow citizens (Whiteneck et al, 1993; Clarke et al, 1996).

Before 1990 much of the literature focused on the importance of emergency and acute care, mainly because SCI had been viewed as a 'static' disability (Hammell, 1994). Knowledge of the long-term effects of ageing with a SCI is sparse, and this is mainly because of the fact that healthcare professionals are only just experiencing people 30–50 years post-injury. However, since the 1980s many authors have identified a number of long-term consequences of living with a SCI including an acceleration of the ageing process, which in some instances has resulted in functional decline, indicating an increase in physical dependence (Trieschmann, 1987; Zarb et al, 1990; Whiteneck et al, 1993) (*Tables 30.1* and *30.2*). For many individuals with SCIs, most would appear to develop problems 20 years after injury, suggesting ageing may be related to duration of disability rather than to chronological age (Menter, 1993).

Spinal injuries is a specialist area, and expert advice regarding patients' care and ongoing management is limited outside of specialist units. This problem is recognized by the Spinal Injuries Association (SIA) whose response is set out in *A Charter for Support* (SIA, 1997). The Charter recommends that spinal injuries centres provide a system of open access and ongoing support so that the welfare of individuals with SCI is maintained, and prevention and/or detection of problems is addressed at an earlier stage in order to reduce the chances of hospital admission (SIA, 1997).

Patient review is aimed at assessing the patient holistically. This can include addressing a number of specific issues relating to neurological dysfunction, such as bowel, bladder and sexual dysfunction, as well as social and psychological issues. The review is usually undertaken by a member of the medical team (senior house officer (SHO) to consultant), although the consultant's knowledge and experience within this field is more extensive than the more junior medical staff.

Table 30.1: Age-related changes

Introduction	As individuals with spinal cord injuries age, a number of physiological and social changes occur. Menter (1993) suggests there are three major areas that, although distinct, interweave with each other
Physiological	Loss of muscle mass resulting in decreased strength
	Osteoporosis (resulting from decreased movement and activity), pain and reduced function, increased risk of fractures
	Alteration in skin tissue — more susceptible to development of pressure ulcers
	Deterioration in function of genitourinary and gastrointestinal systems affecting management of continence
	Deterioration in respiratory function (increased risk of pneumonia in higher level lesions)
	Decreased cardiovascular capacity, endocrine changes
	Decreased resistance to infection and increased problems associated with the immune system
Sociological and psychological	Changes in social status as a result of retirement, death of a spouse or parent
	Personal psychological growth may see a shift of values and ethics, resulting in a reduction in the negative impact of the social and physiological changes
	This view has been supported by a number of life-satisfaction surveys, which have highlighted that life satisfaction has been found to increase with advancing years and duration of spinal cord injury (Whalley Hammell, 1994)

Table 30.2: Neurological changes

- Post–traumatic syringomyelia — an ascending myelopathy occurs as a secondary cavitation in spinal cord in at least 4% of patients (Grundy and Swain, 2001). Symptoms may appear as early as 2 months after initial injury, although the average latent period is between 8–9 years (Grundy and Swain, 2001)

- Treatment is often decompression and drainage of the syringomyelic cavity; this helps to relieve pain and reduce symptoms

- Late interventions may result in reduced neurological recovery following surgery. Without any intervention further deterioration could result in a paraplegia becoming a tetraplegia

- Therefore, earlier detection of symptoms is essential to prevent irreversible damage

This fact had become apparent to the nurses working on the spinal unit, who often reported that patients visited the ward following their check-up to seek help and advice relating to specific care issues from the more experienced nursing staff. When challenged as to why they had not discussed this with the doctor in clinic, most reported that the junior doctor lacked practical advice or simply did not ask.

An inhouse audit carried out by the ward manager to identify a profile of admissions and referrals revealed an increasing number of patients were being referred for admission to review or resolve specific issues associated with skin, bladder and bowel problems. Unfortunately, a lack of available beds on the unit often resulted in patients waiting a number of months before being admitted, which again resulted in the development of more complications that sometimes resulted in longer periods in hospital. This not only had financial implications, but also often restricted the availability of admission beds for newly-injured patients.

Nurse-led initiatives

The Government paper *Making a Difference* (Department of Health (DoH), 1999) advocated nurses extend their skills and knowledge and adopt different ways of working, and strongly supported the development of nurse-led initiatives. *The NHS Plan* (DoH, 2000) highlights the challenges that lie ahead and promotes nurses as change agents to improve service and deliver a more patient-centred service. Another significant driver for changing current practices is the implementation of the European working time directive (DoH, 2003). The reduction in junior doctors' working hours may have a significant impact on service delivery. A review undertaken by Richardson and Cunliffe (2003) to identify the accelerated development of nurse-led services highlighted a number of influences, ranging from NHS policy, practice environment, to local need 'service gap'. The author recognized that a service gap was compromising patient care and a solution was sought to rectify the problem.

The proposal

Before embarking on any proposal to introduce a new concept such as a nurse-led clinic, it is beneficial to identify potential barriers to effective change. Lewin's (1951) force-field analysis is a useful model to review these issues (*Table 30.3*), and this was used in preparing the proposal to present to the directorate manager and rehabilitation consultant to gain approval for the project.

Research cites a number of threats to the development and success of nurse-led initiatives, ranging from a lack of funding, poor planning, doctors' reluctance to relinquish aspects of their role (Cable, 1995) and, in some instances, resistance to the new working practices may be experienced. An additional and realistic risk is associated with ineffectiveness in care, resulting in patient complaints and litigation (Miles et al, 2003). This highlights the importance of nurses working within the boundaries of their professional knowledge and competence in line with the *Code of Professional Conduct* (Nursing and Midwifery Council (NMC), 2002). It was discussed and agreed by the specialist nurses to coordinate the six clinics together, thus providing ongoing support and professional development. Richardson and Cunliffe (2003) advocate supervised practice to prevent isolation.

Table 30.3: Force-field analysis

Forces	Forces that push the system towards change are referred to as 'driving' forces, whereas the forces that pull the system away from the change are referred to as the 'restraining' forces. Lewin (1951) maintained that for change to occur, the balance of driving and restraining forces must be altered. The driving forces must be decreased to alter the present state of equilibrium; change will not be possible until this occurs
	The level of resistance to change generally depends on the type of change proposed
Driving forces	Recognizing the need for change: ward manager's initiative
	Lack of resources: lack of beds to facilitate inpatient review
	High incidence of poor clinic attendance
	Developing nurse-led initiatives (DoH, 1999)
	Support from the directorate manager and consultant to trial initiative became a driving force once obtained
Restraining forces	Limited specialist nurses to run clinics
	Limited staffing and financial resources to release nurses from the ward to run clinics
	Threat to status of medical staff

The directorate manager requested that a written proposal with specific objectives be submitted for consideration (*Table 30.4*) as there would obviously be implications for costs and staff. This would also enable effective evaluation of the new service to explore if there was scope to extend it past the 'project' phase.

Table 30.4: Aims and objectives for the clinic

Aim	To provide professional guidance and support for individuals with spinal cord injury
Objective one	To provide advice on ongoing care issues, relating to bladder, bowel and skin problems, and identify and address problems at an earlier stage to prevent hospital admission/or reduce length of hospital inpatient status, as a result of admitting the patient earlier to hospital
Objective two	To identify what additional input from the spinal rehabilitation team is required
Objective three	To assess if a nurse-led service improved attendance figures

Although the consultant in rehabilitation was enthusiastic and keen to support the initiative, the nurse-led clinic sessions would run parallel with the regular 'medical' spinal clinic sessions, as this would use the medical support available when indicated. For example, the specialist nurse could request medical input if patients presented with significant or new changes in neurology status. Following submission of the objectives, a joint meeting with the consultant in rehabilitation and directorate manager was convened to agree the objectives and develop operational policies.

The project

In preparation for the clinics, a number of 'medical' reviews were observed in order to explore how medical staff assessed the patient and what problem-solving approaches were adopted. The approach varied depending on the doctor and his or her level of experience. While more junior doctors asked the patient if there were any specific problems, it appeared that the more experienced doctor structured the questioning around how the patient managed specific aspects of his or her care or if his or her functional abilities had altered. Once again it was evident that there was a lack of a practical problem-solving advice.

Following these sessions, the patient's medical and nursing notes were obtained and reviewed with the consultant to discuss and agree suitable patients that may benefit the most from a nursing review. At this stage previous poor attendees could also be identified, as this would be useful to see if a different approach might improve attendance rates. Once a suitable list was completed, clinic appointment letters were posted, and it was considered important to highlight to the patients that during their appointment they would see the specialist nurse instead of a doctor. To reassure patients, it was also highlighted that should there be a need to see a doctor one would be available at the clinic. Following a meeting with the clinic coordinator, it was requested that if patients cancelled or re-arranged their appointment, the team would be alerted and the patient would be asked if the reason related to being seen by a nurse instead of a doctor.

Once the project was established, the ward manager and discharge liaison sister (G grade) held a series of clinic sessions that commenced in June 2002. Two fortnightly clinics were held that month, and monthly clinics held thereafter until October 2002.

Evaluating the service

The project was evaluated through an audit of patients' comments. Patients were invited to comment on the effectiveness of the nurse-led service.

Objective one

All patients received a holistic nursing assessment, with a focus on specific problem areas (*Table 30.5*).

Table 30.5: Profile of patients' problems (continued on next page)

Problem type	n	Type of input required	Further interventions required	Specialist nurse follow-up	Additional discipline input indicated
Bladder management	10	Advice on bladder control programme Continence products	Referral to urologist (n=6) Liaise with continence services (n=4)	0 All	Urologist (n=6) Continence services (n=4)
Bowel management	7	Advice on bowel management programme/constipation Medication and technique	Follow-up suggested advice	All	
Changes reported in neurological symptoms	8	Medical assessment	CT/MRI scans/X-ray	0	Rehabilitation consultant
Skin problems	9	Treatment of pressure ulcers Referral for seating assessment and review of pressure-relieving cushion Advice on skin care/pressure relief/dietary intake	Progress review of pressure ulcers and seating assessment	All	District nurse ALAC services
Ineffective pain control	4	Discussion on medication and non-pharmacological interventions	Referral to pain team	0	Pain team
Psychological problems	4	Discussion on coping mechanisms	Highlighted problem to GP and requested to clinical psychologists (no outpatient service available for SCI patients)		Clinical psychologist

ALAC=Artificial limb and appliance service; CT/MRI=computer tomography/magnetic resonance imaging; SCI=spinal cord injury; SIA=Spinal Injuries Association

Table 30.5: Profile of patients' problems continued

Problem type	n	Type of input required	Further interventions required	Specialist nurse follow–up	Additional discipline input indicated
Psychological problems *continued*	4	Advice/support of SIA Referral to clinical psychologist	Highlighted problem to GP and requested to clinical psychologists (no outpatient service available for SCI patients)		Clinical psychologist
Sexual dysfunction	2	Discussion on range of treatments available	Referral to SCI sexual dysfunction clinic		
Review of support services	3	Identification review indicated	Discharge liaison sister to review and liaise with local social services/social worker	All at home by discharge liaison sister	Social worker Occupational therapist
Mobility problems	3	Problem-solving approach to address specific problems identified	Referral to physiotherapist for assessment		Physiotherapist
Educational update	31	Advice and education on: — new products — updated practices in management of bladder/bowel and sexual dysfunction — role of SIA			

SCI=spinal cord injury; SIA=Spinal Injuries Association

A number of patients reported that they benefited particularly from the nurse's up-to-date knowledge of specific bowel and bladder problem-solving approaches. In addition, much-needed new and up-to-date written information on a number of issues, such as changes in approaches to bowel management, new products and samples products, e.g. catheters, were distributed to patients for them to assess.

Of the patients reviewed in clinic, a small core particularly benefited from this form of review. These patients all presented with pressure ulcers (grade 3–4). Raghavan et al (2003) highlight pressure ulcers as possibly the commonest medical problem in chronic spinal-injured individuals. While these patients would normally be admitted to the unit for treatment, at the time of this study one of the wards was closed, which prevented this admission. Consequently, management of care was conducted through the outpatients clinics, involving carers to supplement the lack of district nurse input. Within a short timescale, all ulcers had successfully resolved and hospital admission had been averted, much to the patients' delight and at a financial saving to the NHS.

Pressure ulcers and wounds absorb a considerable chunk of the NHS's budget. However, it is difficult to actually cost in financial terms as a number of areas would need to be scrutinized (such as length of hospital stay, uptake of resources, additional nutritional intake and use of topical dressings). In 1994, an independent survey carried out by Touche-Ross estimated the cost to be in the region of £60–420 million. However, more recent research suggests today's cost is closer to £1.4–2.1 billion annually, and constitutes 4% of the total budget (Bennet et al, 2004).

There were also a few isolated episodes where it was discovered that patients still appeared to be waiting for further investigations or treatments. Such delays could have contributed to the patient developing further problems. An audit of patients' comments and responses to the service indicated that patients and carers were both impressed and confident in the care they received from the nurses. All patients declined when asked if they would prefer to see a doctor instead of a nurse.

There are limited outlets where individuals with SCIs can acquire information specific for their condition other than within a specialist unit. Therefore, the SIA peer-support group was invited to the clinic to be available for patients to talk to, and this also received a positive response.

Objective two

The pilot 'nurse-led' clinic sessions have highlighted both the value and need of this service, which now needs to be extended to meet the continuing needs of this group of patients. The profile of patients' problems (see *Table 30.5*) has highlighted the type and level of input required by the patients attending the clinics, and it has also indicated that additional input is required by other members of the interdisciplinary team. The profile of patients' problems revealed a need to involve disciplines such as physiotherapy, occupational therapy and psychology to address these issues. A community-based interdisciplinary team, which incorporates specialist nurses, physiotherapists, occupational therapists and clinical psychologists, is advocated to meet those needs.

Unfortunately, the issue of increasing the number of qualified nurses on the unit will need to be addressed before any existing experienced nurses can be released to facilitate specialist nurse clinics. This is because experience of the kind required to facilitate this type of service can only be obtained through working on a specialist spinal unit.

Objective three

In reviewing outpatients' attendance figures there appeared to be a large percentage of non-attendees within this group of patients. However, despite this a 75% attendance was achieved (*Table 30.6*); in those patients who required further follow-ups at the nurse-led clinic, a 100% attendance record was achieved. In relation to poor attendance figures, some comments made by patients attending the clinic provided a better insight into this issue. A large percentage of patients commented that they never saw the same doctor twice, and they also felt that there was inconsistency in some of the advice given and that the more practical problem-solving advice was severely lacking. When patients usually attend clinic they may be seen by a senior house officer, who has only spent a small time within this specialist field (3 months), or a specialist registrar on rotation within the field of neurosciences.

Table 30.6: Nurse-led clinic

Clinic date	Number of appointments sent out	Number of DNA	Cancellations by patients	Total seen
11 June 2002	11	2	1	8
25 June 2002	5*	0	0	5
23 July 2002	10	2	2**	6
20 August 2002	6	1	0	5
17 September 2002	5***	2	0	3
22 October 2002	4***	0	0	4
Total	*41*	*7*	*3*	*31*

*25 June 2002 only one nurse available for clinic, hence reduced number of patients sent out

**23 July 2002 cancellations owing to patients' holiday commitments

***17 September 2002 and 22 October 2002 morning clinics only, hence reduced number of patients sent out

DNA=did not attend

Although the outpatient facility provides sound expert medical advice, the audit of referrals and admissions revealed that these mainly required nursing management of skin, bladder and bowel problems. It could therefore be argued that if this input was provided by a specialist nurse in clinic then numbers of readmissions may have been considerably reduced.

Benefits of the service

The profile of admissions and readmissions to the unit has indicated that patients during the post-initial injury/rehabilitation phases do continue to require a service from the spinal unit. However, the number of readmissions affects the number of beds available to admit new injuries, and the delay in admitting patients with new injuries can predispose them to acquiring complications as a result of being managed in a non-specialist unit, and therefore increase their length of stay in hospital (Glass, 1999; Ash, 2002).

There are currently about 850–900 individuals with a SCI that receive ongoing support and reviews by the team at this regional specialist centre; aside from readmission to the unit, there are a lack of facilities to support, review and manage these vulnerable patients in the community. The early intervention from a SCI community liaison nurse could have a significant impact on reducing the number of readmissions to the unit. This would allow the unit to admit more new patients much earlier, and thus improve their potential and reduce the incidence of developing more serious problems from being managed in a non-specialist unit (Harrison and Thomas, 2000).

When retrieving feedback from patients as to the value and usefulness of the nurse-led clinic, the patients perceived the nurses to be more understanding and better informed than their medical colleagues and felt that the nursing sessions were more informative, practical and helpful. A number of patients required further follow ups in the community; one of the two specialist nurses was able to facilitate this within her role as liaison nurse.

Although the nurse-led service was only trialed for a relatively short period (5 months), it had proved effective from both an individual (patient perspective) and a service perspective. However, a number of issues prevented its continuation, ranging from a change in management to one of the key drivers of the initiative leaving the trust. In addition, funding and staffing would be required to secure and develop the service further, and this was not available.

Conclusion

Trieschmann (1987) highlighted the issue of ageing with a disability as a new phenomenon, and one for which the current healthcare system has not planned. As figures for spinal injuries grow annually and successful recovery and rehabilitation improve, so will the need to provide the continued support necessary to assist patients as they age. Spinal injuries rehabilitation units were initially built to address the acute and rehabilitation phase for these individuals, with limited consideration regarding their ongoing management into 'old age'. Although it may not be possible or appropriate to admit some referrals to the unit, it is reasonable that a specialist centre is able to support, advise and educate in their management.

The development of a nurse-led outpatient service has demonstrated not only the effectiveness of this additional service, but also the value of the role of the specialist nurse.

The *National Service Framework for Long-Term Conditions* (Department of Health, 2005a) aims to transform the way health and social care services support people to live with long-term neurological conditions, and the strategy for achieving this, *Supporting People with Long-Term*

Conditions (Department of Health, 2005b), acknowledges that people with neurological conditions have complex conditions that inter-relate and therefore require an approach that promotes the choices of the individual and independent care, through multi-agency/multi-professional working. If the vision for the future is for nursing roles to be aligned with the needs of the patient, then changes are required in both service provision and delivery, and a nurse-led spinal injuries clinic may provide the most effective route to meet those needs.

References

Ash D (2002) An exploration of the occurrence of pressure ulcers in a British spinal injuries unit. *J Clin Nurs* **11**(4): 470–5

Bennet G, Dealey C, Posnett J (2004) The cost of pressure ulcers in the UK. *Age Ageing* **33**(3): 235–39

Cable S (1995) Minor injury clinics: dealing with trauma. *Br J Nurs* **4**(20): 1177–82

Clarke T, Abbenbroek B, Hardy L (1996) The impact of a high-dependency unit continuing education programme on nursing practice and patient outcomes. *Aust Crit Care* **9**: 138–42

Department of Health (1999) *Making a Difference. Strengthening the Nursing, Midwifery and Health Visiting Contribution to Health and Healthcare*. DoH, London

Department of Health (2000) *The NHS Plan: A Plan for Investment, A Plan for Reform*. DoH, London

Department of Health (2003) *Protecting Staff: Delivering Services. Implementing the EU Working Time Directives for Doctors in Training*. DoH, London

Department of Health (2005a) *National Service Framework for Long-Term Conditions*. DoH, London

Department of Health (2005b) *Supporting People with Long-Term Conditions*. DoH, London

Glass CA (1999) *Spinal Cord Injury: Impact and Coping*. British Psychological Society, Leicester

Grundy D, Swain A (2001) *The ABC of Spinal Cord Injury*. BMJ Books, London

Hammell KRW (1994) *Spinal Cord Injury Rehabilitation*. Nelson-Thornes, London

Harrison P, Thomas S (2000) *Bowel Management Problems Outside of Specialist Units*. Spinal Injuries Association, London

Lewin K (1951) *Field Theory in Social Science*. Harper Row, London

Menter RR (1993) Issues of ageing with spinal cord injury. In: Whiteneck GG, Charlifue SW, Gerhert KA, eds. *Ageing with Spinal Cord Injury*. Demos, New York: 1, 4–5

Miles K, Penny N, Power R, Mercey D (2003) Comparing doctor and nurse-led care in a sexual health clinic: patient satisfaction questionnaire. *J Adv Nurs* **42**(1): 64–72

Nursing and Midwifery Council (2002) *Code of Professional Conduct*. NMC, London

Raghavan P, Raza WA, Ahmed YS (2003) Prevalence of pressure sores in a community sample of spinal injury patients. *Clin Rehabil* **17**: 879–884

Richardson A, Cunliffe L (2003) New horizons: the motives, diversity and future of nurse-led care. *J Nurs Manage* **11**(2): 80

Smith M (1999) *Making the Difference: Efficacy of Specialist Versus Non-Specialist Management of Spinal Cord Injury*. Spinal Injuries Association, London

Spinal Injuries Association (1997) *A Charter for Support. Recommendations Regarding NHS Treatment of People Confirmed or Suspected of Experiencing Spinal Cord Injury*. SIA, London

Touche-Ross (1994) *The Cost of Pressure Sores*. Touche-Ross and Co, London

Trieschmann RB (1987) *Ageing with a Disability*. Demos, New York

Whalley Hammell K (1994) *Spinal Cord Injury Rehabilitation*. Chapman and Hall, London

Whiteneck GG, Charlifue SW, Gerhart KA (1993) *Ageing with a Spinal Cord Injury*. Demos, New York

Zarb GJ, Oliver ML, Silver JR (1990) *Ageing with a Spinal Cord Injury. The Right to a Supportive Environment?* Thames Polytechnic and Spinal Injuries Association, London

Chapter 31

Caring for the carers: Measuring quality of life in Huntington's disease

Aimee Aubeeluck

Huntington's disease (HD) is a chronic, progressive dementia of the brain that causes movement abnormalities (i.e. chorea and dystonia), cognitive deterioration and affective disturbances (Folstein, 1989). Symptoms begin on average between the ages of 35–45 years (Quarrell, 1999) and can vary widely from person to person. Patients become severely demented, motorially dilapidated, unable to care for themselves and eventually bedridden.

There is no cure for HD, with the treatments available being purely palliative or experimental and death occurring on average 15–17 years after onset (Bates et al, 2002). HD is a genetic condition inherited as an autosomal-dominant trait with complete lifetime penetrance. Therefore, each person whose parent has HD is born with a 50:50 chance of inheriting the gene (Gusella et al, 2000).

HD is often characterized by progressive involuntary choreiform (dance-like) movements. However, many patients manifest behavioural changes before the onset of the movement disorder. Early symptoms may include a lack of concentration combined with short-term memory lapses, depression and changes of mood that may lead to aggressive and/or antisocial behaviour as well as slight choreic movements, stumbling and clumsiness (Harper, 1996). Later on in the illness, earlier symptoms become exacerbated and patients often experience other symptoms, such as constant involuntary movements, difficulty in speech and swallowing, severe weight loss, emotional changes resulting in a fixed mindset, frustration, mood swings and depression (Quarrell, 1999).

Figure 31.1 shows the affect of Huntington's disease on the brain. In the later stages of HD, full nursing care is required and secondary illnesses, such as pneumonia, are often the actual cause of death rather than the disease itself. Moreover, for every HD patient it is reported that there are another 20 people, including those who are at risk, who suffer the consequences of HD (Hayden et al, 1980). This may be in relation to care giving, genetic inheritance or the sheer burden that such a devastating disease places upon a family.

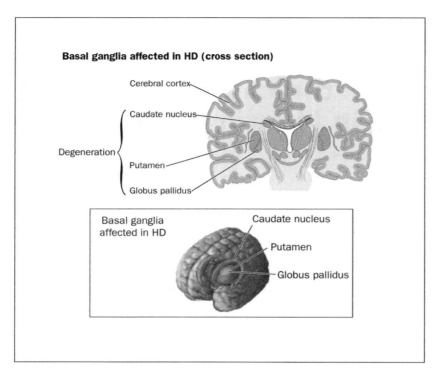

Figure 31.1: The effect of Huntington's disease (HD) on the brain

Family care-giving in Huntington's disease

In HD the immediate family usually takes on the responsibility of caring for an affected individual, and often the primary carer is the spouse (Kessler, 1993). Although there is a wealth of literature investigating the role of dementia family care-givers (e.g. Maslach, 1981; Flicker, 1992; Murray et al, 1997), a number of salient factors demonstrate that HD, as a dementia, imposes a unique burden on family and, especially, on spousal carers (Aubeeluck and Buchanan, 2006a). For example, the genetic implications and chronic nature of HD may mean that family carers experience more intense problems than dementia carers *per se* when caring for a relative with HD.

Tyler et al (1983) examined the relationship between HD disease state and family breakdown and stress in a sample of 92 patients. Tyler and colleagues found that violence, promiscuity, bizarre and slovenly behaviour (i.e. behavioural manifestations of HD) were often reported to be the cause of marital breakdown in HD. Behavioural problems were also cited as one of the main causes of stress within the family, with dangerous and aggressive behaviour reported in nearly half of all patients, and 82% of primary carers reporting feeling stressed. Wives also reported feelings of conflict in choosing between caring for their HD-affected spouse and their children over the duration of the illness. Therefore, such mood and behavioural changes associated with HD can drastically alter family, and especially spousal, relationships.

Hayden et al (1980) established that in HD the non-HD spouse has unique concerns and needs in terms of chronic isolation. They found that the antisocial behaviour associated with HD might cause social embarrassment to the carer and rejection by friends. Moreover, in a qualitative study of 15 wives of individuals with HD, Hans and Koeppen (1980) found that partners frequently describe how they feel they have ended up married to a different person, and perhaps not the sort of person they would have chosen. Feelings of regret, anger and ambivalence are commonplace, and often marriages come under extreme pressure. They also note that none of the partners knew of the presence of HD in the family before marriage, and they reacted with disbelief and denial on hearing the diagnosis. Furthermore, as the partners became aware of the steady progression of the disease process and the threat of disease transmission to any children, they became resentful and hostile. The strain on members of the family is, therefore, further intensified by the impact of the unique implications stemming from the inherited nature of the disease (Williams et al, 2000).

Owing to the genetic implications, HD repeats itself in successive generations; once a patient with HD and their spouse have had children, the impact on the family may span over a number of generations if any children are found to have the disease. The availability of a predictive test to identify offspring who are at risk of developing the disease also brings its own problems in terms of the psychosocial impact it has on both the patient and his or her carer (e.g. Kessler, 1988; Sobel and Brookes Cowan, 2000). Often those who are 'at risk' or know they carry the gene are involved in the care of their parents or other members of their family, and are constantly reminded of the reality of HD. It is not uncommon for a person to nurse his or her parent, then an older sibling and finally succumb to HD themselves, while worrying all the time that they have transmitted the disease to their children (Kessler, 1993).

Hans and Gilmore (1968) note the major emotional, social and financial problems that care-giving in HD creates for the family, and that such issues are made worse because of the lack of attention that HD has received from public health services in terms of interventions. This may be because the physical, neurological, psychiatric and genetic elements of HD mean there are no boundaries between the medical disciplines in relation to who should care for these patients. Therefore, HD sits uncomfortably within the structure of community-based services. This can have implications for the professionals involved and also HD families. Patients and their families find enormous difficulty in gaining access to specific services, and professionals may not always be trained to deal with such family dynamics. Service provision for HD families is therefore often poor and unsuitable, so families are mostly burdened with the main responsibility of care (Shakespeare and Anderson, 1993).

The role of the healthcare provider

Generally, the healthcare professional's role in HD has traditionally been one of assessment, management, evaluation and research into the disease processes and the sufferer themselves rather than the carer. Numerous scales are used to assess the severity of symptoms (e.g. Stroop, 1935; Nelson, 1976), which can demonstrate very early changes in attention, ability to learn and so on, enabling diagnosis often before the onset of chorea. These are clearly useful in preparing control and experimental groups in research, but are of less practical value to the sufferers themselves and their family. Therefore, HD-affected families may experience a lack of expertise and specialism from health professionals on practical aspects, such as therapeutic interventions, advice on genetic counselling or continuity of care.

As with many diseases where there is no cure, focus is quite rightly and obviously placed upon finding a successful treatment. Since the discovery of the Huntington gene (Gusella et al, 1983, 2000), patient care has changed quite dramatically in terms of both searching for a cure and developing more appropriate and specialized care facilities. However, carer issues still appear to remain constant, with the current literature highlighting problems that were being raised in the first part of the 20th century (Davenport and Muncey, 1916). It is, therefore, clearly important to put resources into establishing methods of alleviating the carer burden in HD by successfully addressing carers' needs.

Using quality of life as a therapeutic measure for carers

Since the 1960s, quality of life (QoL) has been emerging as a useful outcome measure by which to judge the efficacy of interventions (Rapley, 2003). Using QoL as a measure of outcome focuses on the impact of a condition or situation on the individual's emotional and physical functioning and lifestyle. As such, QoL indicators can ultimately help to answer the question of whether an intervention leads to an increase in wellbeing by providing a carer-led baseline against which the effects of an intervention can be evaluated. With this in mind, Aubeeluck and Buchanan (2004) have developed a disease-specific measure that brings together theoretical constructs and practical application to produce a user-friendly QoL measurement for HD spousal carers that can be used to implement and assess therapeutic interventions.

The Huntington's Disease Quality of Life Battery for Carers (HDQoL-C) (Aubeeluck and Buchanan, 2003, 2004, 2006b; Aubeeluck, 2005), has been adapted from the Comprehensive Quality of Life Scale for Adults (COMQoL-A5) (Cummins, 1997) to systematically investigate the factors that may enhance and compromise the lives of HD spousal carers by using the theoretical construct of QoL. The HDQoL-C takes about 10–20 minutes to complete and is intended to be self-administered. It contains 34 questions contained within four components:

- Demographic and objective information
- Aspects of caring
- Satisfaction with life
- Feelings about life.

The first component requests demographic and objective information from the client, and each question is treated independently. This information can be used in research to investigate the factors that may predict QoL in care giving. Alternatively, it may be used by the practitioner to build up an overall picture of a client. As this component does not in itself constitute a scale, the researcher/practitioner is able to omit questions or include additional questions that may be of interest in this section.

The other three components all comprise differing aspects of disease-specific and subjective QoL. Each individual component demonstrates good internal consistency, test–retest reliability and congruent validity. Moreover, each component has a moderate to strong correlation with the others, allowing researchers/practitioners to use any combination or all of the components to investigate either specific issues surrounding the QoL of the HD-spousal carer or overall QoL scores.

The HDQoL-C has been established as a multidimensional and psychometrically sound, disease-specific and subjective QoL-assessment tool that incorporates the individual's physical health, psychological state, level of independence, social relationships, personal beliefs and relationship to salient features of the environment. It is important to note that the symptoms and genetic nature of HD make the spousal carer role distinct from other HD family carer roles (e.g. Kessler, 1993) and, as such, the HDQoL-C may not be a valid and reliable tool for use with other HD-specific carer populations. However, it is thought that the HDQoL-C may also prove useful in assessing the QoL of other HD family carers (e.g. child carers, carers who are at risk or carers who are HD positive), and further validation is currently being conducted with these specific populations.

How useful is the HDQoL-C in providing care for the carer?

The purpose of assessing the HD spousal carers' situation is to gain an understanding of their role that may help to prevent or to ameliorate QoL-related problems, enabling the carer to maintain a good standard of life quality while continuing to provide care comfortably for his or her relative. The basis of successful intervention, therefore, lies in gaining an informed understanding of the individual case. As such, using the HDQoL-C may provide helpful ways of organizing the information that is gained during assessment. For example, the HDQoL-C will provide the healthcare professional with the carer's objective QoL information, such as financial situation or the practical suitability of the home, as well as subjective QoL information, such as feelings of stress or depression. As such, the HDQoL-C will demonstrate possible areas for intervention at the level of increasing both objective and subjective QoL in spousal carers of HD patients.

Furthermore, anecdotal evidence that has been gathered during the development of the scale has suggested that just completing the HDQoL-C may have therapeutic and cathartic benefits for HD carers. Carers wrote notes of thanks at the end of the validation study reporting how much they had benefited from filling out the HDQoL-C. They commented upon how it had allowed them to think about their situation from their own perspective rather than thinking about the patient all of the time. They also noted that the mere existence of the questionnaire had made them feel that someone cared about them, and furthermore, that someone might listen to them and be able to help them. From the clinician's or healthcare professional's viewpoint, even using the HDQoL-C at this level may be beneficial to his or her relationship with the HD carer.

References

Aubeeluck A (2005) The Huntington's Disease Quality of Life Battery for Carers (HDQoL-C). *Health Psychol Update* **14**(1): 2–4

Aubeeluck A, Buchanan H (2003) Developing a quality-of-life measure for spousal carers of Huntington's disease patients. Poster presented at the BPS Division of Health Psychology Annual Conference, University of Staffordshire, 8–10 September, Stafford

Aubeeluck A, Buchanan H (2004) *The Huntington's Disease Quality of Life Battery for Carers*. University of Derby, Derby

Aubeeluck A, Buchanan H (2006a) Capturing the Huntington's disease spousal carer experience: A preliminary investigation using the 'Photovoice' method. *Dementia* **5**(1): 95–116

Aubeeluck A, Buchanan H (2006b) A measure to assess time impact of Huntington's disease on the quality of life of spousal carers. *Br J Neurosci Nurs* **2**(2): 126–33

Bates G, Harper P, Jones L (2002) *Huntington's Disease*. Oxford University Press, New York

Cummins RA (1997) *The Comprehensive Quality of Life Scale (CoMQoL-A5) Manual*. Toorak, Deakin University, Deakin

Davenport CB, Muncey EB (1916) Huntington's chorea in relation to heredity and eugenics. *Eugenics Record Office Bull* **17**: 195–222

Flicker L (1992) The effects of caregiving for the demented elderly. *Aust J Ageing* **11**: 9–15

Folstein SE (1989) *Huntington's Disease: A Disorder of Families*. John Hopkins University Press, London

Gusella JF, Wexler NS, Conneally PM et al (1983) A polymorphic DNA marker genetically linked to Huntington's disease. *Nature* **306**: 234–8

Gusella JF, Wexler NS, Conneally PM et al (2000) Disclosure of Huntington's disease to family members: the dilemma of known but unknowing parties. *Genetic Testing* **4**: 359–64

Hans MB, Gilmore TH (1968) Social aspects of Huntington's chorea. *Br J Psychiatry* **114**: 93–8

Hans MB, Koeppen AH (1980) Huntington's chorea: its impact on the spouse. *J Nerv Ment Dis* **168**: 209–14

Harper PS (1996) *Major Problems in Neurology: Huntington's Disease*. 2nd edn. WB Saunders, London

Hayden MR, Ehrlich R, Parker H, Ferera SJ (1980) Social perspectives in Huntington's chorea. *South Afr Med J* **58**: 201–3

Kessler S (1988) Psychological aspects of genetic counselling. A family coping strategy in Huntington's disease. *Am J Med Genet* **31**: 617–21

Kessler S (1993) Forgotten person in the Huntington disease family. *Am J Med Genet* **48**: 145–50

Maslach C (1981) *Burnout: The Cost of Caring*. Prentice Hall, New York

Murray JM, Manela MV, Shuttleworth A, Livingstone GA (1997) Caring for an older spouse with a psychiatric illness. *Aging Ment Health* **1**(3): 256–60

Nelson H (1976) A modified card sorting test sensitive of frontal lobe defects. *Cortex* **12**: 313–24

Quarrell O (1999) *Huntington's Disease: The Facts*. Oxford University Press, New York

Rapley M (2003) *Quality of Life Research: A Critical Introduction*. Sage, London

Shakespeare J, Anderson J (1993) Huntington's disease — falling through the net. *Heath Trends (England)* **25**(1): 19–23

Sobel SK, Brookes Cowan D (2000) Impact of genetic testing for Huntington's disease on the family system. *Am J Med Genet* **90**: 49–59

Stroop J (1935) Studies of interference in serial verbal reactions. *J Exp Psychol* **18**: 624–23

Tyler A, Harper PS, Davies K, Newcome RG (1983) Family breakdown and stress in Huntington's chorea. *J Biosoc Sci* **15**: 127–38

Williams JK, Schutte DL, Holkup PA, Evers C, Muilenburg A (2000) Psychosocial impact of predictive testing for Huntington's disease on support persons. *Am J Med Genet* **96**: 353–9

Further information

For further information and free copies of the Huntington's Disease Quality of Life Battery for Carers (HDQoL)-C, please contact: Aimee Aubeeluck, Derby Education Centre, School of Nursing, The University of Nottingham, Derbyshire Royal Infirmary, London Road, Derby DE1 2QY.

Index

G

GABA 189, 208, 209
gabapentin 51, 228, 229
gamma knife 210
gastrostomy tubes, motor neurone disease 289–90, 292
gate control theory of pain 77–9, 80
general medical service quality outcomes framework 194
general practitioners, information seeking in motor neurone disease 312–15
Glasgow Coma Scale (GCS) 5–6, 21–2, 131–2
glatiramer acetate 222, 234
glenohumeral joint
    arm hemiplegia after stroke 322, 323–4, 325–7
    palpitation 327
glioma 12
gliosis, multiple sclerosis 267–8
glucose, abnormal blood levels 8–9
Glut-1 glucose transport protein 61, 62
glutamate 78, 209
glycerine suppositories 145
glyceryl trinitrate 139
grieving process, spinal injuries 146
Guillain–Barré syndrome 44, 45

H

haematocrit, head injuries 133
haemodilution, blood viscosity 133
haemofiltration 11
halo traction 137
handling techniques, stroke patients 323
head injuries, management 7
head injuries, traumatic 109–17
    blunt 110–11
    cardiovascular system 133
    communication 135
    environment 135
    excretion 134
    falls 112
    hydration 133
    infection 115
    mobility of patient 135
    neurological status 131–2
    nursing 127–35
    nutrition 133
    positioning of patient 135
    respiratory system management 132–3
    seizures 132, 202
healthcare providers, Huntington's disease 379–80
hearing
    age-related changes 19
    loss in meningitis 103–4

heat therapy 86
hemiplegia, arm 319–29
    associated symptoms 322
    complication prevention 322–4
    decreased tone 321
    flexor patterning 321
    increased tone 321–2
    optimal positioning of arm 324–7
    passive non-activity 327–8
    shoulder pain 322, 323–4, 327
    shoulder support 325–7
    stages 320–2
hepatic encephalopathy 9–10
heroin 11
    seizure risk 207
herpes simplex meningitis 13
homeostasis disruption by pain 80
Hospital Anxiety and Depression Scale (HADS) 151, 153–4, 156, 157, 158
human immunodeficiency virus (HIV) 65
Huntington gene 380
Huntington's disease 377–81
    choreiform movements 377
    community-based services 379
    family care-giving 378–9
    genetic implications 379
    healthcare providers 379–80
Huntington's Disease Quality of Life Battery for Carers (HDQoL-C) 380–1
hydration, head injuries 133
hydrocephalus 14
hyperalgesia 80
hypercapnia 7, 8
hyperglycaemia 9
hyperosmolar, hyperglycaemia non-ketotic coma (HONK) 9
hyperthermia, spinal injuries 134
hypnosis for pain 86
hypoglycaemic coma 9
hyponatraemia 11
    dilutional 10
hypoperfusion, spinal cord injuries 124
hypothalamus 76
hypoventilation 8
hypoxaemia 7, 8
hypoxia
    head injury 132
    neuronal 8
    spinal cord injuries 124

I

ibuprofen 87
ileal conduit 250

N